A STUDY OF CHILD VARIANCE

VOLUME 2

INTERVENTIONS

Edited by

William C. Rhodes and Michael L. Tracy

Conceptual Project in Emotional Disturbance
**The Institute for the Study of
Mental Retardation and Related Disabilities of
The University of Michigan**

Ann Arbor   **The University of Michigan Press**

Third printing 1980
Copyright © by The University of Michigan 1974
Copyright is claimed until May, 1984. Thereafter all portions
of this work covered by this copyright will be in the public domain.
This work was developed under a grant from the U. S. Office of Education,
Department of Health, Education, and Welfare. However, the opinions and
other content do not necessarily reflect the position or policy of the
Agency, and no official endorsement should be inferred.
All rights reserved
ISBN 0-472-08759-2
Published in the United States of America by
The University of Michigan Press and simultaneously
in Rexdale, Canada, by John Wiley & Sons Canada, Limited
Manufactured in the United States of America

PREFACE

The papers collected in this volume were, for the most part, written over the 1971-1972 academic year. They represent the second stage of an ongoing series of studies on topics related to emotional disturbance and other forms of child variance. This is the second of four volumes included in the Project plan.

The current papers were written by staff members of the Conceptual Project, who were graduate students representing several disciplines. The papers have been circulated as preprints to a national audience of professors and state personnel in the education of the emotionally disturbed, and have benefitted from the helpful criticism returned by many individuals in this audience.

The Conceptual Project in Child Variance, under the directorship of Dr. William C. Rhodes at the University of Michigan, was initially funded as a Special Project by the Bureau of the Education for the Handicapped under the United States Office of Education. Its prime purpose is to order and organize the vast but scattered literature on emotional disturbance and other types of variance in children. A second purpose is to serve as a prototype for combining the functions of graduate training and professional research.

A major aim of the Project's activities has been to maintain a comprehensive approach. Some clustering of related but not identical ideas and schools of thought has occurred, however, with a resultant omission of detail. This clustering has served our purpose of dividing

1

up the research labor in an orderly fashion, but is only one of many possible schemes of categorization. We have attempted to cover most important ideas and authors; some items of importance may have been left out due to space limitations, others undoubtedly by simple omission. To the extent that the product, of which this volume is a part, is felt to be useful, we hope that others might expand on either the graduate training model underlying it, or on the research itself.

Research Stages and Organizing Schemes

The research topics bearing on child variance were approached in three stages, focusing first on theory, then on interventions, and finally on service delivery systems.

Theory. (The results of this state are collected in Volume I of A Study of Child Variance.) The first stage of research focused on theories, models, and systematic viewpoints. The criteria for determining a domain of thought, or model, were as follows:

1. Related theories should employ the same basic methodology for any exploration and construction (e.g., learning or behavioral theories share the experimental, laboratory investigatory method. Psychodynamic theories share the clinical approach to explanation and exploration).

2. Related theories should share a common orienting outlook in examining and explaining human behavior (e.g., for the sociological theorist all behavior has a social basis).

3. Related theories should acknowledge a controlling pre-emptory principle of behavioral genesis (e.g., unconscious motivation, conditioning or learning, biogenesis). This principle is heuristic, demonstrable in many contents, and ubiquitous in the explanatory system built around it. This principle might be called the basic paradigm of the cluster.

4. Related theories should agree regarding basic ameliorating approaches. (The psychodynamic theorists see psychotherapy and its derivatives as indicated; the learning theorists are biased toward behavior modification.)

5. Each should have a common ambience within its cluster group. These dimensions come together to form a basic model which places a stamp upon any single, isolated theoretical fragment. While it is possible to identify various combinations and permutations of these schools, each has an overriding identity of its own.

On the basis of these criteria, we established the following five categories of traditional theory:

(a) Biophysical,

(b) Behavioral,

(c) Psychodynamic,

(d) Sociological,

(e) Ecological.

3

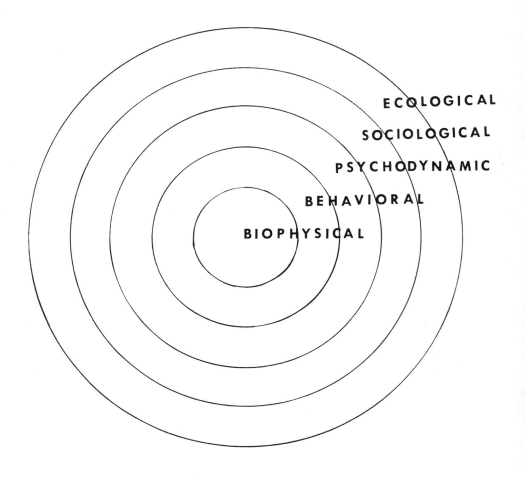

Figure 1. Theoretical domains used by the Conceptual Project.

To cover a large group of "others" who in one way or another disagree with the traditional models, a sixth domain was included:

(f) Counter-theory,

The logical relationship between these domains of thought is schematized in Figure 1, with the innermost circle representing the most individual and physical focus, and the outermost circle representing the most universal and complex focus. This representation is not intended to imply mutually-exculsive territories belonging to the various domains, but rather to suggest the aspects each domain has emphasized and has developed most fully.

Interventions. (The results of this stage are represented by this volume.) The second stage of research focused on the techniques and practices used in intervening into the lives of children. Although many practitioners tend to be eclectic, and although the connection between theory and specific practice is often tenuous and unclear, nevertheless, the same organizational scheme used for theories seemed a best fit to the variety of interventions reviewed. While many specific intervention applications are described in these papers, an overall effort was made to emphasize the generic characteristics of the interventions.

Service Delivery Systems. (The research for this stage will be collected in Volume III of the series.) This stage focuses on the variety of systems that deliver intervention services to variant children. Separate papers are being written to cover

a) the history of the systems (within the United States),
b) the current (national) structure and functioning of the systems,
and c) a case study of the way these systems deal with variant
children in a particular local community. The systems being reviewed,
which are seen as society's major behavior-regulating institutions,
are:

     (a)   the educational system,

     (b)   the legal-correctional system,

     (c)   the mental health system,

     (d)   the social welfare system,

     (e)   the religious agencies,

     (f)   the emerging counter-institutions.

Overview. (This is projected as Volume IV of the series.)
In this final research stage, the previous research efforts will be
reviewed with attention to current events, trends, and potential
developments in the treatment of child variance in the United States.
Based on the previous research, an attempt will be made to assess
the directions of the education of variant children, to assess the
impact of possible fundamental changes in the systematic handling
of these children, and to develop a statement of alternative desirable
changes in such handling, in the light both of new technologies and
ideologies and of ethical concerns being voiced by today's
professionals.

Other Aspects of Project Research

Video Tapes. At every stage of the research, the Project has selected a leading expert in each of the fields to participate in a two-day conference on current issues touching on child variance. Each of these experts was interviewed individually and selections from both the interviews and the conferences are available from the Project on a lending-library basis.

The video tapes are organized in a form suitable for use in classrooms or in workshops, and have been used in undergraduate, graduate, and post-graduate settings. The series includes an introductory tape covering the theory and intervention research and introducing each of the fourteen experts listed below.*

The conference on theories and models took place in Ann Arbor in May, 1971. The experts participating in this conference were:

Dr. Jay Birnbrauer, Professor, Department of Psychology, The University of North Carolina, Chapel Hill, North Carolina (behavioral area)

Dr. Jane Kessler, Professor, Department of Psychology, Case-Western Reserve University, Cleveland, Ohio (psychodynamic area)

Dr. Bernard Rimland, Director, Institute for Child Behavioral Research, San Diego, California (biogenetic area)

Dr. Thomas Scheff, Chairman, Department of Sociology, University of California at Santa Barbara, Santa Barbara, California (Sociological area)

---

*(For further information, contact the Conceptual Project, ISMRRD, The University of Michigan, 130 South First Street, Ann Arbor, Michigan, 48108.)

7

Dr. Edwin Willems, Professor, Department of Psychology, The University of Houston, Houston, Texas (ecological area)

The conference on counter-theories took place in Ann Arbor in November, 1971. Participants included:

Dr. Everett Reimer, Professor, University of Puerto Rico, San Juan, Puerto Rico

Dr. Peter Knoblock, Professor, Syracuse University, Syracuse, New York

Dr. Herbert Grossman, Professor, Tuskegee Institute, Tuskegee, Alabama

Dr. Matthew Trippe, Professor, The University of Michigan, Ann Arbor, Michigan

The conference on interventions took place in Ann Arbor in October, 1972. The participants included:

Dr. Allan Cott, Psychiatrist, New York, New York

Dr. Lamar Empey, Professor, Department of Sociology, The University of Southern California, Los Angeles, California

Dr. Carl Fenichel, Director, The League School, Brooklyn, New York

Jeannine Guindon, Director, Ecole de psycho-education, Universite de Montreal, Montreal, Quebec

Peter Marin, Former Director, Pacific High School, Santa Barbara, California

Dr. Humphry Osmond, Director, Bureau of Research in Neurology and Psychiatry, Neuropsychiatric Institute, Princeton, New Jersey

K. Daniel O'Leary, Professor, State University of New York, Stony Brook, New York

Graduate Training Model. Each of the authors of the papers in this series wrote his paper while a graduate student. The disciplines represented include Anthropology, Sociology, Psychology, Biology, General and Special Education, History, Law, Philosophy and

8

Education, and Medicine. The students were employed half-time over
the academic year for their participation, and each of the departments involved was asked to consider the position as a supervised
research placement. The students met in a weekly seminar, for which
the various departments allowed three hours per term of course credit
to be applied toward their degrees. A great deal of autonomy was
allowed students in the research of their topics; each student was
responsible for establishing contacts with experts outside of the
University of Michigan for early guidance and advice. These experts
also provided a formal review of their papers. The video taped panelists
mentioned above were selected from this advisory group, and each
research assistant was responsible for conducting the interview with
the expert representing "his" system. As a model for graduate training,
this one is unusual in both the depth and the breadth of the exposure
involved.

Authentication Process. The review and revision process for
the papers in this series is important both in terms of the resulting
quality of the product and in terms of the experience of the authors.
As such, it has been somewhat standardized. The basic outline is
shown in Figure 2. In the initial stages, the author establishes a
starting bibliography, drawing upon his own resources, various abstrac-
ting and citation indexes, and on suggestions from others advising
him. At the same time he initiates contact with authorities in the
subject field, both locally and nationally, for other references and

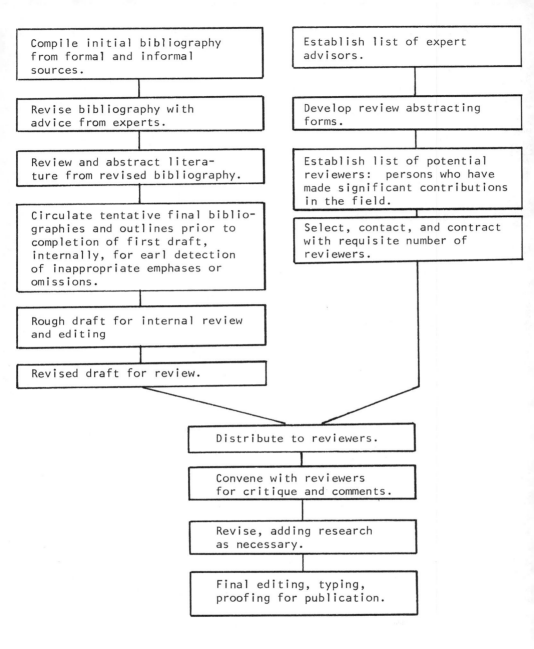

Figure 2.   Authenticated review process model.

general guidance. The bibliography is expanded and refined through suggestions from advisors, through citations and cross-references in the initial bibliography, and through informal and "accidental" sources. Before writing is begun in earnest, a tentative outline is discussed with the other authors and with the Project's directorial and support staff. At this point a tentative bibliography of works to be explicitly covered in the paper is also brought under scrutiny. When the first draft is completed, it is edited, reproduced, and distributed to a small audience of general Project advisors, to local experts, and to others whom the author has contacted, for the purpose of eliciting general critiques. Meanwhile, one particular reviewer is singled out and paid for an intensive review in written form, followed by a telephone discussion with the author. On the basis of the combined critiques, the paper is revised and re-edited for distribution as a preprint. The use of a single major reviewer eliminates some of the logistic difficulties and delays associated with larger groups of reviewers. All of the experts represented in the Project's video tapes were also reviewers of the papers.

Dissemination Model. The basic dissemination model used by the Project for its theory materials has been described in Volume I of this series. In brief, it consists of the active presentation of the total set of materials in a series of national workshops for teacher trainers and state personnel in emotional disturbance. The workshops are run with the assitance of regional leaders, and the

11

materials are used as a stimulus and a backround to elicit personal responses and personal experiences from the participants. A wider dissemination effort includes the mailing of the materials to a larger audience of professionals in psychiatry, sociology, psychology and community psychology, other related fields in education, and to various agencies dealing with variant children.

For the current materials, including the contents of this book and the associated video tapes, an effort is being made to utilize existing regional activities and to encourage entirely local workshop developments. The Project has developed a workshop package which requires approximately seven hours, and which can be organized and run locally. The package is available for a nominal fee; for groups meeting certain requirements of participation and evaluation, the cost can be underwritten by the Project. The package includes a telephone discussion between the workshop participants and the Project staff.*

Other Utilizations. The Conceptual Project materials have been used in a number of ways that have come to our attention. A modification of the basic division of theories and interventions has been used as an organizing scheme for a seminar of graduate students; a video tape representing the basic concepts of one of the categories of theory was then prepared as a term project. The categories of

---

*Inquiries about this package are welcome.

12

theory were used as a background for the observation of children; students chose a particular theoretical position and analyzed their observations in terms of it. In another program, students have developed critiques of one of the papers, with an ultimate purpose of later producing a paper that meets any criticisms. Several professors have reported that they have used the bibliographies incorporated in the papers to develop or update their libraries. Others have modified the Project categories, or have added several distinct ones including diagnostic-remedial, psycho-educational and child developmental models, using the whole set to structure graduate experience at several levels, from introductory to advanced.

Acknowledgements

It is no secret that many people are involved in the production of a book. The authors of the individual papers, of course, formed the backbone of the Project's efforts.

Dr. Matt Trippe, now a Senior Advisor on the Project, provided continuous support to the Project and was instrumental in initiating it at the start.

The reviewers and expert panelists, listed previously, provided a great service both in their critical reviews and suggestions on the papers themselves and in their stimulating contributions through the conference.

Advisors who have come to Ann Arbor to review the Project and provide consultation on its activities have made a large impact on

the Project's functions. We would like specifically to thank
Dr. Frank Bruno, Dr. Paul Graubard, Dr. Peter Knoblock, Dr. Wilbur
Lewis, Dr. Glenn Ohlson, Dr. James Paul, Dr. Herbert Quay, Dr. Richard
Whelan, and Dr. Frank Wood for their help and guidance.

We would also like to thank those professionals who, in
addition to their advice and reviews of the materials, have provided
local leadership in Conceptual Project workshops: Dr. Evelyn Adlerblum,
Dr. Joyce Broome, Dr. Henry Boudin, Dr. Judith Grosenick, Miss Beverly
Kochan, Dr. Theodore Kurtz, Dr. Claude Marks, Dr. Robert McCauley,
Dr. John Mesinger, Ronald Neufeld, Dr. A. J. Pappanikou, Dr. Phyllis
Publicover, Dr. Edward Schultz, Gabriel Simches, and Dr. Loyd Wright.

We are particularly grateful for the collaboration of
Dr. William Morse in the preparation of the psychodynamic interventions paper. Our early efforts to cover this area were unsatisfactory and without his substantial help the present paper could never
have been included.

The tremendous load of work performed by the Project's support
staff must be gratefully acknowledged. The entire editorial responsibility for the individual papers and for the production of the book
was in the hands of Judith M. Smith, who also contributed much to
the ongoing seminar in which the authors hashed out and shared their
developing ideas. Sabin Head, serving first as the Project Evaluator
and now as the Project's Principal Investigator, contributed to the
organization and implementation of the many Project activities.
John Evans, as the Project's Dissemination Coordinator, competently

14

organized this phase of the Project's activities and contributed to the planning and preparation of the video tapes. Anne Nemetz Carlson assumed the difficult job of indexing the concepts and terms used in this volume. Catherine Drob capably formulated, edited and assisted in the planning and preparation of the video tapes which supplement this volume. Mary Morrison, as Head Secretary, managed what at times seemed a small army of other secretaries and typists through the many revisions of the materials, while capably handling other administrative functions.

We are deeply indebted to Dr. Herman Saettler of the Bureau of the Education of the Handicapped, Office of Education, whose help and support has made the entire Project possible.

We are also indebted to the Institute for the Study of Mental Retardation and Related Disabilities, under the direction of Dr. William M. Cruickshank, for the use of the facilities of the Institute and for continued consultation and support.

We would like to express our sincere thanks to Spencer Gibbins for the great amount of time and effort he devoted to the Project.

W. C. R.

M. L. T.

Ann Arbor, Michigan, 1973

15

TABLE OF CONTENTS

OVERVIEW OF INTERVENTION

William C. Rhodes

TABLE OF CONTENTS

I. A FRAMEWORK FOR VIEWING INTERVENTION

Ideas, Actions and Outcomes

It is the intention of the Conceptual Project on Child
Variance, that this volume on Interventions be anchored within
ideational framework.   It is not enough to present a simple
compendium or catalogue of major intervention methods, practices
and   techniques.   That would be like presenting an individual with
a pile of boards and a keg of nails and asking him to build a
house, with no conceptualization of space and shape, no blueprints
of the ways in which space and shape should come together into a
whole.

In an intervention, ideas, actions, and outcomes are all
tied together and greatly affect each other.   Ideas, in and of
themselves, are inert unless active energy is added to their influence.   Active energy, in and of itself, is meaningless and
chaotic unless it is directed.   In an intervention, the conceptual
framework directs and channels the action, by providing an analysis of the nature of the problem which dictates the intervention,
and by suggesting the outcome toward which the intervention is
directed.

One form of intervention, carried out within two different conceptual frameworks can have radically different meanings
and lead to radically different experiences and outcomes for the

participants. A case in point is the method of teaching reading employed by both Sylvia Ashton-Warner and Paulo Freire. Both attempt to "pull" the words to be taught from inside the students. Both interveners derive words from the experiences and emotions of their students and then give these words back to the students to learn. Since Sylvia Ashton-Warner works with children and Freire works with adults, the words are somewhat different, but the intervention technique is largely the same.

In spite of the equivalence of actions, however, the ideational contexts within which the action is embedded are strikingly different, and the effects upon the recipient are quite different. The energy involved in the intervention action seems to be qualitatively transformed by the conceptual framework. Sylvia Ashton-Warner's concept is "organic teaching," in which she uses the "stuff" of the child as a bridge to reading. Paulo Freire, on the other hand, uses literacy to transform the numbed peasant into a free man. The same action becomes "teaching" in one case, and "freeing" in the other.

Furthermore, the same action embedded in strikingly different conceptual models, is intended to lead to radically different outcomes. Sylvia Ashton-Warner's long range goal for the Maori child is to circumvent deviance, and to integrate the child into the prevailing New Zealand culture. For Paulo Freire, however, the expected outcome is revolution. He expects literacy to free the South American so that he will take control of his own destiny, and rise up in revolt against the control of the prevailing culture. Therefore, the trajected paths of apparently identical intervention methods, are guided to achieve quite different outcomes. One is "integration," the other is "revolt."

This may be the reason why people argue theories so vehemently. The framework of ideas within which the action is carried out can add a significant qualitative change to the energy as it is discharged into an intervention. The conceptual framework channels the energy, harnessing it and giving it form and direction, and, thus, influences the quality of the action itself.

Conceptual Models

With this in mind, and for the sake of unity of product, this volume is organized in much the same way as the volume on theoretical models. The general groupings of (a) biophysical, (b) behavioral, (c) psychodynamic, (d) sociological, and (e) ecological are employed. In addition, as in the last volume, we tried to take into account current voices of dissent and reform as they concern themselves with the proper relationship between society and those whom society dubs its variants. For lack of a better description, we have called this grouping "counter theoretical."

The reader will notice that since environmental interventions are common to both the sociological and ecological models, they have been grouped together in one intervention paper. However, in spite of the similarity between many of the sociological and ecological interventions into the lives of children who are seen by the community as variant, the action-channeling frameworks are different. As indicated previously, the conceptual framework does influence the quality of the energy involved in the action interventions and in the outcomes.

Ecological theory is an encompassing framework, an umbrella, rather than a particularized theory. It is a wholistic model, or model of models. It can be seen as a unifying framework, capable of embracing the biophysical, the behavioral, the psychodynamic and the sociological bodies of knowledge. While it shares with the sociological point of view the notion that a human congregation is a composite whole which has its own unique destiny, separate from the whole of which it is a part, it is also vitally concerned with the way in which the life and death of the individual affects the whole. Ecological theory can contain the aggregate historical view of Durkeim that "currents" of cultural influence upon individuals in a specific geophysical area (such as suicidogenic currents), can be transmitted, independent of a total changeover in individual members of that area; but it also can include the "great man" theory of Freud that the repressive forces in the superego of a specific community are the residue of the impact of some great individual figure from the past whose influence still exerts itself in the present.

In being concerned with the reciprocal relationship between individuals and their ocumen, with the transfers of energy and influence between them, the conceptual framework of ecology can influence the focus of behavioral, psychodynamic, or biophysical theory. Thus, conditioning theory can be employed either to bring the individual under the influence of the environment, or to counteract the influence of the environment so that there is more reciprocal influence from the individual. Paul Graubard, for instance (1971), has taught children behavioral principles to counteract teacher and peer influence. Marcuse (1961), has employed psychoanalytic principles to suggest ways in which changes in individuals can influence society to tolerate wider and wider ranges of human differences. In the same vein, biophysical concepts have been employed by physicians in very interesting ways upon the "environment" surrounding children seen as variant. These physicians have prescribed tranquilizers for the parent and the teacher in order that they may tolerate wider ranges of differences in others and, perhaps, in themselves.

What is Intervention?

In this volume we are talking about professional interventions into child variance. Such intervention is a mediational process which enters into the variant reciprocity between a child and his world, to affect that reciprocity, and to promote a different outcome than would have been expected without such interposing.

When action is taken to alter the child's variant experience of the world, this is intervention. Any action performed

27

upon the child's variant behavior, intended to alter that behavior in a particular setting, toward a particular outcome, is an intervention. Any action upon significant people in the child world, intended to bring about directional alteration of variant exchanges, is an intervention. Any action upon child-oriented decision-makers, taken to alter their experience of deviance, is intervention. Any directional alteration of an environment of deviance, either in the child's immediate behavioral setting, or in the larger environment, is intervention. In short, any directed action upon the deviance predicament between child and community is an intervention. Events, persons, things, space, and time are all bound together in the deviance predicament; and any extraneous action entering between these components to change the predicament, is an intervention.

Included are such practices as therapeutic or psycho-educational teaching, psychotherapy, case-work, counseling, community organization, consultation, environmental modeling, etc. Children involved include those who are publicly listed as delinquent, retarded, deprived, underachievers, disabled, etc.

Intervention is an energy in-flow. It is a flow which comes from outside a balanced energy-exchange system. It is an input that is added to an on-going energy field as an increment which makes a difference in the stabilized energy exchange between individual and environment. As an extraneous energy source it comes from outside to enter between events and occurrences to affect, modify, or prevent the current deviance action pattern. It is something different which interrupts fixed energy patternings between individuals and community, and allows for re-groupings and re-patternings of such an energy complex. As related to continuity, it is an interruption. As related to environment, it is an inter-position. As related to instrumentality, it is mediation.

When we look at interventions which now take place in agencies serving exceptional children, we can group them into clusters. There are behavior-focused interventions which aim the energy in-put at the behavioral field, at the action-exchange pattern taking place between child and world. The major agency pattern which gives preference to such behavior-focused interventions is the judicial-corrections system. The in-put attempts to prevent certain kinds of behavioral exchanges from taking place, to contain or con-strain them, or to stop them. Within correctional institutions, these behavior-focused in-puts rarely try to transform or modify the behaviors upon which they are focused. The general public seems to expect interventions within the correctional framework to con-tain, constrain, and punish; not to re-form or transform the be-haviors into something different. When viewed through the cor-rectional framework, bizarre behaviors are experienced by the public as deliberate threats against society. Therefore, they must be repulsed, or surrounded and contained. If such intervention is not successful, the next level of public defense requires destruction of target behaviors and the producer of those behaviors. This extreme level of intervention can be seen in jury-directed death sentences.

Behavior-focused interventions can take other, less defensive forms, as they sometimes do in intervention systems other than corrections. In such cases, behavioral interventions seek an outcome such as behavior transformation or behavior modification. The general public allows this more benign intervention to take place through institutional systems such as education or mental health. Apparently, the use of these more sanguine forms of behavior-focused in-puts, is confined to those behaviors which do not carry the same loading of threat as do behaviors which are referred by the public to the correctional system. Perhaps one of the tasks for future interventionists is to separate that part of the threat which is fanciful in the public mind from that part which may be a real community threat; in that way, the community would need to devote less of its energy and resources to defend against behavioral differences. The effort now being made by many experts in the legal-corrections system to decriminalize "crimes-without-a-victim" may be an example of rationally defusing public fears and anxieties about behaviors, thus releasing professional and agency resources to concentrate less on incarceration and containment and more on behavioral transformation.

As we look further at programs of intervention which now take place in public agencies, another cluster can be discerned. The term "personal interventions" might be used to cover them. This includes interpersonal and intrapersonal interventions as they are now practiced by several community systems of intervention. Two of these, which overlap greatly, are teaching and psychotherapy. These interventions **focus** primarily upon personal exchanges which take place in a deviance predicament. They attempt to involve the individual in commerce with himself and with others; and try to re-form the energy pattern at that level. The public sanctions these types of interventions in those cases in which it experiences unacceptable or painful differences in community members, but in which the threat of such differences is not considered extreme. The individual difference is not perceived as a behavioral crisis for the collective in which the behavior has to be immediately controlled or eliminated. The outward behavior is viewed as more personally restrictive than collectively destructive; and therefore the community can be more tolerant and succorant. More leisurely methods, more embracive explorations and mediations are allowed, and even encouraged.

In this case the particular outward bits of behavior which claim community attention are accepted as surface manifestations of a more generalized personal condition which has to be investigated at a deeper level. The methods designed for such investigation depend on a human-to-human exchange of energy. It becomes necessary for the receiving individual to accept and collaborate in the exchange, which is not true in the more extreme forms of behavioral control.

Another cluster of interventions which are practiced under public auspices involve environmental modeling and environmental transfers. These environmental interventions assume a wide range of forms, although all are carried out to affect, modify, prevent, or treat a deviance action pattern. The approach has historical precedent in various forms of "in-door" and "out-door" relief, and in special colonies created for predicament populations. Under the concept of indoor relief, special problem populations were collected and exiled from the community into "asylums" such as into almshouses, orphanages, prisons, mental institutions, etc. Under the concept of out-door relief, such populations were either placed with village families and supported by the community, or financially supported by the community in their own homes. Another precedent is special colonies for predicament populations. One form of such special environmental arrangement can be seen in the colonies created by Makeranko after the Russian revolution to house and socialize roaming bands of youths uprooted by the upheaval. To some extent, the Kibbutzem in Israel seems to have served the same purpose in handling the rapid flood of children into Israel. A

32

related development was the gradual evolution of an open community into a protective colony, like the Gheel Colony in Belgium, which took upon themselves as a raison d'être the care of special populations like the mentally ill and retarded.

Interventions classified as environment modeling might include the "new towns" in Europe, or the residential communes in Denmark, which took whole populations of "slum" dwellers and placed them in a new intentional community, especially constructed as a total salutary habitat. In the United States, "slum clearance" and "urban renewal" fits under this rubric.

Many new forms of this approach are appearing across the country today. Institutional alternatives for the retarded and the mentally ill, such as "half-way houses," sheltered workshops, etc. are being developed by the state. Special populations, such as drug-addicts, are themselves creating their own intentional communities, such as Datop Village.

Other examples of environmental modeling and environmental transfers are contained in the chapter on Environmental Interventions.

Such interventions are much less familiar to the public than are behavioral or personal and interpersonal interventions. There is a general public uneasiness about this approach unless the special environment is a carefully guarded, enforced-incarceration facility, for individuals who are viewed as requiring separation from the community. The gathering of variant individuals into special, self-contained clusters seems to present a threat to the established power structure of the community, particularly if the group is a foreign cultural group. Perhaps this is why the public school became such an important instrument of socialization during the early flood of immigrants to this country. Pluralistic "foreign" groups, setting up small ethnocentric conclaves within the environs of large cities were experienced as a threat to the established community of American culture-bearers. Therefore, the public school was activated as the site of a culturally unifying intervention into the lives of children inhabiting those enclaves, to assure that they would be absorbed into the pre-established culture.

It is also possible that environmental molding is not usually a public choice because there is not yet a general grasp of the part which the "public" itself plays in the deviance predicament. It is certainly difficult for the public to gain insight into the general uses which society makes of deviance. It is much easier to grasp the concept of individual change through individual intervention. It is much easier to conceive of one-by-one solutions, than general communal solutions to the deviance dynamics of communities.

Still another cluster of interventions might be grouped under the heading of medical interventions. There has been a recent historical shift in Western Civilization completely away

from the religio-magical interventions into deviance predicaments
of communities (the Inquisition, the Witch Trials), toward naturalistic or scientific interventions. As a result, medical interventions have become of tremendous importance in the public mind.
The growing conviction that more and more human predicaments can
be solved medically has given control of the mental-health system
to medicine, transformed some correctional facilities into psychiatric centers, and has laid the groundwork for efforts to control
individual differences in the classroom through behavior-suppres-
sant drugs. It has also given rise to such practices as genetic
counseling and megavitamin therapy.

The Disability, Deviance, and Alienation Views

The choice of interventions to be undertaken depends very
much on whether the problem is viewed as disability, deviance, or
alienation. Disability is the absence of physical, intellectual, or
moral competency. Deviance refers to a noticeable difference from
the average. It is characterized by departure from the norms of
behavior in a given society. Alienation is the state of indifference
or hostility, where devotion or attachment formerly existed. In
Latin "alienatus" means to alienate from oneself, to be insane or
deranged but alienation may also imply estrangement from society.
We see that there is something in common in all of these definitions;
and yet, each has a decidedly different shade of meaning. It is for
this reason--the differences in shade of meaning--that different types
of interventions are predominantly favored by each approach.

35

This is not to say that both the definitions of, and actions upon child variance, do not have common historical roots. The bio-physical interpersonal and intrapersonal (psychodynamic), the behavioral and the environmental (systems) interventions can be found to co-exist in all stages of the history of Western civilization.

If a child carrying the label of mentally retarded, disturbed, delinquent, etc. is characterized as disabled, the approach of the intervener is heavily biophysical. The major techniques employed may involve psychopharmacology, psychosurgery, macrobiotics, convulsive therapies, etc. However, the disability conception can also incorporate intrapersonal and interpersonal therapy, as in many of the psychiatric and meta-psychiatric interventions. Occasionally, behavioral and systems approaches are also incorporated.

When the concept of deviance is employed, one is much more likely to find interpersonal, intrapersonal and systems interventions-- such as, for example, education and psychotherapy. All types of education can be classed as interpersonal and intrapersonal, whether or not they are therapeutic in nature. Within the deviance rubric, psychotherapy becomes educational rather than medical.

In terms of alienation, interpersonal and intrapersonal interventions, such as education and psychotherapy, are utilized. However, if the alienation is not from oneself, but rather from society, then the logical intervention is into the social system or ecosystem which has caused the estrangement. It is quite likely that alienation is a mutual process; that it is a true mutual divorce between the individual and society. If this is so, then the appropriate intervention would be a composite of systems intervention and personal intervention.

Therefore when you, as a reader, are examining the separate papers which catalogue the interventions as biophysical, behavioral, psychodynamic, environmental, or counter-theoretical, you should keep in mind the point of view (disability, deviance or alienation) which seems most logical and helpful to your work.

II.   THE DEVIANCE PREDICAMENT

The Nature of the Predicament

One interpretation of the phenomenon of intervention is a threat-convergence postulate (Becker, et al., 1964; Szasz, 1970; Menninger, 1968; Platt, 1969; Kvaraceus, 1959). According to this postulate, the community converges certain of its fears and collective disorders upon the person of distinctive members who differ in some way from the prototype for the group. This distinctiveness could be a physical stigma, a difference in conduct or manner, a lack of certain common skills, a difference in behavior or appearance, or any of several other possible departures from the norms of the collective or of the dominant group in the collective.

According to various conceptualizations along these lines, threat can either be stimulated by, or discharged through, observable or imagined differences in members who deviate from established prototypes of the collective. The threat which is stimulated by deviation of individual members is felt to be directed against the established order or well-being of the community:

> because of their weak minds or their diseased minds,
> [individuals] are making our country a dangerous place
> to live in. We are breeding defectives, we are making
> criminals (Goddard, 1921, p.iv).

Another version of the deviance predicament suggests that any intolerable or prolonged threat to the community will be converted into a "personal" source, and discharged through that source. The cause and the cure will be attributed to certain individuals who

38

stand out in the group. They will be singled out and used as a proxy for collective threat.

In this interpretation of the deviance predicament, the threat actually originates in some impersonal, outside source, such as war, natural disaster, economic depression, racial conflict, etc; alternatively, the source may be in the psychic make-up of the collective members (repressed hostility, sexual desire, etc.). In this "scapegoat" version of the deviance predicament, particular members are selected to bear the burden of the threat to the collective.

The notion that we can transfer our guilt and suffering to some other being who will bear them for us is familiar. Sir James G. Frazer, in the Golden Bough has collected numerous examples of this phenomenon from many cultures and many ages. In the past, whole communities have employed the mechanism of transference to escape the diverse evils that afflict them. The mishaps, the losses, the pains, the harassments and torments which are part of all communities are transferred in a particular ritual, onto the person of one of the community members. Usually the person chosen is different, in some way, from the rest of the community. He can be stronger and handsomer, poorer and uglier, orphaned or widowed, etc. He is chosen as the receptacle into whom the evils will be expelled and then he will be driven out of the community so the evils go with him (Frazer, 1950, p.655).

For example, from time to time, the gods used to warn the King of Uganda that his foes, the Bunyoro, were working magic against him and his people to make them die of disease. To avert such a catastrophe the king would send a scapegoat to the frontier of Bunyoro, the land of the enemy. The scapegoat consisted of either a man and a boy or a woman and her child, chosen because of some mark or bodily defect, which the gods had noted and by which the victims were to be recognized. With the human victims were sent a cow, a goat, a fowl, and a dog; and a strong guard escorted them to the land which the god had indicated. There the limbs of the victims were broken and they were left to die a lingering death in the enemy's country, being too crippled to crawl back to Uganda. The disease or plague was thought to have been thus transferred to the victims and to have been conveyed back in their persons to the land from which it came.

Anthropological studies of simple human communities have demonstrated various aspects of the deviance predicament discussed above (Frazer, 1963; Milland, 1973; Mead, 1963; Driver, 1961; Selegman & Selegman, 1932).

The "deviance predicament" is a complex, constant, interactive process, endemic to all forms of collective life. The process of threat and release through deviation is a basic, natural, universal predicament of communities. It can be found in insect nests, in fish schools, in bird flocks, in deer herds, in baboon colonies, in primitive tribes, and in modern communities. Consternation is an inevitable part of the deviance predicament. Konrad Lorenz (1967), for instance, reports that in huge communities of social insects such as bees, termites and ants, the members of the clan recognize each other by unique patterns of smells, conduct, etc. which are characteristic of the particular collective. A stranger

40

wandering into the collective and producing strange smells, conduct, etc. will be ejected and destroyed. This capacity for deviation to product violent disturbance can also be seen in fish schools. Jacques Cousteau, in one of his films, has shown how drugging an individual fish, or placing him in a floating glass bowl, alters his behavior and produces attack by predators and flight of the rest of the school. Lorenz (1967) also reports findings of studies of rats which describe disturbance to the whole colony resulting from the entry of a stranger with a strange odor. Eventually, the colony converges upon the stranger to destroy him. However, if he is rubbed with the dirt and nesting materials of the colony, he does not disturb the tranquility of the unit.

It is not only the fact of being a stranger to the collective that creates a community predicament, but any observable departure from the accustomed pattern of self-signals or manner of self-presentation seems to establish a disturbing predicament to the society. In Hebb's (1949) studies of fear, he produced general consternation by drugging a chimp or presenting a disembodied head to the colony.

Ways of Resolving the Predicament

Intervention such as is described in this volume, is one way of coming to terms with the experience of collective threat associated with deviance. At least two other avenues have appeared in the literature (Benedict, 1934; Szasz, 1970). Since the community's predicament revolves around assimilation of differences into the total collective, most of our interventions attempt to make the individual more like the group. Instead of trying to do away with, preventing, or modifying an individual's strange behavior, strange feelings, strange life-styles, etc., and modeling him into a normative member of the group--or, instead of trying to radically modify social structures, systems, or environments, etc.--we may have recourse to two universal cultural solutions. One method of assimilation is to incorporate the difference into the mores of the group by institutionalizing it; in this way, visions, trances, hallucinations, etc. have been incorporated into the culture of American Indians, The Catholic Church, and religions of India.

Another possible method of assimilation is to establish a national ethos for toleration of wide ranges of group and individual differences. The nation that prides itself on wide variation in both groups and individuals, or that extols eccentricity, has reduced its intervention problem considerably. When human differences are prized, de-differentiation becomes less important in the affairs of that nation. The strange, the different, the unusual, become an occasion for celebration rather than cause for intervention.

This could be a viable solution for a nation that developed around cultural plurality, and whose major harbor entrance for refugee citizens symbolized its ideal with a national monument on which is inscribed, "Give me your tired, your poor, your huddled masses yearning to breathe free, the wretched refuse of your teeming shore. Send these, the homeless, tempest-tost to me..."

A Balanced View

Although the postulation of deviance as a community predicament has focused here on threat and threat-discharge, such a view of intervention does not exclude the idea of true differences among certain members, nor the idea that true caring impulses are involved in intervention. Some individual members do differ from the rest of the community in ways that require care. There is a constant dialectic of impulses in community care giving. Threat and caring seem to be opposite sides of the same coin in almost all community interventions. Sometimes these conflicting impulses are expressed simultaneously in community reactions to its deviance predicament. Sometimes threat and defensive responses predominate in the total collective, or particular segments of the collective. Sometimes caring predominates in collective expressions, or in the expressions of certain segments of the collective.

Just as there is considerable evidence in the behavior of collectives that deviation is either threat-provoking and/or invites threat projection and discharge, the evidence also points to deviation as care-provoking, and caring is projected onto unfortunate or helpless members of the society. Insect, bird and animal studies also document a collective "caring" response to signs of tragedy or helplessness in individual members of a colony, a flock, or a herd (Tinbergen, 1960; Chauvin, 1968; Etkin, 1967; Murie, 1944).

Furthermore, most conceptualizers attribute the basic motivation of communities to caring. The very terms used for intervention systems (i.e., caretaking agencies), or for interveners (caretakers), or for community benevolence in providing care (care giving) indicates the extent to which this type of motivation is perceived as crucial to the intervention complex of communities.

III.   THE INTERVENTION STRUCTURE

From this discussion of deviance and intervention, we might conclude that intervention always implies:

a.   a trained, socially sanctioned intervener;

b.   an intervention target;

c.   a set of assumptions, attitudes, and perceptions about deviance which make up the world view of society;

d.   a set of specific rituals and structured contacts between the intervener, the intervenee, and their cultural binding;

e.   a circumscribed set of contracts between the power structures and the intervener-intervenee contacts.

The Intervener

The trained, sanctioned intervener, whether in a primitive tribe or a modern society, receives his authority from the official governing body. In our society this authority comes from the state, and is in the form of licensing, certification or merit systems. This sanction is extended by the state only after the individual has completed a prescribed course of socialization and indoctrination in his intervention art. For instance, the doctor must go through a certain prescribed course of training before he is eligible for licensing; the teacher must also spend so many years in a specific training program before he can be certified. A tester must have had certain courses and certain experiences before he is certified, etc.

This type of training and social sanctioning for the intervener's role is also common in more "primitive" societies. As pointed out by Frank (1961), modern interventions date from two historical traditions: the religio-magical and the naturalistic or scientific. The religio-magical regards certain forms of alienation as caused by supernatural or magical intervention (e.g., possession of soul). Intervention consists of suitable rites conducted by an intervener who combines the roles of priest and doctor to restore the victim to health and re-strengthen his ties with his group. The shaman or sorcerer within the religio-magical tradition also goes through a carefully prescribed, arduous path of sequential training, indoctrination and socialization before assuming the role of intervener (Casteneda, 1968), just as does the professional in today's society. His functional role as an intervener exists because it is sanctioned, believed in, and operationalized by his society.

The naturalistic intervener is much more a product of "civilization." However, even in civilized countries such as China, India, and the Western societies, there was much of the religio-magical in the naturalistic interventions. Doctors, teachers, tutors, etc. have been very much a part of that tradition. They may play much the same role in their society as does the shaman in his, but there is an attempt to divest the process of the religious and magical assumptions and trappings.

The Target

The ultimate target of intervention is, of course, a person or persons. As indicated earlier, this person is either alienated from the assumptive group or is the representative proxy for the group. In the first case, he is seen as having a disjunctive relationship to the world of the group of which he is a part. In the religio-magical tradition, he is under a spell of some sort; foreign forces or foreign bodies have somehow entered into him. These intrusions have to be routed or dispelled. In the second case, he is seen as a transference proxy for the evils suffered by the group.

Assumptions

All interventions, in whatever society, are based upon an assumptive system of that society. The framework within which the intervention takes place is a self-consistent, assumptive world shared by that society. The powers of the intervener are explained in terms of the society's assumptive world and are unquestionably accepted as genuine. The assumptive world of the Ugandans above contained malevolent foes who could work magic against them, and cause the people to die of disease. This force was as real to the Ugandan as schizophrenia is to the American. It was a world in which evil could be warded off by a sacrificial goat. Szasz (1970, p.239) in comparing diagnosis of mental illness with diagnosis of witchcraft says:

47

The faithful christian hunting witches and the devout
mental health worker ferreting out cases of undiscovered
mental illness must rely on the covert signs, or hidden stigmata, of witchcraft and mental disease. These
supposed signs are not evident to ordinary persons, or
even to the person who allegedly exhibits the sign. This
is what justifies, indeed requires, the employment of
specialists--witch-finders and psychiatric diagnosti-
cians--to discover heretical and insane members of the
community. The result is that in both the Inquisition
and in Institutional Psychiatry, the well-doers must
first gain social authorization for his "case-finding"
before being permitted to practice his "therapy."

Szasz (1970, p.260) further says:

I have argued that both the medieval witch and the
modern mental patient are the scapegoats of society.
By sacrificing some of its members, the community
seeks to "purify" itself and thus maintain its integrity and survival.

In the assumptive world of our own society there are con-

ditions of disability such as emotional disturbance, retardation,

delinquency, which can be prevented, modified or cured through

appropriate interventions. There are more or less absolute conditions

of normality and abnormality and the individual who departs from

normality can be helped to come closer to that standard. The vari-

ous naturalistic or scientific elaborations of that assumptive world

are more clearly spelled out in the previous volume of the Conceptual

Project dealing with theories. However, in terms of public beliefs

and convictions there are assumptive systems existing side-by-side

in the society. All of them have been carried over from other his-

torical periods and have the same legitimacy as the more scientific

and naturalistic translations of these assumptions. The religious

concept of "bad" or "possessed" still has credence in many circles

48

and in many communities of the United States. The belief in poor genes or bad genes, not only survives, but has recently received renewed support in this country. The concept of craziness and juvenile criminality is very much a part of society. [Juvenile delinquency as a public concept did not come into existence until the early 1900's (Platt, 1969)]. Each of these explanatory systems have been and are still being applied to the same conditions and even the same persons. Acting-out behavior in the psychiatric sense, is the same thing as unadaptive conditioned behavior in the psychological sense, is the same thing as social maladjustment in the educational jargon, and is the same thing as delinquency in correctional terminology. In every case, a variety of naturalistic explanatory systems can be used to account for and characterize the child who exhibits such behavior.

These elaborated views of the world have brought a variety of interventions and interveners into existence in our society. More "primitive" societies, on the other hand, rely on fewer forms of intervention, fewer rituals and fewer structured contacts with the intervenee.

Contract

In addition to operating within an assumptive world shared by the society, and to some extent by the intervenee, the intervention is a cricumscribed, structured contact between intervener and intervenee. The specific forms which the contact may take are

spelled out in the individual intervention sections of this volume.
The particular strategies, methods and practices operationalize the
contact. In some of the cases, the contact is deep and powerful
requiring that the intervener experience the other through himself,
as though he were part of the phenomenology of the other. This
type of contact, required in the psychodynamic interventions, the
existential and counter-theory interventions, places great demands
upon the intervener and brings him very close to the religio-magical
state existing between shaman and client. Other types of contact,
such as the behavioral and biophysical, do not put this requirement
upon the intervener. Such contacts fall much more into the naturalistic and scientific mode of intervention. They encourage the intervener to clearly separate himself from the intervenee so that he
can maintain an objective stance. Instead of the I-thou relationship of the existentialists, it is a subject-object relationship,
like that employed by the physicist or the chemist toward his subject matter. This latter type of contact places much more emphasis
upon prediction and control of the deviance complex, rather than
upon understanding and experience of the deviance phenomenon.

All of the components of intervention which have already
been mentioned--the "world-view" of the community, the target of
intervention, the deviance assumptions of the society, and the
specific rituals or structured contact between intervener and
intervenee--can only occur within a specific set of social contracts

or legitimations. In our own society these contacts are legitimized in some very circumscribed ways.

First of all, there is the contract between intervener and society. In our own intervention systems, society is represented primarily by governmental bodies, and secondarily by professional guilds. The major intervention delivery systems are governmental, and are administered by governmental bodies at the national, state, and local level (i.e., the mental health system, the educational system, etc.). Sanctioning of intervention into the lives of children is assured both through governmental funds and governmental "ownership" of the service agencies. In addition, the specific techniques of intervention, such as special education teaching and psychotherapy, are licensed or certified by the state. The state legislates who may practice the interventions, and the course of indoctrination which the professional must complete in order to obtain formal sanctioning. The professional guilds themselves, further regulate the use of the intervention practices by their own professional bodies under state laws.

It can be seen, then, that society carefully controls the legitimization of the practice of interventions. One of the greatest struggles in professional history has been over the professional ownership of psychotherapy. With the growth of alternative forms of schooling, this struggle may also develop over the right to teach.

51

Another level of the intervention contract is between the intervener and the intervenee. In order for the intervener to be able to practice upon the intervenee, there must be some sharing of the legitimacy of such contact. The intervenee must, at some level, consent both to the assumptive system being imposed upon him--that is, that he is in the state or condition that society is perceiving him to be--and must also assent to the power of the intervener to affect this state.

In the case of the shaman, for instance, the village member receiving his ministrations must have some belief in and be somewhat acquiescent to what the shaman is doing with him. When the intervenee either loses the faith, or when he questions the legitimacy of the intervener, the structured contact is broken.

This is true to a considerable extent in our own society. The professional and his charge must be bound in a mutual covenant in order for the psychotherapy, the teaching, the counseling, etc. to take place. Where there is a failure to share in the belief system framing the professional contact, or when the intervenee is a reluctant captive of the intervener and the intervention system (such as school, clinic, etc.), the intended action does not take place. This may be one reason why teachers are not able to bring about socially expected levels of achievement in poverty schools, why testers seem to get such unreliable test results in those same geophysical areas, why psychotherapy doesn't work very well in correctional facilities, or even in state mental hospitals.

In discussing the contract between intervener and intervenee we have also implicitly and explicitly treated the contract between power structures and the intervener-intervenee contact. Even reluctant intervenees are frequently required by law to go through the intervener-intervenee rituals. Subjecting oneself to the ministrations of the school is compulsory. Subjecting oneself to the incarceration institutions is frequently compulsory. Power structures such as school boards can force the intervenee to undergo the intervention prescribed by the school. Neither a child nor his parents can refuse to be tested within the schools without bringing all of the power available to the school down upon their heads. In terms of the rituals of interventions, then an individual who has been publicly labeled deviant (declared insane, adjudicated a delinquent, classified as retarded by the schools, etc.) has little choice except to go through the ritual of the contract. However, he can abort the intervention contract, as suggested above, by not really believing or cooperatively participating in the contract.

IV.   THE RENAISSANCE OF CARING

Cultural Resurrection

Every intervention carries with it a particular view of the situation of condition that invites intervention. It carries a notion of the source of the problem, what the outcome of entry should be, and what the intermediary should cause to happen. Intervention is value-oriented and value-directed. Without implicit or explicit values, interventions would not be undertaken.

In a world in which there is general consensus about the nature of values, there is an acceptance of established interventions. Studies of earlier forms of society, or of "primitive" societies existing today, show that particular kinds of interventions and interveners are accepted as part of the givens of life, like the weather and the physical surroundings. A shaman or a medicine man is assumed to be as natural as a drink of water, and as necessary as the air that is breathed. In the same way, in our society, until recently there was little questioning of "fixed" intervention processes such as teaching, therapy, counseling and testing. Teachers, therapists, counselors and testers were considered necessary fixtures in a society which had maintained a consensus with respect to the right relationship between the individual and the society. However, in the current period of rapidly shifting values this agreement is dissolving. There is no social consensus about the right relationship between men and between man

and society. Hence, men are not in agreement about human interventions or intervention structures. The whole area of human care-
taking is under careful scrutiny and reexamination from many diverse
segments of society. Many of the social and institutional arrangements for care-giving and care-receiving are being sharply questioned.

It is not surprising that at this time in history there
should be so much concern with the beliefs, practices and conven-
tions of public caring. Man has been so forceably confronted with
the technical perfection of his destructive tendencies, that he is
desperate to find a way out before he destroys himself. In all
areas of private and public life, radical efforts are being made
to break through to his deeper layers of caring. The experienced
meaning of care was lost to individuals by the formalization of
care structures and processes which isolate the care-receivers
from the general populace. Now, like returning feeling in a cramped
limb, we are experiencing the pain of direct caring. A new awareness seems to be developing that the caring experience is a necessary
ingredient in the preservation of community life.

Many groups of individuals, formerly uninvolved in the functions of care-giving institutions, are suddenly aware of the part
they play in the process. Such groups are taking stances vis-a-vis
these institutions, and are examining what they do, and whom they
serve. Many of these groups are opening up previously closed conceptions of the place of these in public life. This applies to the

whole range of care-taking institutions, from public schools to
mental hospitals. Groups of professionals, of scientists, of care
recipients, of various political fraternities, of social critics,
of youth groups, etc. are all involving themselves in the life and
ways of such social institutions.

Criticisms of the Care Giving Function

Most of the psychosocial criticisms of intervention and the
intervention professions being raised today view with great clarity
and wisdom the ignoble aspects of care giving. The critics see the
self-serving, the defensive, the naked power politics of intervention
and intervention instruments. They view a continuity between the
Inquisition and witch burning and modern-day care giving (Szasz, 1970).
Such egregious human search and destroy activities were carried out
in the name of love, in the name of saving the deviant in spite of
himself. These critics point out that the neurotic twisting of the
inborn succorrance urge results in the destruction of men by fellow
men, the projection of evil, of pain and pestilence, of threat and
horror onto some poor, defenseless, masocistic target. They point
to the tendency which man has had across cultures and across eons
of history to band together in a congeries, denying their pain,
their evil, their involvement in their own misfortune, or their
helplessness in the face of adversity, and wishing it all onto a
poor sacrificial lamb.

The critics see in sharp relief, that facet of the succor-
rance-aggression dimension which man feels toward his fellow man,

and then discharges upon a proxy, a hostage to the collective. The hostage becomes a receptacle upon whom they unburden their ills, their pain, their fear. And they do this in the name of love; because love is also there. Love for the sufferer. Love for the tormented one who takes upon himself their torment; actually, love for their tormented selves.

In most of its institutional forms, care giving is a parody on love. It frequently encompasses the aggression, the fear, the desire to purge oneself of that difference that might separate one from the collective. In order to maintain unity, the collective frequently gives a special name to the one singled out as different. This one is called disabled, or deviant, or alien. At the very moment he is labelled, the rest of the group suffer, and they yearn to take the name away from him, to make him conform to their ideal-- perfect, without blemish, without differences. At that moment they know his pain and try to give it back to him and rid themselves of it. But they are feeling with him and seeing themselves on the other side, his side, the side that is separated from the masses.

Furthermore, as we examine some of the greatest of the "scapegoats," such as Christ, we see direct evidence of powerful positive values such as "love." Such historically important scape- goats may be said to have taken ills upon themselves, according to generally accepted, shared beliefs. They expressed great succorrance and demonstrated care values as a model for all who observed and all who heard about this act.

And so, there is a medley of emotions, a blend of aggression and succorance, of revulsion and love. And the other one sees and feels it, and assumes these feelings as characteristics of himself. He cannot separate their caring and their hating, nor can he separate the qualities of himself from their caring and hating. And so he takes onto himself the scorn, the pity, the conditions of life, which they impute to him as though they were his own. He becomes the disabled, the deviant, the alien one--so different from the others.

It doesn't matter whether he yields to their ministrations or fights them off. In either case, intervention will be undertaken. If he accepts the projections of the collective as justified, he becomes the retarded, the delinquent, the disturbed. Most of the critics see this institutional violation of human rights, and conclude that only they sympathize and feel the pain and suffering of the sacrificial goat. Somehow the care and the succorrance are not actualized in the institutions and bureaus set up for care giving. Care and love elude the concrete forms of the institutions, and those who observe the intervention institutions, assume that there is no care or love for the collective proxy.

The critics see the act of intervention as a hostile act, one which serves to exile the collective proxy from the whole, from the body politic. And, in many ways, it may be. If we see the

natural collective in action, we see many of the same actions and
behaviors as we observe in our institutional care giving today.
A strange bee, entering a beehive, is attacked and extruded because
he is different. A fish whose swimming behavior departs even slightly
from the school is swiftly abandoned by the school and attacked by
other predator fish. A drugged chimpanzee, introduced into a colony
of chimpanzees, arouses consternation in the colony because of his
sensed difference. A rat, who is removed from a rat colony and
cleansed of the colony smell and the nesting materials in his hair,
aroused colony-wide upset when re-introduced into the collective body,
and is eventually searched out and destroyed. Behavioral ethologists
say that this is the attempt of the herd, the hive, the colony, the
school, to protect itself and ensure its own continuity. In some
cases, the differentiated member is abandoned so that predators can
destroy him, and thus remove the source of disease, etc., which could
contaminate and wipe out the collective group. In other cases, the
collective itself either drives out the "offending" member or destroys
him. In reading the reports of some naturalists, this writer finds
accounts in which one sees a concert of possible emotions being expressed
in the group behavior. In the case of the drugged chimpanzee, the behaviors are either flight from the drugged member, attack of the drugged member, or a medley of attack and flight. According to accounts
of bird behavior, when one of the members is wounded, the group circles
around and around the wounded member, sounding cries. The observer

can read into this behavior any emotions he wishes. It depends upon the value which he imputes to the group behavior. The medley of behaviors reported in animal studies are also reported in human studies.

Recent students of institutional care giving, particularly studies of professions such as psychiatry, psychology, and teaching, have evolved a social-deviance theory which compares the treatment of deviants to the ancient and pan-cultural practice of scapegoating. Szasz's thesis in Manufacture of Madness (1970) is compelling and powerful. He sees institutional psychiatry as a direct continuation of the Inquisition and of witch hunting, with the modern-day concept of mental illness image taking the place of the witch image. Becker (1964), Scheff, and other sociologists have also presented powerful arguments that the society needs deviants for its own purposes, and when there is no obvious candidate for that role, it creates deviants.

One draws from this literature a rather bleak picture of man's caring for man, of man's nuturance efforts, of man's service acts toward his fellow man. The message which these investigators convey is that they are opposed to such "de-humanization." They demand that we should feel as they do: we should be repulsed and demand a humanization of our institutions. Their emotions, their values, are humanistic; and since they bother to write to us, they must assume that there may be a resonating value in those who read their works.

Revolt Against Care Giving Metaphors

The care giving metaphors themselves, such as retardation, mental illness and disturbance, delinquency and criminality; culturally disadvantaged, etc. are coming into question (Szasz, 1970; Scott, 1958; Mercer, 1970; Menninger, 1968; Kvaraceus, 1959). The theoretical bases of such attacks differ from investigator to investigator, but the essential argument is that the attribution of any of the above conditions to individual members of the community involves, in some degree, psychological projection, scapegoating, or arbitrary labeling. These authors frequently examine the function that such assignments serve for society and present sound arguments and documentation that human caring is either absent or distorted in the assignment process. The very tone of their arguments, however, the very substance of their case is empathy, sympathy and concern; it is an implicit statement that the authors know their audience is capable of caring, is capable of revulsion at its own use of labeling to extrude some of its own members.

The technical process by which these metaphors are assigned, the instruments themselves, are being successfully challenged and legal decisions are being handed down against them. Such litigation and the resulting decisions indicate a willingness to use the legal process to review and renew the care giving and care taking process.

At the same time, general revolt is taking place among the labeled groups against public stereotypes of themselves; and at the same time, these groups are emancipating themselves from their own acceptance and incorporation of such public stereotypes. Individuals and groups, boxed in to such narrow niches as "homosexuals," "criminal," "addict," etc. are beginning to liberate themselves from these all-embracing social incantations. They are counterattacking both the metaphors being imposed upon them, and the barriers to social participation which the metaphors erect. They not only challenge public authority to impose such barriers, but they are angry at their own previous acceptance of these barriers as natural and justified. They are angry at their previous self-rejection and are beginning to care for themselves.

Revolt Against Care Receiving Investiture

Challenges are also coming from many quarters of society to the social dominance of care givers _vis-a-vis_ care receivers. There is deep probing into the "investiture of care receiver" bestowed by society upon certain of its members. This probing goes beyond the labeling process and investigates the institutionalized procedures by which we carry out early-identification and then program certain individuals through a series of funnels, into narrow care-giving niches, pre-ordained by society. Investiture of an official care receiving title, role, and function in society is being demonstrated to be frequently arbitrary and capricious (Mercer, 1970).

The term "investiture" is used here to refer to the broader ecological actions of collectives, not only in singling out candidates

for labeling, but also in moving candidates through a set of institutional decision structures and critical junctures, to the exclusion
niche. Jane Mercer's description (1970) of the stages through which
a child passes in becoming officially "retarded" in the school system
is an example of this type of action structure.

Again, as in the case of disputation of the labeling process,
the questioning of the investiture procedure expresses a new level
of caring, a new willingness to act upon one's empathetic concern
for fellow members who become victims of such care-taking investiture.
The reaction of society, the avid interest which the general public
shows in buying books and popular magazines which report such scientific
investigations is an indication of a new aliveness, a new consciousness of caring in the society.

Revolt Against Care Givers

There is another important movement occurring in the midst
of these other evidences of a new consciousness of caring. The
credentialized care takers themselves are being questioned with respect
to their qualifications and capacity to intervene in the lives of
those to whom they give care. The challenge of the "indigenous"
mental health workers in the Lincoln Mental Health Center against
the administration and professional staff, the revolt of parents in
inner-city neighborhoods, such as the Oceanhill-Brownsville area,
against the professional authority of the school system, are examples
of this questioning. This challenge of the professional intervener
is occurring on two grounds; one is the inability of someone so

63

totally removed from the life and culture of the intervenee to be
able to care, understand, and deal with his crushing problems; the
second is on the questionable legitimacy of the interveners' special
expertness. Teaching, psychotherapy, counseling, etc. the argument
goes, is a talent widely shared in the population. It does not
require a special credentialing process, and elite schooling to be
effective in such interventions.

Furthermore, this challenge to the unique authority of the
professional intervener is tied to a broader examination of the
use and abuse of care giving, care taking and care receiving.

Revolt Against the Economics and Politics of Care

There is a serious probing of the economics of care giving
and the social politics of care giving. There is a growing conviction that those whose careers are based largely upon care giving
and decision making about care receivers, are in an advantageous
position, economically and politically, in society. The official
care taking institutionalization of health, education, welfare, etc.
has grown to be a very powerful part of domestic life in the United
States. These institutional forms have become mammoth governmental
monopolies which reach into many parts of life. Legislators, informal power groups, scientists, university faculties, etc. have a
tremendous stake in such care taking monopolies. A Presidential or
gubernatorial candidate frequently offers some form of care taking
as a major plank in his platform. Special industries such as book-

publishers, test-publishers and test services, equipment manufacturers, etc. accumulate their wealth and prestige from the care giving industry. The huge government research institutes, major professional schools and departments in universities are directly tied to the care giving institutions. The mammoth care taking cartels are clearly the source of great power and wealth.

There is a growing concern about the size of these institutions and about their political and economic importance in this country. After all, the power and wealth of the church, founded to a large extend upon the monastic movement, and enlarged by the Inquisition, shows the powerful advantage of the care giving intervener. The investigation of the National Institute of Mental Health by Ralph Nader (Chu, et al., 1972), the questions being raised by the poor and the minority groups, the criticisms by authors such as Thomas Szasz (1970), Franz Fanon (1968), John Holt (1964) and Ivan Illich (1971), all demonstrate the new probing into the economics and politics of care.

Behind such powerful re-examinations is a strong concern for the real meaning of care, a desire to strengthen the sentiment of caring, to attempt to disentangle it from some of the overlay of power and economics, so that it might be made clearer and free of some of its contaminants.

Revolt Against Care Taking Institutions

There is another curious set of events taking place across

the country and across institutional lines. It is occurring in relation to educational institutions, correctional institutions, mental health institutions, and welfare institutions. These events have to do with questioning the legitimacy and power of these institutions to regulate, control, or intervene in behavior. It is interesting, of course, that the care receivers themselves are raising questions about their mandated interactions with these institutions. It is even more interesting, however, that some of the professional and scientific groups aligned with these institutions, and increasingly large segments of the general populace are also joining forces with the compulsory care receivers. The events at Attica prison, being repeated in less dramatic fashion all across the nation, are an example of this trend. The various forms of student unrest in public schools and universities is another example. The wide questioning and searching for alternatives to mental institutions is still a third example.

In general, the criticism is against the way in which these facilities deal with their resident populations, against the quality of relationships, against the lack of compassion and relevance. Some recent experiments raise even more serious concerns. One is a university experiments in replicating a prison atmosphere and the simulation of inmate and custodian roles. This simulation had to be halted after a few days because of the violent changes taking place in the feelings, attitudes, and behaviors of the role players.

66

The other was a study by a Stanford University psychologist (Rosenhan, 1973), in which eight colleagues successfully feigned symptoms of schizophrenia, hoodwinking doctors at all twelve hospitals they visited in a five-state area. Diagnosed as schizophrenic, the pseudo-patients were admitted as in-patients. They were not released until an average of nineteen days had passed, even though every one dropped the phony symptoms upon admittance. There were a number of very interesting evaluations indicating serious pathology in these "sane" pseudo-patients. Although the hospital staff were frequently benign in their treatment of these phony patients, the relationship was depersonalized.

These attacks on institutions from many quarters suggests that our major caretaking solutions are being declared irrelevant and non-human. Providing care for deviant populations is no longer a sufficient reason for existence in today's society. New measures have to be found, new care-relating structures have to be created.

Underclass Revolt

Along with the self-caring reaction of individually labeled groups such as homosexuals or prisoners, we are also witnessing a significant growing community-sense among the underclass groups who now see themselves as the major recruiting pools from which the individual care-receiving categories are drawn. Their strengthening sense of community grows from their developing conviction that their own self-denigration of their underclass status such as poor, or black, or Chicano, or Indian, makes them particularly susceptible to the social-contagion of such roles as mentally ill, alcoholic, addict, prostitute, pimp, etc. They are declaring to their fellow-members that self-denigration makes it easy for mainline culture-bearers to assign them such roles. Therefore, they argue that as a group, they must counteract self-denigration, and foster self-respect and self-caring by assuming the exact antithesis of the public denigration of their ethno-cultural status. "Black is beautiful," is a typical expression of this attitude, or "Political Prisoners," or "racism," or "chauvinism."

Therefore, any attempt of the intervention structures of society to focus their case-finding, diagnostic, corrective, reha-bilitative or remedial services upon their special ethno-cultural groups is increasingly being met with active resistance, and counter-control efforts.

Revolt Against the Melting Pot Myth in Caretaking

Along with this new perception of the care-receiving segment of the general population, a more generic concern has begun to surface. The many specific examinations of care giving philosophies, attitudes, and structures in society have led to a re-thinking of the melting pot homogeneity assumption which has been so significant in the history of this country. The question is being raised as to whether this conventional belief system has not always been based upon a myth. "Is it not true," the query goes, "that the real motif of this country has always been ethno-cultural pluralism?" "Does not the melting pot assumption militate against group and individual rights and differences?" "Does it not sustain a fantasy of an 'ideal type,' an 'inherent cultural normality,' a single standard of behavior to which all could and should adhere. Isn't this essentially what all of our care giving interventions attempt to insure? Are not many of our care-giving efforts of treatment, remediation, education, rehabilitation, etc. aimed toward achieving in all members of the society some attainment of this vaguely hypothesized "healthy, happy, normal, individual?" So goes the new dialogue.

The Gathering Force

At the present time, each of these separate movements, actions, and voices are unorganized and lack any central unifying focus. However, each of them can be perceived as a new emergence of caring, a re-experiencing in new depths the new dimensions of a strong force, relatively inactive over a long period of history. It is as though our society has gone through a long period of a collective neurotic fugue, in which the strong drive of man to succor his fellow man, has become submerged and covered over by strong, impersonal, structures of institutional care taking and mechanical professional care giving. It is as though these murky layers of impersonal institutionalization had so obscured the individual caring drive, that it was rendered impotent and passive

69

by the mammoth structures of intervention which came between the drive and the objects of caring. It is as though we defused the caring force, and separated man from his caring affections by intervention structures.

But, the strength of the above-mentioned efforts indicates that it has become a deep force in the social order today, and promises to gain strength and power as it advances. The voice of Thomas Szasz (1970), questioning institutional psychiatry and psychiatric interventions, the voice of Ivan Illich (1971), Christopher Jenks (1972), or John Holt (1964) questioning institutionalized education are solo efforts at the present time rather than a united chorus. The various legal attacks of special interest groups upon psychological and educational testing, the legal attacks upon incarceration in mental and correctional institutions as a form of intervention, the legal attacks upon "special" education, and the rights of "exceptional children," are typical of these scattered counterattacks upon our present forms of caretaking.

No matter where you look in the society today, there is this new awareness of the consciousness of caring, and of its significance in counteracting the forces of technical destruction let loose in the world by the perfection of a nuclear holocaust. This has led to a total examination of the right relationship between men and between men and community; and in the process the whole fabric of our caring apparatus and assumptions is under scrutiny. Any thought about future interventions has to take this force into account.

70

Alverdes, F. *Social life in the animal world.* New York: Harcourt, Brace, & Company, 1927.

Ardrey, R. *The territorial imperative: A personal inquiry into the animal origins of property and nations.* New York: Atheneum, 1967.

Ashton-Warner, S. *Spearpoint.* New York: Alfred A. Knopf, 1972.

Ashton-Warner, S. *Teacher.* New York: Simon and Schuster, 1963.

Becker, H. *The other side.* New York: The Free Press, 1964.

Benedict, R. Anthropology and the abnormal. *Journal of General Psychology,* 1934, 11, 59-80.

Carpenter, C. R. *Naturalistic behavior of nonhuman primates.* University Park, Pennsylvania: The Pennsylvania State University Press, 1964.

Chauvin, R. *Animal societies from the bee to the gorilla.* Tr. by G. Ordish. New York: Hill and Wang, 1968.

Castenada, C. *Journey to Ixtlan.* New York: Simon and Schuster, 1972.

Castenada, C. *Separate reality.* New York: Simon and Schuster, 1971.

Castenada, C. *The teachings of Don Juan.* Los Angeles: University of California Press, 1968.

Chu, F. D., Trotter, S., Simon, G., & Wolfe, S. M. *The mental health complex: Part 1. Community mental health centers.* Washington, D. C.: Center for Study of Responsive Law, 1972.

Driver, H. E. *Indians of North America.* Chicago: University of Chicago Press, 1961.

Durkheim, E. *Suicide.* New York: Free Press of Glencoe, 1951.

Etkin, W. *Social behavior from fish to man.* Chicago: University of Chicago Press, 1967.

Fanon, F. *The wretched of the earth.* Tr. by Constance Farrington. New York: Grove Press, 1968.

Frank, J. D. Persuasion and healers. Baltimore: Johns Hopkins Press, 1961.

Frazer, J. The golden bough. New York: Macmillan, 1950.

Freire, P. Pedagogy for the oppressed. New York: Herter & Herter, 1970.

Freud, S. Civilization and its discontents. London: Hogarth Press, 1958.

Graubard, P. S., Rosenberg, H., & Miller, M. B. Student applications of behavior modification to teachers and environments: Ecological approaches to social deviance. Presented at Second Annual Invitational Conference on Behavior Analysis in Education. Department of Human Development. Lawrence, Kansas: University of Kansas, 1971.

Harlow, H., & Harlow, M. The young monkey. Readings in Psychology Today. Del Mar, California: CRM Books, 1969.

Hebb, D. O. The organization of behavior. New York: Wiley, 1949.

Holt, J. How children fail. New York: Pitman, 1964.

Holt, J. How children learn. New York: Pitman, 1969.

Illich, I. Deschooling society. New York: Harper & Row, 1971.

Jenks, C. Inequality. New York: Basic Books, 1972.

Kvaraceus, W. C., & Miller, W. Delinquent behavior: Culture and the individual. Washington, D. C.: National Education Association, 1959.

Lorenz, K. On aggression. New York: Bantam Books, 1967.

Makarenko, A. S. The road to life (an epic of education). Moscow: Foreign Language Publishing House, 1951.

Marcuse, H. One dimensional man. New York: Beacon, 1964.

Mead, M. (Ed.) Cooperation to competition among primitive peoples. Boston: Beacon Press, 1961.

Meggitt, M. J. Desert people: A study of the Walbiri aborigines of central Australia. Sydney, Australia: Angus & Robertson, 1962.

Melland, F. H. In witch-bound Africa. London: Seeley, Service and Company, 1923.

Menninger, K. The crime of punishment. Saturday Review, Sept. 7, 1968, 21-55.

Mercer, J. Sociological prespectives on mild mental retardation. In H. Haywood, Social-cultural aspects of retardation. New York: Appleton-Century-Crofts, 1970.

Murie, A. The wolves of Mt. McKinley. Washington, D. C.: U. S. Government Printing Office, 1944.

Platt, A. The child savers: The invention of delinquency. Chicago: University of Chicago Press, 1969.

Poole, T. B. Aggressive play in polecats. Symposia of the Zoological Society of London, 1966, 18, 23-44.

Rosenhan, D. L. On being sane in insane places. Science, 1973, 169 (4070), 250-258.

Scott, W. A. Research definitions of mental health and mental illness. Psychological Bulletin, 1958, 55, 29-45.

Selegman, C., & Selegman, B. Pagan tribes of the Nitale Sudan. London: George Routhledge and Sons, 1932.

Szasz, T. The manufacture of madness: A comparative study of the Inquisition and the mental health movement. New York: Harper & Row, 1970.

Tinbergen, N. The herring gull's world: A study of the social behavior of birds. New York: Basic Books, 1960.

Webster, H. Taboo, a sociological study. Stanford, California: Stanford University Press, 1942.

Williamson, P. W. The social and political system of central Polynesia, VII. Cambridge: The Cambridge University Press, 1929.

Wood, M. M. The stranger: A study in social relationships. New York: Columbia University Press, 1934.

BIOPHYSICAL INTERVENTIONS IN EMOTIONAL DISTURBANCE

L. I. Kameya

TABLE OF CONTENTS

I. INTRODUCTION

In the following review of the biophysical substrates of behavior and of interventions that are based upon these biological mechanisms, no assumption is made that these mechanisms account for <u>all</u> differences in behavior. The nature-nurture question is not at issue; it is posited that both environmental and innate factors <u>interact</u> to influence the behavior of any organism. However, the exact nature of these interactions cannot be understood without some background knowledge of environmental agents as well as biological mechanisms. Environmental influences are now generally understood and taken for granted, especially since Locke's notion of the <u>tabula rasa</u>.

However, in the education and special education fields there has been a dearth of knowledge of biophysical theories, and of the mechanisms that relate to human behavior. In this review, three general areas are covered. First, genetic factors are discussed. Genetic anomalies, while not always related to emotional disturbance, are useful in illustrating heritability and specific gene effects. Also included are discussions of genetic counseling and of the ethical implications of genetic manipulations that are possible and imminent. The second section deals with neurological factors and interventions. Included are drug therapy, retraining methods, and environmental restructuring for biologically-based behavioral syndromes. The third section is concerned with biochemical factors and interventions. Included are orthomolecular approaches (e.g. megavitamin treatments) and nutritional considerations.

79

A.   Background Information

"Genetics may be broadly defined as the study of relations between genotypic and phenotypic levels of biological organization." The phenotype   includes all morphological, physiological and behavioral traits;   the genotype refers to the complete endowment of genes and chromosomes.   It is assumed that the phenotype is the result of an interaction between the genotype and the environment, and that individual differences are a function of both genetic and environmental differences (Murray and Hirsch, 1969).   Some general terms and concepts shall first be defined. The material in this section is drawn largely from Redding and Hirschhorn (1968), Townes (1968), E. B. Ford (1968) and Volpe (1971).

Chromosomes (from the Greek for colored bodies, because of their affinity for certain dyes), each with a specific sequence of genes, are the structures in each cell which determine heredity; the genes are the specific unit which transmit this information.

Except for reproductive cells (sperm and ova) every cell in the body has 46 chromosomes. A karyotype (an arrangement of the chromosomes by pairs, according to size) shows 22 pairs, called autosomes, each of which is identical to its partner, plus 2 sex chromosomes, called X and Y. Normal males have an X and a Y chromosome and normal females have two X chromosomes in addition to the normal complement of autosomes. The karyotype can be studied for abnormalities in either number or structure of the chromosomes and these deviations may be related to phenotypic traits.

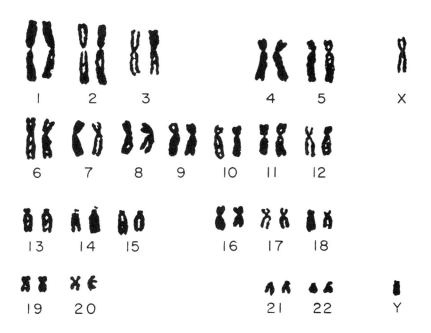

Fig. 1. Karyotype of the Chromosomes of a Normal Male. Notice that the 22 paired chromosomes (the autosomes) are arranged in descending order according to size and shape. The X and Y chromosomes, which determine the sex of the individual are easily recognized as different from the autosomes.

(Redding and Hirschhorn, 1968, p. 92)

The fertilized human egg carries in its 46 chromosomes all of the genetic information that is necessary in the cellular differentiation that is to follow. All females have at birth 100,000 to 600,000 immature egg cells (oocytes) within their ovaries. During the fertile years, about 400 of these egg cells ripen and are released (ova). These ova and the sperm (reproductive cells from the male) contain only 23 chromosomes (22 autosomes and an X or Y chromosome). Hence when an ovum and sperm fuse, they carry the 46 chromosomes of the new organism.

These mature egg cells are produced through a process call meiosis. In simple terms, meiosis is a process whereby the cellular material divides twice while the chromosomal material, after duplicating itself, divides once. The end result is that each immature reproductive cell results in 4 cells, each of which contains one-half of the chromosomes of the parent cell (haploid number); when it combines with another reproductive cell, the resulting organism has the full complement (diploid number) of chromosomes.

The somatic division of cells (by which the organism grows and replaces lost cells such as skin and blood cells) occurs through the process of mitosis. In this cellular division, the chromosomal material duplicates itself and the cellular material, divides once, with the chromosomes evenly divided between the daughter cells (see diagram). Hence the daughter cells have the same chromosomal count as the parent cell.

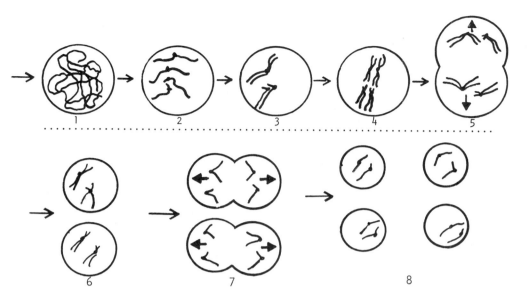

Fig. 2. Meiosis. The type of cell division which results in sperm
and ova with only 23 single chromosomes rather than the 46 (22 pairs
plus two X's or an X and a Y) which are found in other cells. Only
two pairs of chromosomes are shown in this diagram for simplicity.
1) The resting cell is between divisions, its chromosomes not visible
at this point;
2) preparing to divide, the chromosomes are now recognizable as
separate structures;
3) the chromosomes form pairs;
4) the pairs line up across the center of the cell and have duplicated
themselves;
5) the pairs now separate, forming....
6) two cells, each with a single member of each pair of chromosomes;
7) the chromosomes in these cells split in half, resulting in....
8) a total of four new offspring cells, each with one chromosome
from each original pair.
                        (Adapted from Redding and Hirschhorn, 1968, p. 93)

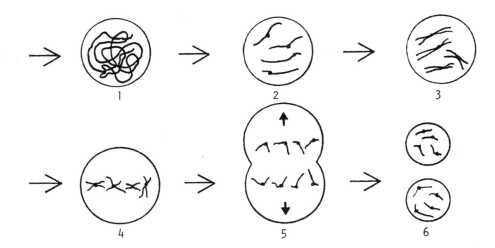

Fig. 3. Mitosis. The division of normal body cells
takes place as follows:
1) Resting stage; the cell is between divisions;
2) the cell is preparing for division and the chromosomes
are now visible (for simplicity, only two pairs of
chromosomes are shown);
3) each chromosome duplicates itself;
4) the duplicated chromosomes line up across the center
of the cell;
5) in the last stage of cell division the duplicated
chromosomes pull apart and move to opposite ends of
the cell; we now have twice as many chromosomes as in
a normal resting cell;
6) two complete new cells have been formed, each with
the same number of chromosomes as the original cell.
   (Adapted from Redding and Hirschhorn, 1968, p. 100)

The importance of understanding these two processes will

become clear as the discussion proceeds to syndromes that can be

attributed to dysfunctions in the chromosomal divisions during

meiosis or mitosis.

Human genetic researchers have utilized two methods

(Parsons, 1967). The first method is a determination of traits controlled by a single gene. This includes studies of behavioral consequences of abnormal karyotypes. The second method is a determination of the heritability of quantitative traits, such as intelligence or personality traits, using correlations and twin studies.

A history and discussion of mongolism, Down's syndrome, or 21-trisomy (Lejeune, 1964) could serve as an illustration of the first method.

The syndrome was first identified by Seguin (1846) and his description of what he called "furfuraceous idiocy" is as complete as many modern day accounts. The term mongoloid was introduced by Langdon-Down as part of his racial hypothesis of mental deficiency (Langdon-Down, 1866).

Twin studies (in which at least one twin was mongoloid) indicated a genetic basis for the disorder. Dizygotic twins (originating from 2 separate egg cells) were generally discordant (i.e., only one of the twins was afflicted) whereas monozygotic twins (originating from one egg cell which separated to form 2 complete organisms) were always concordant (i.e., when one was afflicted, so was the other). This ruled out intrauterine environmental effects as primary agents.

An accurate etiological analysis was not possible until the technological advances of the fifties. In 1956, the diploid number of man was established as 46 rather than 48 as previously believed. Studies published 2 to 6 years later definitely established that mongoloid children of all races possessed an extra chromosome, (47 diploid number). Karyotypic analysis showed this to be an extra 21 chromosome (21-trisomy). Ninety-five percent of all individuals with this syndrome have a 21-trisomy. The trisomy arises during the production of the reproductive cells (meiosis). A pair of chromosomes fail to separate at the appropriate time (meiotic non-disjunction) producing one daughter with both sets of one pair of chromosomes (the other cell produced has none of that pair). If this cell should unite with a normal cell the result would be an individual with 47 chromosomes with a trisomic chromosome. The cell with none of the chromosomal material of that pair would produce, if fertilized, an organism that would be monosomic (with only one of that pair) since it would receive one-half of the material from the other reproductive cell. This individual would have 45 chromosomes rather than the normal 46.

Trisomy-21 produced through nondisjunction is generally related to maternal age and not to paternal age. Hence the nondisjunction probably occurs during the formation of eggs. The probability of delivering a trisomy-21 baby for 20 year old mothers is 1/3,000 and for 45 year old mothers it is 1/50 or higher (Parsons, 1967). This maternal age effect probably is the reflection of the degeneration of the oocytes present in the female from birth as mentioned earlier (Volpe, 1971).

The trisomy-21 syndrome was also found in individuals whose karyotype had the normal 46 chromosomes. This apparent contradiction was resolved when it was determined that the extra chromosome had affixed itself to the 15th chromosome (translocated). At times, small bits of chromosomal matter is deleted (lost) in the process. Of course, if the deleted matter is important or of large quantity, the organism is non-viable. In general, most translocations occur in the chromosome groups 13-15 and 21-22. Although translocations are possible within any group of chromosomes, such abnormalities in the larger pairs (e.g., pairs 1 & 2) are more likely to be lethal since they contain many more genes (Volpe, 1971).

Translocations are not related to maternal age and tend to run in families. The carriers of the translocation can be either male or female, but tend to be female (Redding & Hirschhorn, 1968). There are two types of translocation carriers (phenotypically normal). The first type has a centric fusion translocation where the long arms of the two chromosomes are joined at their centromeres (the point at which chromosome pairs are fused). The short arms of the chromosomes are lost with no deleterious consequences. A reciprocal translocation results when genetic material is exchanged between two chromosomes. The translocation carriers can have normal and afflicted children. For example, if one parent is a carrier with a centric fusion translocation he or she will have (if we concern ourselves with

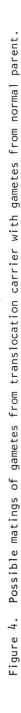

Figure 4. Possible matings of gametes from translocation carrier with gametes from normal parent.

the affected chromosomes) only 3 chromosomes: a 15, a 21, and a
15/21 which is the other two chromosomes fused together. The possible
matings of the gametes from the translocation carrier with the
gametes from the normal parent are represented in the diagram below
(Volpe, 1971; Redding & Hirschhorn, 1968). See Figure 4.

The child who has the 15, 15/21, 21, 21 complement of
chromosomes, because of the three 21 chromosomes will have the Down's
syndrome.

Chromosomal abnormalities can also occur during the process
of mitosis, that is during the normal cell division which occurs when
the fertilized egg begins to divide. Chromosomal material may be
lost in the mitotic process (anaphase lag) or may fail to separate
when the cell divides (mitotic nondisjunction).

If this occurs in the one of the first few cell divisions,
the cells in the individual's body may have different chromosome
counts; some may be normal or trisomic and some may be monosomic.
This condition is call mosaicism. (See Figure 6). Mosaic trisomy-
21 children, for instance, may have normal cells, trisomy-21 cells,
and monosomic 21 cells. The severity of their symptoms is a function of the proportion of trisomy-21 cells in their bodies.

It is not clear exactly what genetic messages are carried
in the 21 chromosomes, since the trisomy-21 has such widespread effects, and it is not clear which effects are interactive with environmental agents. Other phenotypic traits, besides the well-known distinctive facial appearance and mental retardation of the trisomy-21

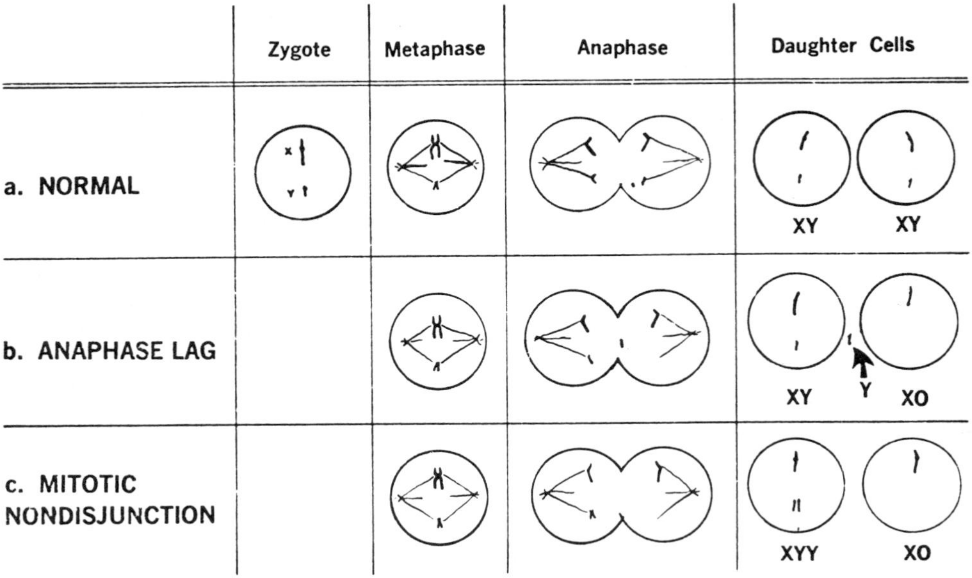

	Zygote	Metaphase	Anaphase	Daughter Cells
a. NORMAL				XY XY
b. ANAPHASE LAG				XY Y XO
c. MITOTIC NONDISJUNCTION				XYY XO

Fig. 5. Methods of Formation of Mosaicism. Only the X and Y chromo-somes are shown in these three diagrams (read horizontally) which illustrate: a) Normal mitosis; b) Anaphase lag; and c) Mitotic non-disjunction in representative male cells (XY-carrying).

Anaphase lag and mitotic nondisjunction can occur in the autosomes as well as in the sex chromosomes. A <u>zygote</u> is a fertilized ovum (the result of a sperm cell and egg cell having mated). This one cell now proceeds to duplicate itself--the first step in creating a complete individual. <u>Metaphase</u> is the point in cell division at which the chromosomes line up across the center of the cell; <u>anaphase</u> is the stage during which the duplicated chromosomes pull apart just before the separation of the zygote into two <u>daughter cells</u>. The term "daughter" does not have any sexual connotations; daughter cells are merely the result of any one cell splitting into two.
(Redding and Hirschhorn, 1968, p. 100)

individuals, include distinctive dermatoglyphic patterns (skin ridge), a high incidence of leukemia (twenty times higher than the general population) and low blood calcium levels.

Another behavioral syndrome that has been recently associated with a specific chromosomal pattern is the aggressivity of males with XYY or XXYY chromosome constitution (Price, 1969a; Volpe, 1971; Redding and Hirschhorn, 1968). This syndrome was first reported in the early sixties and it was noted that the incidence of XYY males in prisons and mental institutions was higher than expected (although the incidence of the XYY chromosomal pattern in the general population is purely a matter of conjecture). The XYY males were usually taller than average (six feet or more) and of average or below average intelligence. The XYY males, compared with a control group of criminal patients, were predisposed to crimes against property rather than against the person, began delinquent behavior at an earlier age, and had fewer siblings who were convicted of criminal offenses. Moreover, the XYY patients had no significant history of mental illness within their families. These last two factors, especially, argue for the case that the extra Y chromosome is responsible for the antisocial behavior (Price, 1969a).

Other genetic abnormalities reflecting trisomy and monosomy conditions of other gene pairs have been discovered; discussions of these numerous syndromes are beyond the province of this paper but will be found in works such as those by Volpe (1971) and E. B. Ford (1968), and Roberts (1970).

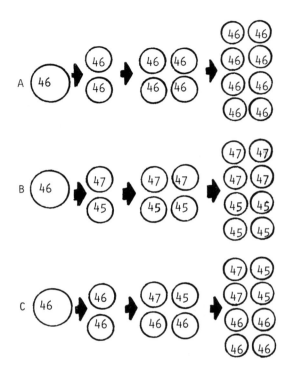

Fig. 6. Relationship of Timing of Division Error to Type of Mosaicism.
a) Normal cell division: all resulting cells contain 46 chromosomes
b) Error occurring during first cell division after conception: two types of cells are present in the developing individual (half containing 47 chromosomes, half containing 45).
c) Error occurring later in cell division: three different cell lines are present (half of the cells with the normal 46 chromosomes, a quarter of the cells with 47, another quarter with 45).

(Adapted from Redding and Hirschhorn, 1968, p. 101.

The second general method utilized in genetic research is the study of twins to determine the heritability of quantitative traits. If monozygotic (originating from one egg or ovum) twins were concordant (both affected by a certain condition) more frequently than dizygotic twins (originating from two separate ova), then it was assumed that heredity played a role in the etiology of that condition. Twin studies, however, have many pitfalls and biases (Roberts, 1970; Clarke and McConnell, 1969). It must first be established that the syndrome under study is similar for twins as for single-borns. For instance, cerebral palsy and cancer are much more frequent in twins than in single-born and, hence, any conclusions from twin studies of these two diseases may not be applicable to the general population (Clarke and McConnell, 1969). Moreover, the diagnosis of zygosity, especially in earlier studies, is open to question since conclusive comparisons (e.g. extensive blood matching) were not made; frequently the determination of zygosity was based upon appearance and family testimony. Other features (e.g. common placenta) were not usually noted. Secondly, adequate sample sizes of twin populations with the desired syndrome are difficult to obtain, especially with rare diseases, and biases in sample selection are common unless an entire population is combed (Roberts, 1970; Clarke and McConnell, 1969). With these cautions in mind, we shall review briefly a portion of the literature on the transmission of schizophrenia.

In general, twin surveys have shown a higher concordance

rate among monozygotic twins (as high as 86 per cent) than among dizygotic twins (Price, 1969a; Kaplan, 1969; Sagor, 1971). Moreover, the concordance rate between dizygotic twins is no higher than between siblings; this tends to argue against environmentalist theories.

Also consanguinity studies (Price, 1969a; Sagor, 1971) indicate that a positive family history of schizophrenia increases the probability of being affected by that disease; this holds even for children adopted a few days after birth. Furthermore, this probability increases with the closeness of the relationship with the schizophrenic relative (Slater, 1961).

The disagreements in these investigations have centered around the specific genetic transmission hypotheses advanced to account for the data (e.g. single or multiple-gene theories) as well as the acknowledged role of non-genetic factors in the etiology of schizophrenia. Recently, great strides have been made in isolating the biochemical mechanisms of schizophrenia; these will be discussed in a subsequent section of this paper.

B.   Treatment of Genetic Disorders

A hereditary disorder is not by nature untreatable.
Rimoin (1970) and Lynch (1970) list current therapeutic methods
for disorders of demonstrable genetic origin. Some of these
are:

(1) Elimination diets. In many inborn errors of metabolism, a
specific enzyme deficiency may lead to an accumulation of a
specific compound. A restriction of the dietary intake of this
compound or its precursors may prevent or modify the disease
symptoms. This has been applied to phenylketonuria, galactosemia and fructose intolerance, among others.

(2) Replacement of the missing gene product. This is a direct
method employed in certain hormone deficiency states, as in the
use of insulin in diabetes mellitus, and growth hormone in
pituitary dwarfism.

(3) Organ replacement. Once organ rejection problems have been
solved, heart transplants for those with congenital heart defects would be a possible curative method. Such organ transplantation may also be a means of producing an enzyme or protein
in an individual genetically incapable of its synthesis; for
example, a liver transplantation would benefit a patient with
phenylketonuria.

(4) Genetic engineering. This covers all methods which manipulate
the genetic apparatus directly. The various techniques falling
under this rubric will be discussed in greater detail.

C. Genetic Engineering

The day of the biological manufacture of an organism
according to desired specifications is not yet at hand, but recent
technological and scientific advances have brought a few of the
intervening steps closer to reality. The specification of the
genetic constituents of an organism would be, from the medical
point of view, an ultimate method of preventing genetically-
based illnesses, although ethical and legal issues would have to
be resolved. The Journal of the American Medical Association
(1972) covered in recent issues the methods concerned with the
transmittance of life (as opposed to the creation of life).
Artificial insemination, the laboratory introduction of sperm,
is widely practiced in the livestock industry. This technique is
also gaining increasing acceptance in use with humans (e.g.,
frozen sperm banks). Artificial in vitro fertilization, the
union of sperm and ovum outside the body has been accomplished
with human gametes and the fertilized ovum has been maintained
through several divisions. The artificial implantation of the
embryo resulting from in vitro fertilization into a uterus has
been accomplished with laboratory animals with normal offspring.
This has not been attempted with humans. Ectogenesis, or the
total gestation outside of the human body, would produce a true
test tube baby. This is not yet possible. Cloning, (the transmittance of the exact genetic material of one organism to a

developing one) is accomplished by replacing the nucleus of an ovum with the nucleus of an asexual cell (e.g., skin cell) from a donor. The ovum develops with a genetic makeup identical to the donor. This method makes the preservation of a species possible even with only carriers of mature ova. This has been accomplished with frogs. The final stage of genetic engineering would be the specification and manufacture of an organism. This procedure is not yet possible.

Although these procedures have rarely been applied to humans, laws concerning eugenics, both positive and negative, have been on record for many years (Parker, 1970). Some laws promote negative eugenics by reducing the birth of infants with "undesirable genes". Such laws deal with voluntary and involuntary sexual sterilization, and with prohibition of marriage between mental defectives, criminals, close relatives and individuals of different races. On the whole, these laws reflect social rather than eugenic goals. Positive eugenics is promoted by laws seeking to increase the number of births of individuals with "desirable genes". Laws regarding artificial insemination are the most important in this area, although the practice of artificial insemination usually reflects the desire to have children rather than eugenic aims (for example, as in marriages where husbands are impotent, or where vasectomies are planned but a safeguard is desired to accommodate any change in heart).

The laws are fairly restrictive in the case of therapeutic abortions where the fetus is known to be defective; the criterion for such an abortion is usually the physical health of the mother. However, once techniques for determining the genetic make-up of a fetus are improved and a defective fetus can be identified with certainty, the pressure to liberalize abortion laws will undoubtedly increase.

D. Genetic Counseling

Since the present state of genetic knowledge and technology does not permit the elimination of genetic defects, the one preventive program available is genetic counseling. This counseling is usually sought by an individual who is concerned about the possible genetic etiology of a trait or disease (Lynch, 1970). Many of these ailments have secondary behavioral symptoms (e.g., mental retardation).

Genetic counseling involves providing an estimate of probablity of occurrence (or recurrence) of a disease or defect for a particular individual. It also includes an interpretation of the risk, guidance for the family, and referral to an appropriate individual or agency (Rimoin, 1970; Roberts, 1970; Fraser, 1970; Lynch, 1969).

The probability estimate is obtained by first establishing the diagnosis of the individual in question. Then a complete family history of the proband or propositus (the individual who, in seeking counsel, brings the family under study although not necessarily the one with the disease) is obtained. Depending upon the disease at hand, specific tests, such as dermotoglyphic analyses, karyotype studies, and enzyme analyses are performed. All of the above information, along with the current literature on the etiology of the disease, is used in estimating the probability requested.

In light of the information imparted by the genetic counselor, the individuals seeking counsel must make the ultimate decision regarding their course of action--be it to attempt to have more children, practice birth control, or adopt a child.

Genetic counseling is usually sought by couples after the birth of an afflicted child and the probability of recurrence of the affliction in subsequent children is of concern. The diagnosis should be confirmed, especially in the less common diseases. A careful listing of symptoms is useful since they may provide clues to the mode of transmission. (For example, Roberts (1970) points out that gargoylism may be recessive or sex-linked, but corneal opacities do not occur in the sex-linked form. Similarly, in muscular dystrophy, the age of onset and pattern of development may help in distinguishing between recessive and sex-linked forms.)

The family history is a pedigree of the proband. Full facts on all normal and abnornal relatives are included including data on all pregnancies of the proband, information on immediate relatives including spouse, siblings, parents, grandparents, cousins, aunts and uncles (Roberts, 1970).

On the basis of the family history, diagnosis, and any necessary lab tests, the disease strain can be classified by type [e.g. mutant gene, a chromosomal aberration, a major environmental agent, or a multifactorial group with genetic and environmental factors (Fraser, 1970), or be percentage of recurrence (Townes, 1970)].

High-Risk Families

High-risk families are those with a recurrence risk of 25% or more. Although risks exceeding 50% (but less than 100%) do not follow any accepted genetic model, cases are found of exceptional families whose empiric recurrence risk appears to exceed fifty percent (Townes, 1970).

When a dominant autosomal trait is involved, 50% of all progeny (male and female) of the affected person can be expected to inherit the disorder. The unaffected progeny have no increase in risk for their offspring. However, it is possible for the gene to have a low expressivity (degree of manifestation of a given gene) in one generation and a high expressivity in a succeeding one, hence appearing to skip generations (Townes, 1970; Rimoin, 1970; Roberts, 1970). That is, the gene may have incomplete penetrance (the percentage with which a gene produces its corresponding characteristics in the organisms having that gene).

If the affliction in question is an autosomal recessive disorder, and both parents are unaffected but heterozygous (and hence carriers), the recurrence risk is 25 percent. Unlike the autosomal dominant traits, the autosomal recessive trait is not likely to show up in the family history. All individuals carry three of four harmful recessive genes (Roberts, 1970), but these are not likely to be manifested unless there is a union with another carrier of those same harmful genes. Phenylketonuria and galactosemia follow this pattern.

Sex-linked disorders are for all practical purposes X-linked disorders. Y-linked disorders are rare and usually lethal, and will not be discussed. Hemophilia, red-green color-blindness, and one form of muscular dystrophy are examples of X-linked disorders. If the mother of the affected child has a positive family history (i.e., an affected brother or maternal uncle) then she is a carrier, in which case there is a 50 per- cent chance of having carrier daughters and a 50 percent chance of having affected sons. If there is no maternal history of the affliction, the child may represent a new mutation, in which case the recurrence risk would be slight. Fortunately, methods for detecting carriers of the X-linked traits are being im- proved; this will allow a more definite statement of probablities in the future.

Low-Risk Families

The low-risk group includes many of the congenital malformations such as cleft lip, club foot, hydrocephaly and un- translocated 21-trisomy; the inheritance patterns are unclear and hence empiric risk figures must be relied upon. These risks are in the 5 percent to 10 percent range (Townes, 1970; Rimoin, 1970). Congenital malformation affects from 2.5 to 7 percent of children and eight defects account for three-fifths of these malformations. Of these eight defects (club foot, cardiac anomalies, mongolism, hydrocephaly, anencephaly, spina bifuda,

102

clefts of lip and palate, polydactyly) only polydactyly has a high risk of recurrence. The greater portion of the other disorders are not easily preventable through genetic counseling or other means (Townes, 1970).

The presentation above belies the enormous complexity of the biophysical technicalities and the moral, philosophical and legal issues involved in mechanisms of genetic transmission and in the process of genetic counseling. New advances in the study of etiology of diseases may someday make it possible for all parents of children whith an anomaly to be informed of their risk; the significance of genetic information is such that it could and should be brought from the recondite to the comprehensible.

In this chapter, psychopharmacology (drug therapy) will be discussed--especially as it is applied to children who have been diagnosed as "minimal brain damaged", or "hyperkinetic", or as having a "learning disorder". A discussion of neural transmission, drug action and a listing of some of the major classes of drugs will precede an examination of evaluative studies.

Following the section on psychopharmacology is a description of interventions based upon suspected perceptual-motor impairments. Included is the work of Cruickshank, Kephart, Frostig, and Doman and Delacato. While the target population of these interventions is not usually labeled "emotionally disturbed", it does constitute a variant group, that is, deviant from the larger group through labelling or segregation in special programs.

Neural Transmission

Since it is assumed that the brain is the site of action of many of the drugs under consideration here, it may be worthwhile to review some principles of neural transmission. Few studies have been done on neural transmission within the brain itself; most of the information we have has been the result of experiments with peripheral nervous tissue. It is assumed that similar processes occur within the central nervous system.

A junction refers to the space between the termination

of an axon of a nerve cell and an adjacent cell. If this space is between two nerve cells, it is called a synapse, and if it is between a nerve cell and a muscle or a gland cell, it is a neuroeffector junction. The stimulation of the prejunction nerve cell may generate a response in the adjacent cell (nerve, muscle, or gland cell). The exact nature of the activation process was not clear until experiments in the nineteenth and early twentieth century demonstrated that the activation of the postjunction cells was due to chemical mediators such as acetylcholine and epinephrine. Studies with peripheral nervous tissue have isolated two different mechanisms that mediate nerve junction transmission. One mechanism was named cholinergic because the effect was similar to that produced by acetylcholine. Acetylcholine produces responses similar to those which occur with stimulation of the parasympathetic nerves, such as increase in tone and contractibility of smooth muscles, dilation of blood vessels and cardiac deceleration. The other mechanism was named adrenergic because the effect was similar to that produced by epinephrine. Epinephrine effects resemble stimulation of sympathetic nerves, which produce decreases in tone and contractibility of smooth muscles, constriction of blood vessels, cardiac acceleration, etc.

Transmission between all neural junctions appear to be mediated through chemical substances, although it is not known if the chemical mediators (neurohumors) within the central nervous system are the same as those found in the peripheral nerves. It is known that there are concentrations of epinephrine, norepinephrine and serotonin within the brain and that these concentrations can be affected by behaviorally-active drugs; hence, there appears to be a relationship between the concentration of these substances within the brain and the behavioral effect of the drugs (Thompson and Schuster, 1968).

Drug Action

Pharmacology as a science dates from about 1800, although the first record of medicinal agents dates from about 1550 B.C. The early 1800's saw many discoveries regarding the specification of the loci of drug action. The notion of specific sites of drug reaction within the organism was expanded in the early 1900's by Ehrlich and, later, by Clark into a broad receptor theory. According to this theory, the introduced chemical has a selective affinity for different tissues in the body, and enters into a chemical relation with receptors in the cells. Moreover, there exists a relationship between the amount of drug anchored to the receptors and the effect produced. These "receptors" are hypothetical constructs and no specific receptor has been isolated; to this day, the receptor theory has played a vital role in conceptualizing the effects of drugs.

We may characterize drugs as having local effects (such as a local anesthetic) or general systemic effects; the former are rarely important in behavioral pharmacology.

Drugs affect the _degree_ of functioning of the cells but do not change the _kind_ of functioning. Cells may be stimulated

106

(cell functions increased) or depressed (cell functions decreased).

Two drugs present in the organism at the same time can interact in differing ways. The second drug could have no effect on the other drug, diminish the effects of the other drug, (i.e., be atagonistic), or enhance the effect of the other drug. Enhancement may take three forms. Drugs may potentiate each other if the combined effect is greater than the sum of individual effects. They are synergistic if they produce an effect greater than either drug alone, but not greater than the sum of the effects of the two drugs. The drugs summate if the total effect is the sum of the individual effects.

The fate of a drug refers to the transformations that it undergoes after absorption, and the mechanism of its excretion from the organism. By and large, drugs are excreted by the kidneys. Other routes of excretion include the lungs, skin, and the intestines. Some drugs are excreted without change, and others are excreted after a biotransformation (a transformation within the organism of a drug to an inactive form or to a form with different effects).

Types of Drugs

Without any concern for taxonomic purity, a listing of groups drugs of interest and some of their primary effects will serve as a background for later sections. (From Thompson and Schuster, 1968).

Sympathomimetic agents are those which produce responses similar to the stimulation of sympathetic adrenergic nerves. Epinephrine is the natural prototype of this class. The amphetamines (whose various forms include Dexedrine and Benzedrine) are a major group in this class. Behavioral effects include increased motor activity, insomnia, and accelerated and desynchronized encephalograms.

Sedatives and hypnotics were the first drugs used in psychiatric management. Hypnotics produce a greater degree of cerebral and behavioral depression than sedatives; hypnotics induce anesthesia at high dosages, and drowsiness, decreased motor activity at lower dosages. The barbiturates are included in this class; the duration of its various derivatives range from long (e.g., barbital and phenobarbital) to ultrashort (e.g., hexobarbital).

The use of opium in large psychiatric hospitals was at its height in the mid-1800's, to relieve symptoms such as anxiety and depression. Other sedatives and hypnotics were developed to replace opium; bromides were introduced in the 1850's, chloral hydrate was first used in 1869, paraldehyde in 1883 and the barbiturates in 1903 (Tourney, 1969).

The use of behaviorally-active drugs was not widespread until the mid-fifties. At this time chlorpromazine was introduced; it was the first of the tranquilizing drugs and the first of a long line of phenothiazine derivatives. Its effect was to decrease the frequency of aggressive outbursts in psychotics without the confusion, muscular incoordination, and drowsiness

108

that was common with the use of barbiturates and bromides.
Some of the generic names for drugs in this group are promazine,
chlorpromazine, trifluoperazine, perphenazine, and thioridazine.

Further information on drug groups may be obtained from
Thompson and Schuster (1968) or Gordon (1964, 1967).

Effects of Drugs

Bradley (1937), was the first to publish results of
studies of the effects of drugs (amphetamines) on children
with behavioral disorders. Using children in a hospital setting,
he found that the most marked changes in behavior (teacher
ratings) occured in those that had received the drug (Benzedrine).

Increase in interest in school material was noted,
as well as heightened comprehension, accuracy and apparent
motivation to accomplish as much work as possible. No negative
effects were noted although some of the children noted feelings
indicating mild euphoria. Since this initial study, there has
been a plethora of studies, many of questionable design (e.g.,ex-
perimenters were not "blind"), which have evaluated the effects
of drugs upon various behavioral measures including learning,
attention, and activity level. Some of these studies, as well
as the practical and ethical issues that they raise, will be
discussed here.

Two main types of drugs are used in the treatment of
hyperactivity: psychic stimulants (amphetamines, methylphenidate),
and tranquilizers (phenothiazine derivatives).

Bradley (1950), treated children with Benzedrine and Dexedrine to alleviate their behavioral problems. Two hundred and seventy-five children were treated over 12 years. Sixty to 70 percent showed symptomatic improvement (i.e., quieter, increased attention, more cooperative, happier) while 15 to 25 percent showed no change, and 10 to 15 percent showed negative behavior changes (i.e., anorexia, more tense, active, seclusive, and irritable).

Recent time-sampling observations of classroom behavior indicate that the stimulant drugs reduce inattentive behavior, undirected motor activity and tend to increase attention to tasks and the amount of positive teacher-pupil contact (Conners, 1971). Moreover, contrary to the belief that drugs merely dope the youngsters into inactivity, time-stop photography used in free-field activity show that stimulants increase the total amount of activity; it is the quality of the activity rather than the total amount of energy expended that is changed by the drugs (Conners, 1971).

Denhoff, Davids, and Hawkins (1971) provide a recent example of an evaluation of the effects of dextroamphetamine on hyperkinetic children. Methodological issues were considered and a double-blind design was used, although only teacher ratings were used to evaluate changes.

Forty-two pupils attending a private school for children with learning disabilities were the subjects. They were 6- to 13-

years of age, of normal intelligence and had not been referred because of a primary emotional disturbance. The children were from a middle class background and, after complete pediatric neurological, psychiatric and psychological examination, were diagnosed as having a learning disability of visual-perceptual-motor or language-related origin. Most of the children were at least two years behind in school achievement.

The dependent variable was personality and behavioral characteristics as measured by rating scales for hyperkinesis developed by one of the authors (previously tested for validity and reliability). With this scale, the raters are asked to judge the child along the given dimensions, in comparison with other children of the same age and sex ("normal children"). Dimensions include: (1) activity (involuntary and constant overactivity, always on the move); (2) attention span and powers of concentration; (3) variability (fluctuations in behavior); (4) impulsiveness and inability to delay gratification; (5) irritability (low frustration tolerance); (6) explosiveness (easily provoked fits of anger); (7) school work (concentration, participation in school activities, learning difficulties).

All children had medication discontinued during the summer vacations. Three weeks after the resumption of school in the fall (without medication), pretest ratings were made separately by teachers and parents; the parent data was later discarded because of the poor return rate. One-half of the children were randomly assigned to the treatment condition and the others to the control condition. Children in the treatment condition were given a 10-mg capsule of dextroamphetamine sulfate (Dexedrine) each morning by the school principal (the only person who knew the contents of the capsules). Children in the control condition received matched placebos. Three weeks later, the parents and teachers were again asked to complete rating scales for each child. During the final three week phase of the project, the children who had received dextroamphetamine received placebos and those who had been in the placebo group received the dextroamphetamine. A third rating scale was filled for each child after the lapse of another three weeks.

Lower ratings (high scores indicate more hyperkinetic characteristics) were obtained under the drug condition than under the placebo condition. On each of the scales, teachers rated the children as more hyperkinetic after the placebo condition than at the time of the pretest ratings. No differences were found on the rating of school work; the length of the drug treatment intervals may not have been long enough to induce effects that would be reflected in the school performance. Longer treatment intervals could have provided more data in this respect. As the authors point out, other measures, such as direct observations and counting of specific behaviors by observers and measurement of physical movement by mechanical devices, could be considered in future studies, especially where cost is not a limiting factor. This study and others (e.g., Conners, Eisenberg, and Barcai, 1967) provide some evidence that amphetamines can lead to a reduction in the hyperkinetic behavior patterns of young children.

Phenothiazine derivatives (most notably, chlorpromazine) have been used with hyperactive children since the advent of chlorpromazine in 1954. Grant (1962), in examining the studies utilizing this drug, concluded that chlorpromazine was useful and effective in treating hyperactivity. More recently there has been less interest in tranquilizers, although studies comparing tranquilizers and stimulants (e.g., Sprague, Barnes, and Werry, 1970) and studies of the effects of tranquilizers on specific learning tasks (e.g., Werry, et al, 1966) still have general currency. However, whenever comparisons have been made of the effects of stimulants and tranquilizers, the latter have shown an impairment of learning and cognitive functions (Conners, 1971; Sprague et al, 1970). This may be an effect of problems with diagnosis, which are discussed below, or of problems with identifying the specific population for which tranquilizers may be effective (Conners, 1971).

If one assumes that medication of some sort is in fact indicated, the prescribing physician must monitor certain effects (Laufer, 1971). The goal of the medication is to have activity and attention under the individual's control, without over-control and without a total lack of it; the level of medication that accomplishes this end is the desired dosage level. Excessive dosage may be indicated by over-control (soporific behavior) or by stimulation (irritability, tension). Some of the possible side-effects with amphetamines and methylphenidate (Ritalin) include the "amphetamine look" (pale, pinched, facial expression with dark hollows under eyes), anorexia, insomnia, headache and abdominal pain.

At some point in time, the child will no longer require medication to maintain control over his behavior. Recognition of this stage may be accomplished by discontinuing the medication and observing the effects. Or, when the condition is outgrown, the child will display the normal reaction to stimulants rather than the paradoxical response which had previously slowed and controlled his motor behavior. Concurrent with the medication of the child, the family and school must be enlisted to determine the behavioral effects in the class, as well as to modify the environment within the home and school in order to complement the effects of the medication.

Obviously, careful supervision and follow-up are necessary if the drug is to be used effectively. Unfortunately, little re-search has been done on the relationship between drug dosage and behavioral effects in children (DiMascio, 1970); the appropriate child dosage is frequently merely extrapolated from the adult/child weight ratio.

But deeper issues are involved here. First there is the question of diagnosis and classification of the presenting symptoms. Hyperactivity is not a diagnostic entity (Fish, 1969). The target population is a heterogeneous group and there is little agreement

114

in diagnosis, except in the most servere disorders (DiMascio, 1970); the labeling confusion that results is in part a reflection of the disagreements in specification of etiology. A large portion of this confusion is connected with the question of organic brain damage. Labels such as "minimally brain damaged", "brain injured", are used when organicity is not established. The circularity of reasoning is apparent: these labels are used to explain why the child has the behavioral symptoms, when, in fact, the labels were ascribed on the basis of the behavioral symptoms (DiMascio, 1970; Hallahan, 1971). The argument is that since certain types of organic brain injury are sometimes found in conjunction with particular behavioral symptoms and/or neurological abnormalities ("soft" signs), then it follows that the presence of the behavioral symptoms, with or without the "soft" neurological symptoms, is proof of brain injury. In fact there is no necessary, consistent relationship between the three phenomena (DiMascio, 1970; Fish, 1969).

Once the determination of drug dosage and treatment population has been completed, there remains the problem of assessment of drug effectiveness. Early studies relied upon rather global descriptive categories such as "improved". More refined methods such as time-sampling observations have been employed, as mentioned earlier.

Besides the above medical and evaluative considerations, ethical issues must be considered. Should medication be used to effect conformity (and control) within the classroom, to increase achievement (children who are more manageable may not necessarily accomplish more), or to improve the accessibility of other forms of intervention (e.g., psychotherapy, behavior modification). Or, is the drug being advocated to handle only the symptoms of what may be deep-rooted problems in the home, school or in the child? The danger is in considering the tangible and immediate as the preferable mode of treatment for complex problems (Freeman, 1972; Ladd, 1970). Other factors may be relevant to the occurrence of the undesirable behavior, but are usually ignored due to social or political ramifications. These include poor teaching, misinformed or mistreating parents, home problems, and schools with limited budgets and hence without the means to provide for alternative modes of treatment, and even such factors as malnutrition and "the normal ebullience of childhood (Report..., 1971)." An in-ability to cope with these problems promotes a gravitation to the encapsulated panacea.

Another central concern is the long-range effect of drug administration (Ladd, 1970; Freeman, 1972; Laufer, 1971; Solomons, 1971). One common fear of parents and teachers is that the use of drugs with young children will merely accelerate the pill-popping progression among adolescents. In fact, however, middle-class housewives are the greatest consumers of drugs today and are themselves, poor models of drug abstinence. No well-de-signed study of long-range effects of drug use has been carried out. One study (Laufer, 1971) of 66 former hyperkinetic patients treated

116

with amphetamines or methylphenidate, while uncontrolled (i.e., no comparison group), does not support the dire predictions of heavy dependence on drugs and instability which many expect. Better planned and executed studies are needed in this area.

Because of the publicity surrounding the use and misuse of drugs in schools (Ladd, 1970), the Department of Health, Education and Welfare called a conference on the use of stimulant drugs in the treatment of behaviorally disturbed young school children. Portions of the Report of the conference will be summarized here (Report..,, 1971; Freeman, 1972). Conclusions drawn were that stimulants should be employed only with due regard to the problem at hand and after a thorough medical examination. If used with the precautions outlined, the Report states that the drugs may be expected to be effective in one-half to two-thirds of the cases. Moreover, the conference participants concluded that:

    1)   the toxicity of stimulant drugs is not a problem in the dosages employed,

    2)   there is no established risk of later drug dependency,

    3)   it is unlikely that the small amount of drugs manufactured for these purposes would lead to illegal diversion,

    4)   the stimulants permit greater attention to self-initiated probelm solving,

117

5)   parents should not be coerced into seeking

or accepting any treatment, and

6)   the school's role is not to specify a method

of medical treatment but to inform the parents of the

child's behavior.

The drug therapy outlined above is a relatively recent

phenomenon. Historically, the concerns of investigators regarding

children now labelled "minimally brain damaged" or "learning dis-

abled" initially centered on their perceptual-motor (especially

visual perceptual-motor) coordination and development. The seminal

work of Strauss and Werner during the thirties and forties with

mentally retarded youngsters influenced many important figures in

the field, such as Cruickshank, Kephart and Frostig (Hallahan, 1971).

Werner and Strauss, in studying the psychological effects

of brain damage in retarded youngsters, divided the children into

two groups, the exogenous (mental retardation due to neurological

defects) and the endogenous (mental retardation due to familial

factors). In studies comparing the two groups, they found that the

exogenous group had more difficulty than the endogenous group

in making visual- and auditory-motor cross-modal integrations,

maintaining their attention to the task at hand, making figure-

ground discriminations, and making categorical classifications.

The exogenous children were also more impulsive, erratic and un-

coordinated than the endogenous ones (Strauss and Werner, 1942;

Strauss and Kephart, 1940; Strauss and Lehtinen, 1947). Drawing

118

educational implications from their findings, they suggested that treatment may occur by controlling the environment and in training the child to exercise voluntary control (Strauss, 1943; Strauss and Lehtinen, 1947; Hallahan, 1971). Specific tasks to accomplish the latter end were suggested by Strauss and Lehtinen.

The contributions of Strauss and Werner include a concern for: 1) specific disabilities and methods to deal with them, 2) perceptual-motor difficulties and training to alleviate them and 3) the characteristics of hyperactivity and distractability and management procedures to minimize them (Hallahan, 1971).

Cruickshank refined some of the suggestions flowing from Strauss and Lehtinen (1947) and incorporated them into a complete program (Cruickshank, et al, 1961). The brain-injured children were effectively educated through environmental restructuring and the use of new teaching materials. The environmental changes included the use of monochromatic rooms with minimal decor (in contrast to the typical polychromatic classroom) and the utilization of individual cubicles for the exceedingly distractible.

Like Cruickshank, Kephart was associated with Strauss and Werner early in his career. His primary emphasis was on perceptual-motor development (Kephart, 1960), especially the development of laterality (left-right discrimination) and other aspects of motor and kinesthetic development which constitute body awareness, and which he considered prerequisites for visual development. The therapeutic regimen that he recommended for slow learners included exercises for lateral coordination and development (e.g., angels in the snow) and kinesthetic development (e.g., balance beam exercises): progress along these exercises was thought to improve body awareness and directionality, which would be reflected in better achievement since many academic skills (e.g., reading) require directional discriminations.

Another important figure in perceptual motor development and training is Marianne Frostig, who developed the Frostig Development Test of Visual Perception (DVTP) and founded the Frostig Center for Educational Therapy in Santa Monica. The DTVP, which purports to measure five visual motor skills including eye-motor coordination (drawing a line between varying boundaries), figure-ground discrimination (outlining a given figure on a sheet with overlapping figures), form constancy (discriminating geometric shapes varying in size and orientations), position in space (identifying a figure from a number of choices) and spatial relations (copying dot patterns of varying complexity) (Frostig, Lefever, and Whittlesey, 1964). A low score on any of the subtests can be remediated through the training program developed to accompany the assessment device. The DTVP has been demonstrated to be useful in predicting reading readiness (Hallahan, 1971) but the training program, while effective in raising DTVP scores, has not been demonstrated to generalize to academic achievement.

Glen Doman and Carl Delacato's theory of neurological organization (Delacato, 1959; Doman et al, 1960) has provoked much controversy (Robbins and Glass, 1969). The program advocated by the Institutes for the Achievement of Human Potential, founded by Doman and Delacato, calls for rigidly prescribed exercises to which the child must be subjected on a regular basis. These exercises are based on a theory of hemispheric dominance, and or the tenet that ontogeny recapitulates phylogeny. The theory as outlined in Doman et al (1960) calls for (1) training the child on the floor to remediate brain damage (2) manipulating the child into body patterns   appropriate to the level of the damaged brain (3) imposing hemispheric dominance and unilaterality (4) utilizing carbon dioxide therapy and (5) stimulating the senses.

Several national organizations including the American Academy of Cerebral Palsy, and American Academy of Neurology, and the National Association for Retarded Children have officially adopted a statement ("The Doman Delacato Treatment of Neurologically Handicapped Children") which concludes in its summary:

> The Institutes for the Achievement of Human Potential appear to differ substantially from other groups treating developmental problems in (a) the excessive nature of their undocumented claims for cure and (b) the extreme demands placed upon the parents in carrying out an unproven technique without fail.
>
> Advice to parents and professional workers cannot await conclusive results of controlled studies of all aspects of the method. Physicians and therapists should acquaint themselves with the issues in the controversy and the available evidence. We have done this and concur with the conclusions of Robbins and Glass (1969):

There is no empirical evidence to substanti-
ate the value of either the theory or practice
of neurological organization...If the theory
is to be taken seriously...its advocates are
under an obligation to provide reasonable
support for the tenets of the theory and a
series of experimental investigations, consistent with scientific standards, which test
the efficiency of the rationale.

To date, we know of no attempt to fulfill this obligation.

(American Academy of Neurology, 1967; Hallahan, 1971).

IV. BIOCHEMICAL FACTORS AND INTERVENTIONS

This discussion of biochemical interventions has two parts. The first deals with the current state of biochemical theories and with treatment of schizophrenia. Most of the research has been characterized by poor experimental design and poor controls (Coppen, 1967; Wyatt et al, 1971) and the results obtained by different experimenters have frequently been contradictory; experiments with schizophrenics, at the very least, provided research leads and a base for hypotheses-generating. Several theories are now popular; a discussion of these theories may draw together many superficially disparate interventions and serve to illustrate the nature of these investigations.

The second section will consider nutritional factors. While nutrition has not been etiologically implicated in any emotional disturbance, nutritional factors (and malnutrition) have been shown to affect learning and performance, two very important behavior parameters. Because of this, and because nutritional factors can cause, in some sense, deviations from the norm, they are deemed worthy of separate discussion.

A.   Schizophrenia Research

Schizophrenia is one of the oldest recognized illnesses of man, its description being first recorded by the ancient Hindus 3300 years ago. In the last ten years or so with the rapid technological and biochemical advances, support has been uncovered for the theory that schizophrenia is the result of some abnormal factor or substance in the body. Schizophrenia is one of the most serious mental illnesses, accounting for twenty-five percent of all admissions to mental hospitals and one-half of all occupied beds within those hospitals. It strikes one person out of every hundred, usually during late adolescence or early adulthood.

In discussing the biochemical mechanisms of schizophrenia, it must be remembered that the explication of the mechanisms does not in any way specify the etiology. Environmental and psychological events (e.g., stress), as well as hereditary or biophysical factors, may precipitate and maintain the biochemical changes which lead to the disorder. More likely, it is an interaction of these factors which lead to biochemical changes.

Much of the material which follows has been drawn from Coppen (1967), and Wyatt, Termini and Davis (1971) who reviewed the last ten years' work in biochemical and sleep studies on schizophrenia. Some of the difficulties of these studies are important for the proper evaluation of the field (Wyatt, et al, 1971; Coppen, 1967).

124

(1) It is possible that schizophrenia is not a unitary disease but a syndrome with multiple etiologies; several environmental or hereditary factors could lead to the development of the same syndrome.

(2) It is also possible that the disease encompasses several biochemical abnormalities that may not be related and hence any one biochemical theory may not suffice to cover the entire schizophrenic population.

(3) Although schizophrenia is presumed to be an affliction of the brain, no direct measurement of brain biochemical functions are possible. Hence peripheral body fluids (e.g., serum, urine) are used to provide indices of brain functioning. There is no certainty that changes in metabolism in the brain will be reflected in detectable changes in the serum or urine.

(4) In studies of schizophrenia, appropriate control subjects as well as double-blind procedures are important. All subjects should be exposed to similar conditions since such factors as stress, diet and medication may affect the minute biochemical changes which are being assessed.

The Transmethylation Hypothesis

The transmethylation hypothesis postulates that a schizophrenic has an abnormal ability to form, or inability to metabolize, methylated substances. There are several hallucino-

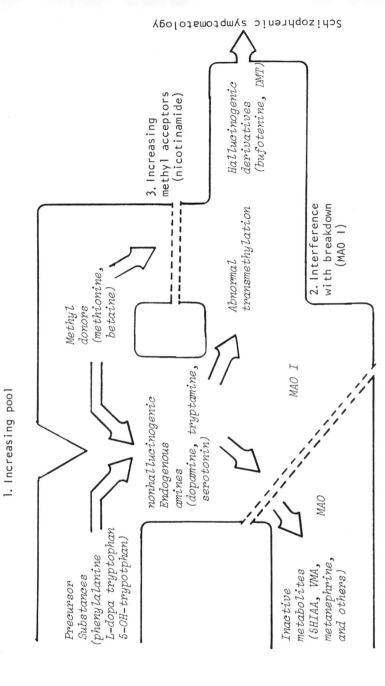

Fig. 7. Strategies used to study the hypothesized abnormal transmethylation in schizophrenia.

1. Increasing available pool of substances thought necessary to process: precursor substances and/or methyl donors. 2. Interfering with normal enzymatic breakdown by use of monoamine oxidase inhibitor. 3. Increasing available pool of methyl acceptors.

(Adapted from Wyatt et al, 1971, p. 14.)

genic substances which are derivatives of endogenous amines. Many of these compounds are methylated derivatives of catechole and indole nuclei. For example, mescaline is a derivative of phenylalanine and bufotenine (believed to be hallucinogenic) is a derivative of serotonin.

Osmond and Smythies noted the similarity between mescaline and norepinephrine and hypothesized that an abnormal transmethylation of norepinephrine might be responsible for some forms of schizophrenia, through the endogenous formation of methylated amines which would function as hallucinogens. This compound, if it did function in the hypothesized manner, (1) should be capable of producing or exacerbating physiological and psychological symptoms found in schizophrenic patients, (2) if it is endogenous, the schizophrenic patient should be able to produce it from precursors; if the production capability is found in normal individuals, its production should be quantitatively different in schizophrenics and normals, (3) if it is an exogenous compound, its metabolism should be quantitatively different in schizophrenics and normals. The enzymes necessary for the methylation of both catechole amines and indoles have been discovered in the human brain (Wyatt, et al, 1971).

If the transmethylation hypothesis is correct and the compounds which increase the supply of hallucinogenic derivatives exacerbate the schizophrenic symptoms, then it follows that a decrease in the amount of schizophrenic derivatives should result

127

in the melioration of the schizophrenic state. To test the hypothesis, therefore, experimenters have sought to exacerbate schizophrenic symptoms by (1) administering precursor substances (e.g., L-dopa, phenylalanine and typtophan) or (2) increasing the number of methyl donor substances available (by use of monoamine oxidase inhibitors), or they have sought to ameliorate schizophrenic symptoms through (3) decreasing the amount of methyl donor substances available by administering methyl acceptors (e.g., nicotinic acid or nicotinamide adenine dinucleotide) (Wyatt, et al, 1971). See Figure 7.

Unfortunately, studies attempting to exacerbate schizophrenic symptomatology by increasing donor substances have not been convincingly successful. This could be because the substances introduced were metabolized before any effect was shown or because the administration of the compounds orally or intravenously did not change their levels in brain tissue (Wyatt et al, 1971).

Studies attempting to aggrevate the schizophrenic symptoms by increasing the supply of methyl donors (e.g., methionine) have been more successful, especially if the methyl donors are given in conjunction with monoamine oxidase inhibitors (MAOI) which would interfere with the normal enzymatic breakdown of the endogenous amines by inhibiting the enzyme catalyzing the reaction. This result tends to support the transmethylation hypothesis, although there is a possibility that what was labelled exacerba-

128

tion of the schizophrenic symptoms was in fact the result of drug toxicity (which is indicated by the high incidence of confusion and autonomic symptomatology evident with methionine administration). This methionine loading should cause differential reactions in schizophrenics and nonschizophrenics (according to the transmethylation hypothesis) but methionine administration to nonschizophrenics has been carried out only twice and hence this aspect cannot be evaluated adequately (Wyatt, et al, 1971).

Nicotinic acid (niacin) and nicotinamide adenine dinucleotide (NAD) are methyl acceptors and hence decrease the amount of methyl donor substances available for transmethylation, which would lower brain concentrations of the abnormal methylated substances. In 1952 Hoffer and Osmond began to treat schizophrenic patients in Saskatchewan, Canada, with large doses of nicotinamide (5-10 g./day). To date, the strongest support for the use of nicotinamide and NAD in the treatment of schizophrenics comes from Hoffer and Osmond and their associates (e.g., Hoffer, 1962; Hoffer and Osmond, 1966; Cott, 1967). Many others have failed to replicate their results (Wyatt et al , 1971).

DMPEA.

A compound 3,4-dimethophenethylamine (DMPEA) was identified in 1952 as a possibly psychomimetic compound relevant to the transmethylation hypothesis. The abnormal methylation of dopamine was presumed to play a role in catatonia since methylated phenethylamines can produce catatonic-like behavior in laboratory animals. In 1962

the presence of DMPEA was established in the urine of 15 of
19 schizophrenics but not in the urine of any of 14 normals.
However, the subsequent research with DMPEA (called "pink spot"
because one assay technique yields a pink spot as a positive
indication) has been marred by (1) failures to replicate crucial
experiments, (2) failure to establish that DMPEA causes schizo-
phrenic-like symptoms in humans and (3) the inability to establish
the in vivo synthesis of DMPEA. It is quite likely that DMPEA
is a metabolite of dietary substances (especially plant substances
and in particular, tea) since schizophrenic patients on restricted
or plant-free diets are DMPEA negative and the presence of DMPEA
is correlated with the addition and removal of tea from the diets.
Moreover, DMPEA-positive chronic schizophrenic patients become
DMPEA negative when placed on a restricted diet for 3 days, and
return to DMPEA-positive when the regular diet is reinstated. All
of this evidence appears to suggest that the DMPEA is of endogenous
dietary origin although findings are not yet conclusive since
different researchers have used assay teachniques of differential
sensitivity and have measured different compounds (Wyatt et al,
1971).

Bufotenine

        Bufotenine is a naturally occurring compound (which occurs
in certain mushrooms and sea anemone nematocysts) which, like
DMPEA, has been implicated in the mechanism of schizophrenia on the
basis that:

(1) Bufotenine (N, N-dimethylserotonin) is a derivative of serotonin;

(2) The enzyme which could convert serotonin to bufotenine has been found in brain tissue of man;

(3) Bufotenine has been found in urine of schizophrenics; but not (or in lower concentrations) in the urine of normals;

(4) Bufotenine has caused schizophrenic symptoms when administered to humans. This is based on the supposition that some naturally occurring compounds (e.g., serotonin) could, through an abnormal methylation, be converted to an hallucinogen (e.g., bufotenine).

However, the research with bufotenine has been marked by inadequate methodology and poor controls. Moreover, conclusive evidence for the differential occurrence of bufotenine in schizophrenics and nonschizophrenics is not available and the verification of the hallucinogenic properties of the compound is incomplete (Wyatt et al, 1971).

Histamine

Histamine (a compound found in animals which causes dilation of the blood vessels and which is implicated in allergic reactions) is of interest to schizophrenia researchers because there is some evidence of an inability of schizophrenics to metabolize it appropriately. Histamine is found in the brain and partially metabolized there. Observations tying histamine with schizophrenia include:

(1) Schizophrenics have a low incidence of allergies.

(2) The onset of schizophrenia frequently coincides with the remission of asthmatic symptoms.

(3) Schizophrenics are relatively insensitive to the effects of histamine (e.g., wheal formation).

(4) Schizophrenics have elevated histamine blood levels.

In spite of the considerable evidence of abnormal histamine metabolism in schizophrenics, the nature of this abnormality has yet to be outlined. Possible mechanisms include: a rapid inactivation of histamine in schizophrenics, excessive amounts of antihistaminic substances in schizophrenics, or a lack of substances which potentiate the effects of histamine. Histamine is partially metabolized by methylation but none of the metabolites are hallucinogens; hence, this is not in concert with the transmethylation hypothesis. One interesting finding: the identification of schizophrenics with high blood histamines and those with low blood histamines suggests that schizophrenia is not a unitary disease but at least two disease complexes (Wyatt et al, 1971).

The Bioassay Technique

A common strategy in schizophrenia research is to develop a bioassay system which is altered by material obtained from schizophrenics and not altered by material from control subjects. The material, once so characterized, is then chemically identified and isolated. The research at Lafayette Clinic in Detroit over the

132

last fifteen years has taken this tack and has isolated a serum protein (alpha-2-globulin) from schizophrenic patients, which does not seem to be an effect of diet or drug usage (Wyatt, et al, 1971). Because of the importance of their work, an extended coverage will be given regarding their findings (Gottlieb, Frohman, and Beckett, 1970; Gottlieb, Frohman, Harmison, 1971; Tourney and Gottlieb, 1971; Link, 1972; Elliott and Truax, 1972).

The biological energy-regulation mechanism depends upon the metabolism of glucose within the cell. The energy from this metabolism is stored and released to drive various body functions. The storage and release depends upon a process of phosphorylation. Adenosine triphosphate (ATP) stores much of this energy. It releases the energy by losing a phosphate. An early discovery was that chronic schizophrenic patients had a much higher turn-over of ATP in the red blood cells than normal individuals or acute schizophrenic patients, suggesting that the cells of the chronic schizophrenics act as though the individual were under constant stress. Moreover, when placed under stress (e.g., through administration of insulin) chronic schizophrenic patients had a drop in ATP turnover, while controls had an increase in ATP turnover; the chronic schizophrenics did not display a ready adaptability to stress, as did controls (Gottlieb, Frohman, Beckett, 1970).

The metabolism of glucose has two pathways, an energy-releasing one and an energy-storing one. The pathway utilized is a function of the energy needs of the organism. When stressed (e.g., with insulin) controls were able to shift from storage mechanism to the energy release mechanism; schizophrenic patients, however,were not able to make this shift. Subsequent experiments showed that the substance effecting the glucose metabolism was located in the plasma of schizophrenic patients.

The bioassay technique eventually developed called for incubating the serum or plasma from schizophrenic patients with red blood cells from chickens, and measuring the uptake of glucose and the production of metabolites (such as lactate and pyruvate). The ratio of lactate to pyruvate (L/P ratio) was elevated significantly when the serum of schizophrenics was used. The substance causing this elevated L/P ratio was eventually isolated and identified as an alpha-2-globulin, one of 100,000 proteins in the blood of a human. The alpha-2-globulin (or S protein) has a molecular weight of 400,000 and is eighty percent lipid (fat). The lipoprotein is in the blood of all humans, and in the same amounts, but in the blood of schizophrenics it has a special function: it affects cell permeability and allows an increased amount of tryptophan (one of 21 amino acids, the building blocks of proteins) to pass into cells. Tryptophan is important since vital neural transmitters (e.g., serotonin) are derived from it. If the metabolism of tryptophan goes awry, psychotic-producing metabolites such as DMT (dymethyltryptomine) could be produced (many psychomimetic drugs have DMT as part of the molecules). These metabolites would affect neural transmission, information processing and could produce

psychomimetic effects   (Gottlieb, Frohman and Becket, 1970).
The schizophrenic is an ambulatory drug-abuse factory.

Serotonin is one of the neural transmitters in the
brain. The brain has both serotonin and norepinephrine pathways,
which are always parallel. If the formation of serotonin is
blocked in rats, they cannot sleep; if one blocks the synthesis
of norepinephrine, the animal sleeps continually. The two
pathways seem to control levels of alertness, with the one tending
to move the organism towards the less alert state and the other
tending toward the more alert state. Serotonin seems vital to
REM (rapid eye movement) sleep (Wyatt et al, 1971) and is found
in high levels in autistic children (Coppen, 1967). Serotonin
is bound to a protein when formed; a nerve impulse releases it,
it serves its function, and it is then destroyed by enzymes (the
MAO, see diagram in the discussion of the transmethylation
hypothesis). One of the effects of reserpine (an early drug
used in the treatment of schizophrenia) and chlorpromazine (a
drug used presently) is to lower the level of serotonin in the brain.

Since the same amount of the S protein was found in
schizophrenics and normals, and the composition (the proportion of
the various amino acids which compose it) of the S protein found
in normals and schizophrenics was similar, what was the reason for
their different functioning? Optical analyses with polarized light
revealed that the S protein in schizophrenics was primarily shaped
like an alpha helix (like a corkscrew) while the S protein of

non-schizophrenics was either like a random coil or in a beta

conformation (pleated).   (See diagram)

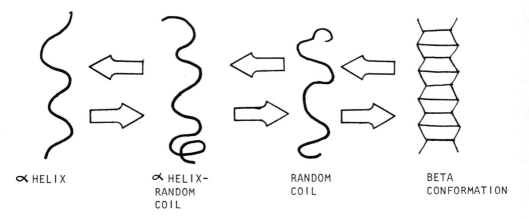

∝ HELIX   ∝ HELIX-   RANDOM   BETA
                          RANDOM   COIL   CONFORMATION
                          COIL

Fig. 8.   Illustration of various components in the conformation
          of the S protein: ∝ -helix (corkscrew shape), random
          coil, β -conformation (accordion shape).
       (Adapted from Gottlieb, Frohman and Harmison, 1971, p. 744).

This finding is important since the shape of a protein

determines its functions; binding with other substances depends

upon the shape.   About 30 to 74 percent of the S protein in schizo-

phrenics had the alpha helix;   the greater the percentage of helix

formations, the greater the amount of trytophan that was pumped

into the cells.

The S protein described above (with the alpha helix)

has been found in only 60 per cent of the schizophrenics examined. The other 40 per cent have abnormal alpha-2-globulin, which is unlike that of controls and unlike that of the schizophrenics with the alpha helix. Although this may suggest that a separate mechanism is operative on the forty per cent without the alpha helix, recent work at the Lafayette clinic and in the Soviet Union suggests that they are schizophrenics in a different evolutionary stage of the illness. Soviet research suggests that the levels of the alpha helix S protein reaches its height during the first year of the illness and gradually declines until it is no longer in evidence (with the present assessment techniques) by the end of the seventh year. Several patients who have displayed the S protein have, after seven years or so, ceased to exhibit any evidence of it without any necessary decrement in symptomatology. Hence the forty per cent who do not exhibit the alpha helix are not evidence of a different mechanism but merely an extension of the pathophysiologic mechanism outlined (Gottlieb, Frohman, Beckett, 1970). Although no mechanism for the phenomenon has been demonstrated, it is hypothesized by the Layfayette Clinic group that leakage of an intracellular enzyme which controls or regulates the alpha helix is responsible for the gradual elimination of the alpha helix.

The biochemical mechanism outlined defines the mechanism and not the cause of the illness. The chain of reactions may be precipitated by   environmental or genetic factors or perhaps by both (such as a genetic predisposition which requires a favorable environment for its expression). An analogy could be made to diabetes: although the underlying cause of diabetes is not understood, an understanding of the mechanism permitted the development of a treatment program with insulin.

Assuming that the role of the S protein in schizophrenia is verified by other experimenters, what are the possible avenues for treatment or cure of schizophrenia? One method would be to develop a drug which would increase the metabolism caused by the S protein through an innocuous pathway before any damage is done. Secondly, a blocking agent could be developed which would prevent the production of the schizophrenic-producing substances, the methylated metabolites of tryptophan. Third, an agent which would correct or control the S protein itself could be used. Such an enzyme has been isolated from the brain. This enzyme (anti-S protein) rids the alpha-2-globulin of the helix shape and hence stops the pumping of tryptophan into cells. An examination of brains of normals and schizophrenics reveals that normals have four times as much of this anti-S protein as schizophrenics; apparently, schizophrenics are not able to keep the S protein in a non-helical shape, as do normals, and, hence, the helical form builds until it reaches levels at which it can affect cell permeability and start the chain reaction of biochemical events leading to the symptoms. Researchers at Layfayette Clinic are currently collecting and stockpiling this anti-S protein preparatory to beginning tests with animals. If it carries out its function of ridding the S protein of the helix without any side effects, etc., it promises to form the basis of a treatment for schizophrenia analogous to the treatment of diabetes; just as a diabetic has glucose that is out of control and is brought to normal levels by insulin, so the schizophrenic with the helical S protein that is out of control, can have it brought to normal levels with the anti-S protein (Gottlieb, Frohman, Beckett, 1970; Gottlieb, Frohman, Harmison, 1971; LINK, 1972). This would not cure the problem but serves, as in the use of insulin with diabetics, as a maintenance therapy.

B. Orthomolecular Psychiatry

Orthomolecular psychiatry (or megavitamin therapy) is the treatment of mental illness by the "provision of the optimum molecular composition of the brain (Pauling, 1968, p. 271)." Basic to this point of view is the supposition that the optimum molecular concentrations of body substances is different from that produced by diet and by the genetically-controlled metabolic mechanisms, and that essential nutrilites (e.g., vitamins, essential vitamins and essential fatty acids) are required in amounts different from that usually recommended for good health. [Theoretical support for a particular aspect of the orthomolecular position (the treatment of schizophrenia) may be found in the trans-methylation hypothesis. See discussion in preceeding section.]

Support for this theory is, in part, based on the fact that in several illnesses caused by dietary deficiencies, associated mental symptoms appear even before the physical symptoms are manifested. For example, the psychosis associated with pernicious anemia may precede the physical symptoms by several years. Other examples citied by Pauling include the mental symptoms (depression) which accompany a vitamin C deficiency, the mental illness caused by a shortage of cyancobalamin (B_{12}), and the psychosis associated with a shortage of nicotinic acid (niacin), which also produces pellagra.

The functioning of the brain and nervous tissue is more sensitively dependent on the rate of chemical reactions than the

140

functioning of other organs and tissues....mental disease is for the most part caused by abnormal reaction rates, as determined by genetic constitution and diet, and by abnormal molecular concentrations of essential substances.

(Pauling, 1968, p. 268)

Substances implicated in the etiology of mental illness by Pauling and others include thiamine, nicotinic acid, pyridoxine (B_6), cyanocoblamin (B_{12}), biotin (H), ascorbic acid (C), and folic acid (Pauling, 1968).

The aforementioned finding that niacin removed symptoms of the associated psychosis, as well as pellagra, prompted some researchers in the thirties to administer niacin in fairly small amounts (0.3 to 1.5 grams/day) to psychotics; a remission of symptoms was reported (Pauling, 1968). Since 1952, Hoffer and Osmond (Hoffer, 1962; Hoffer and Osmond, 1966) have been treating schizophrenics in Canada with either nicotinic acid or nicotinamide adenine dinucleotide (NAD) with a high reported rate of success. They recommend a dosage of 3-18 grams per day of niacin or NAD with 3 grams per day of ascorbic acid. Cott reports success with adults, as well as children, with this method. In one four year period Cott treated 175 children diagnosed as schizophrenic, autistic or brain damaged. Although he reports no exact data, Cott noted dramatic changes within 3 to 6 months in children who had previously been exposed to a host of other therapeutic methods without success (Cott, unpublished manuscript).

141

In a study done with 70 ambulatory schizophrenics Cott (1967) administered niacin and ascorbic acid (3-9 grams daily). Tests for relative hypoglycemia (a syndrome resulting from malfunctioning of the adrenal gland which causes a relative drop in blood sugar level in response to an intake of high carbohydrate foods and beverages containing caffeine) were also run on the schizophrenics, since the symptoms for hypoglycemia (depression, fatigue, exhaustion) are similar to the early symptoms of schizophrenia. Twenty-eight of the 33 patients who took the tests for relative hypoglycemia were positive for the syndrome. Dietary treatment for hypoglycemia (which includes a diet high in protein, fat and fruits and low in carbohydrates and caffeine beverages) was coupled with the niacin and ascorbic acid treatment. Fifty of the 70 patients were "improved" by the treatment (which lasted 3 to 9 months), 19 had "not improved" and one had deteriorated in his condition. The conclusion drawn was that the treatment for hypoglycemia had improved the effectiveness of the niacin-ascorbic acid treatment. This has been corroborated by other researchers (Cott, unpublished manuscript).

An evaluation of orthomolecular treatment is difficult because of the absence of well-controlled, double-blind studies (Oken, 1968; Wyatt et al., 1971). Although theoretical foundations may be given for some of the megavitamin treatments (as in the section on the transmethylation hypothesis), most of the methods

142

have been developed on a trial and error basis, with inadequate validation procedures. However, reported success rates have been high. In part the difficulty may lie in present technological shortcomings. The orthomolecular approach postulates that substances, particularly those in the brain, are not at their optimum levels. It is impossible at the present time to accurately assess the in vivo concentration of any brain substance or compound. On the other hand, those with an orthomolecular bent have not defined, with any theoretical or empirical evidence, the exact "optimum" level for a substance. Nor have they defined the criteria for the compounds or substances of concern to the orthomolecular psychiatrist. Improved laboratory techniques may provide some of the answers, but, for the present, well-controlled experiments are in order.

C. Nutritional Factors In Behavior

This section on nutritional factors, like the preceding section on orthomolecular psychiatry deals with the intake and metabolism of dietary substances; it also deals to some extent with genetic considerations, since some of the syndromes characterized by inappropriate vitamin utilization are due to inborn errors of metabolism (Coursin, 1968). But nutrition is important in and of itself, because it influences behavior. Some of the parameters of this influence will be examined here.

Nutrition (or malnutrition) is defined by the relationship of nutrient intake to bodily needs. The measurement of nutritional status is at best difficult and unsatisfcatory, since input and utilization cannot be defined closely enough to compare individuals. However the gross differences used in human studies provide some suggestive results (Kallen, 1971).

In studying the effects of nutrient intake upon behavior two courses may be followed: (1) observe the changes in learning and behavior over a long period of time, or (2) demonstrate permanent damage to the central nervous system as a result of the nutrient manipulation. Some of the major variables are: species; type of deficiency; age of onset of malnutrition; duration; severity; time and extent of nutritional rehabilitation after malnutrition.

Two-thirds of the preschool-aged children of the world are subjected to enough malnutrition to retard their physical growth and development (Scrimshaw, 1969). It is important to examine some of the effects of this malnutrition especially since we are one of the few nations where obesity is a public health problem. [We could exist comfortably with 15 per cent less food, and could adequately feed ourselves with one-half of the animal proteins now consumed (Garn, 1971).]

Among all of the nutritional diseases of childhood, only protein-calorie malnutrition has been demonstrated to be a cause of a permanent deficit in mental development. Malnutrition has political and social ramifications, but only the biological aspects will be discussed here. [For example, it appears likely that a family picks one member to be under-nourished, just as it picks one to be mentally ill (Kallen, 1971).]

Authorities disagree about separating the syndromes of protein versus calorie malnutrition. Robson (1972), for instance, places them along a continuum ranging from marasmus (severe calorie deficiency) to kwashiorkor (severe protein deficiency with adequate calories), with the symptoms and physiological effects a function of the quality and quantity of the nutrient intake and the timing of the onset of malnutrition. Klein (1971), on the other hand, maintains that the clinical, anatomic, histologic and biochemical changes in the body in response to malnutrition (where protein is limited or of inadequate quality and calories are adequate) are quite different from the bodily responses to undernutrition or starvation (where there is a lack of calories). Severe calorie deficiency (marasmus) is characterized by a slowing of growth and increased susceptibility to infection. Marasmus is frequent in young urban infants, especially of the lower classes, who are weaned early and fed an inadequate milk substitute (Scrimshaw, 1969; Klein, 1971). Severe protein deficiency (kwashiorkor) is characterized by cessation of growth, edema, wasting of muscles, and frequently, apathy and loss of appetite (Robson, 1972).

Protein malnutrition after weaning entails irreversible changes in the brain, while calorie malnutrition during this period does not. To understand some of these effects, some developmental facts are necessary. The amount of desoxyribonucleic acid (DNA) in the nucleus of each cell is constant for a given species, so the total DNA content of an organ gives an estimate of the number of cells within it. Man has two periods during which there are great increments of DNA in the brain (i.e., periods of cell proliferation). The first occurs at 15 to 20 weeks after conception and the second occurs a month later. Apart from these two spurts, the DNA content increases gradually until the fifth month after birth, after which there is little increment. DNA synthesis in the brain ceases entirely after one year of age. In man, the DNA within the cerebrum and cerebellum increases four-fold from

146

birth to one year of age while the brain stem DNA increases only fifty percent (Klein, 1971).

If the restriction in calories occurs during this period of cell proliferation and myelinization, there is decreased myelinization and reduced cellular proliferation. If the malnutrition continues beyond a critical point, the effects cannot be made up by subsequent good nutrition; i.e., some cells are never developed and the brain has fewer cells than normal (Klein, 1971; Scrimshaw, 1969). If the onset of the calorie malnutrition is after the period of cell proliferation and myelinization, there are no apparent irreversible effects which occur (in terms of brain biochemistry, anatomy); the brain in this case will contain cells normal in number although smaller in size.

Protein malnutrition before or after weaning causes a degeneration and loss of neurons. Whereas in calorie malnutrition the cells never develop, in protein malnutrition, the cells are irrevocably lost. This neuronal degeneration is associated with clinical and neurologic abnormalities that are not reversible by nutritional rehabilitation (Klein, 1971).

Studies using malnourished children in the community are subject to confounding variables that make it difficult to specify the contribution that malnutrition makes to the overall effect. For example, Klein (1971) reports a study in which malnourished subjects and well-nourished controls were taken from the same hos-

pital and matched for socioeconomic status, age, sex, race and birth
weight. When compared with the families of well-nourished children,
the families of the undernourished children had lower scores on
parent-child interactions scales, more siblings under age 2 at
the time of the subjects' birth, more marital separations during
pregnancy and after birth, and a higher probability that the subject was the result of an unwanted pregnancy. Depressed developmental scores usually found with malnourished youngsters could
thus be the result of a host of nutritional and nonnutritional
factors.

Assuming that neural damage caused by nutritional deficiencies should be reflected in integration difficulties, Cravioto
and his associates (Cravioto et al., 1966, 1968) worked with malnourished Latin American children on intermodal sensory integration
tasks (i.e., visual-kinesthetic, visual-haptic, and haptic-kin-
esthetic tasks). He found that children in the lowest quartile
for height and weight for age achieve consistently lower scores
on these tasks than children in the highest quartile. (In this
village, height and weight had been found to be unrelated to height
of parents and to the minor social differences among the village
families; hence, they were judged to be primarily due to nutritional
differences). In well-nourished communities (where differences in
height and weight reflect hereditary rather than nutritional factors)
there were no differences in test performance by quartiles for
height and weight.

While the results of some of these studies may be ambiguous because of confounding variables, they are strongly suggestive that malnutrition is one of the primary factors in the retardation of physical and mental development (Ricciuti, 1969; Scrimshaw, 1969 ; Springer, 1970). Moreover, the social and economic concomitants of malnutrition are not subject to change within one generation. Preventive medicine and applied nutrition could, on the other hand, bring immediate and palpable results--especially in underdeveloped countries, and also in the rural and ghetto areas of this nation. Federally-subsidized free lunch programs within "target" areas are a step in this direction; evaluations of the impact of this program upon school achievement are not known to this writer.

It is also of interest that the effects of early malnutrition upon the child are quite similar to those produced by a lack of sensory and social stimulation; whether an enrichment of either factor could forestall or prevent negative effects is worthy of further investigation as possible adjunctive interventions.

Researchers have also explored the consequences of deficiencies in specific nutrients, both in man and laboratory animals, apart from the effects of the gross protein or calorie shortages noted above. Coursin (1968) implicates thiamine, riboflavin, pyridoxine, niacin, folic acid, panothenic acid, and vitamins A, B_6 and C as being especially crucial to appropriate central nervous system activity, energy metabolism, and the synthesis of transmission substances. Vitamin B_6 for instance plays a vital role in the metabolism of serotonin and norepinephrine. Shortages of folic acid during development results in abnormalities in the brain, especially in the hypothalmus. Trace elements are also important for proper biological functioning. Caldwell and his associates (Caldwell et al., 1966, 1967, 1969, 1970) have documented learning impairment in adult rats with an acute zinc deficiency; general lethargy and a reduced weight gain were other consequences. It is believed that zinc plays a role in protein utilization. A similar learning impairment was found in the progeny of rats deprived of either protein or lipids during pregnancy.

After all is said and done, more questions have been raised than have been answered. The issue of the appropriateness of the medical model has been sidestepped, in part because it has been exhaustively covered by others (Szasz, 1961; Rimland, 1969; Begelman, 1971) and in part because even the longest of discussions will serve to elucidate the author's biases rather than the essential issues. One's stance concerning the medical model rests upon whether one regards an organic basis as necessary and/or sufficient in the etiology of "mental illness," behavioral disorder, or deviance. To regard psychological factors and sociological agents as important in the etiology of an illness does not necessarily preclude a recognition of the role of the biological substrates of behavior, just as recognition of the biological agents does not obviate consideration of ecological, psychological and sociological variables. But if one presumes that an interactive model provides the maximum explanatory and exploratory power in the field of deviant behavior, then one must have some knowledge of the contributions the various disciplines have made; this is a small step in that direction.

American Academy of Neurology, Joint executive board statement--the Doman-Delacato treatment of neurologically handicapped children. Neurology, 1967, 17, 637.

Begleman, D. A. Misnaming, metaphors, the medical model and some muddles. Psychiatry, 1971, 34, 38-57.

Bradley, C. The behavior of children receiving Benzedrine. American Journal of Psychiatry, 1937, 94, 577-585.

Bradley, C. Benzedrine and Dexedrine in treatment of children's behavior disorders. Pediatrics, 1950, 5, 24-37.

Caldwell, D. F., & Churchill, J. A. Learning impairment in rats administered a lipid-free diet during pregnancy. Psychological Reports, 1966, 19, 99-102.

Caldwell, D. F. & Churchill, J. A. Learning ability in the progeny of rats adminstered a protein-deficient diet during the second half of gestation. Neurology, 1967, 17 (1), 95-99.

Caldwell, D. F. & Oberleas, D. Effects of protein & zinc nutrition on behavior in the rat. Prenatal factors affecting human development. PAHO Scientific Publications, No. 185, 1969.

Caldwell, D. F. & Oberleas, D., Clarecy, J. J. & Prasad, A. S. Behavioral impairment in adult rats following acute zinc deficiency. Proceeding of the Society for Experimental Biology and Medicine, 1970, 133, 1413-1421.

Clarke, C. A. & McConnel, R. B. Pitfalls and problems in genetic studies. In C. A. Clarke (Ed.), Selected topics in medical genetics. London: Oxford University Press, 1969, 2-21.

Conners, C. K. Recent drug studies with hyperkinetic children. Journal of Learning Disabilities, 1971, 4, 476-483.

Conner, K., Eisenberg, L. & Barcai, A. The effect of dextroamphetamine on children with learning disabilities and behavior problems. Archives of General Psychiatry, 1967, 17, 478-485.

Coppen, A. The biochemistry of affective disorders. British Journal of Psychiatry, 1967, 113, 1237-1264.

Cott, A. Orthomolecular treatment: A biochemical approach to treatment of schizophrenia. Unpublished manuscript.

Cott, A. Treatment of ambulant schizophrenics with Vitamin B_3 and relative hypoglycemic diet. Journal of Schizophrenia, 1967, 1, 189-196.

Coursin, D. B. Vitamin deficiencies and developing mental capacity. In N. S. Scrimshaw & J. E. Gordon (Eds.), Malnutrition, learning and behavior. Cambridge: M.I.T. Press 1968, 289-299.

Cravioto, J. & De Licardie, E. Intersensory development of school-aged children. In N. S. Scrimshaw & J. E. Gordon (Eds.), Malnutrition, learning and behavior. Cambridge: M.I.T. Press, 1968, 252-267.

Cravioto, J., De Licardie, E. & Birch, H. Nutrition growth and neuro-integrative development: An experimental and ecologic study. Pediatrics, 1966, 38, No. 2, Part II, 319-372.

Cruickshank, W., Bentzen, F., Ratzeburg, F., & Tannhauser, M. A teaching method for brain-injured and hyperactive children. Syracuse: Syracuse University Press, 1961.

Delacato, C. H. The treatment and prevention of reading problems. Springfield: Thomas, 1959.

Denhoff, E., Davis, A. & Hawkins, R. Effects of Dextroamphetamine on hyperkinetic children: A controlled double-blind study. Journal of Learning Disabilities, 1971, 4, 491-498.

DiMascio, A. Psychopharmacology in children. Massachusetts Journal of Mental Health, 1970, 1, No. 1. Also in S. Chess & A. Thomas (Eds.), Annual Progress in Child Psychiatry and Child Development, 1971 New York: Brunner/Mazel, 1971, 479-491.

Doman, R., Spitz, E. B., Zucman, E., Delacato, C. & Doman, G. Children with severe brain injuries. The Journal of the American Medical Association, 1960, 174, 257-262.

Elliott, A. & Truax, R. E. Research in Schizophrenia. Ann Arbor News, June 18-21, 1972.

Fish, B. Problems of diagnosis and definition of comparable groups: A neglected issue in drug research with children. American Journal of Psychiatry, 1969, 125, 900-908.

Ford, E. B. Genetics for medical students. 6th ed. London: Methuen, 1968.

Fraser, F. C. Counseling in genetics: Its intent and scope. Birth Defects: Original Article Series, 1970, 4, 7-12.

Freeman, R. D. Drug effects on learning in children: A selective review of the past thirty years. Journal of Special Education, 1966, 1, 17-44.

Freeman, R. D. The drug treatment of learning disorders: Continuing confusion. Journal of Pediatrics, 1972, 81, 112-115.

Frohman, C. E. Biochemical mechanisms. In G. Tourney $ J. S. Gottlieb, (Eds.), Lafayette Clinic studies on schizophrenia. Detroit: Wayne University Press, 1971, 125-162.

Frostig, M., Lefever, D. & Whittlesey, J. The Marianne Frostig developmental test of visual perception. Palo Alto: Consulting Psychology Press, 1964.

Garn , S. M. Nutrition, malnutrition and growth. Lecture presented at the Interdisciplinary Nutrition Seminars, 2 October 1971, Towsley Center, Ann Arbor.

Genetic engineering: Reprise. Editorial in Journal of the American Medical Association, 1972, 220 (10), 1356-1357.

Gordon, M. Psychopharmacological agents. Vol. I. New York: Academic Press, 1964.

Gordon, M. Psychopharmacological agents. Vol. II. New York: Academic Press, 1967.

Gottlieb, J. S., Frohman, C. E. & Beckett, P. G. The current status of the a-2-globulin in schizophrenia. In H. E. Himwich (Ed.), Biochemistry schizophrenias and the affective illnesses. Baltimore: Williams & Wilkins, 1970, 153-170.

Gottlieb, J. S., Frohman, C. E. , & Harmison, C. R. Schizophrenia-- New concepts. Southern Medical Journal, 1971, 64, 743-749.

Grant, Q. R. Psychopharmacology in childhood emotional and mental disorders. Journal of Pediatrics, 1962, 61, 627-637.

Hallahan, D. Learning disabilities in historical and psychoeducational perspective. Doctoral dissertation, University of Michigan, 1971.

Hoffer, A. Niacin therapy in psychiatry. Springfield: Thomas, 1962.

Hoffer, A. & Osmond, H. Nicotinamide adenine dinucleotide (NAD) as a treatment for schizophrenia. Journal of Psychopharmacology, 1966, 1, 79-95.

Kallen, D. J. Malnutrition, learning and behavior. Lecture presented at the Interdisciplinary Nutrition Seminars, 2 October 1971, Towsley Center, Ann Arbor.

Kaplan, A. R. Genetic counseling in mental retardation and mental disorder. In H. T. Lynch (Ed.), Dynamic genetic counseling for clinicians, Springfield: Charles Thomas, 1969.

Kephart, N. The slow learner in the classroom. Columbus, Ohio: Merrill, 1960.

Klein, R. E., Habicht, J. P. & Yarbrough, C. Effects of protein-calorie malnutrition on mental development. In I. Schulman (Ed.), Advances in pediatrics. Vol. 18. New York: Year Book Medical Publishers, 1971, 75-91.

Ladd, E. T. Pills for classroom peace? Saturday Review, 1970, 53, 66-72.

Langdon-Down, J. Clinical Lectures and Reports. London Hospital, 1866, 3, 259.

Laufer, M. W. Long-term management and some follow-up findings on the use of drugs with minimal cerebral symptoms. Journal of Learning Disabilities, 1971, 4, 519-522.

Lejeune, J. The 21-trisomy: Current state of chromosomal research. In A. G. Steinber & A. G. Bearn (Eds.), Progress in medical genetics. Vol. III. New York: Grune & Stratton, 1964, 144-177.

Link. Michigan Department of Mental Health. Vol. II, No. 9, 14, February, 1972.

Lynch, H. T. Dynamic genetic counseling for clinicians. Springfield: Thomas, 1970.

Lynch, H. T. International directory of genetic services. 2nd. edition. New York: The National Foundation, 1969.

Murray, G. & Hirsch, J. Heredity, individual differences, and psychopathology. In S. C. Plog & R. B. Edgerton (Eds.), Changing perspectives in mental illness. New York: Holt, 1969, 596-627.

Oken, D. Vitamin therapy: Treatment for the mentally ill. (letter), Science, 1968, 160, 1181.

Parker, W. C. Some ethical and legal aspects of genetic counseling. Birth Defects: Original Article Series, 1970, 6, 52-57.

Parsons, P. A. The genetic analysis of behavior. London: Methuen, 1967.

Pauling, L. C. Orthomolecular psychiatry. Science, 1968, 160, 265-271.

Price, J. The XYY syndrome: Genetics and criminality. In C. A. Clarke (Ed.), Selected topics in medical genetics. London: Oxford University Press, 1969a, 233-234.

Price, J. Genetics and schizophrenia. In C. A. Clarke (Ed.), Selected topics in medical genetics. London: Oxford University Press, 1969b, 228-233.

Redding, A. & Hirschhorn, K. Guide to human chromosome defects. Birth Defects: Original Article Series, 1958, 4, 91-106.

Report of the conference on the use of stimulant drugs in the treatment of behaviorally disturbed young school children. Journal of Learning Disabilties, 1971, 4, 523-530.

Ricciuti, H. N. Malnutrition, learning and intellectual development. Presented at annual meeting of the American Psychological Association, Washington D. C. , September, 1969.

Rimland, B. Psychogenesis versus biogenesis: The issues and the evidence. In S. C. Plog & R. B. Edgerton (Eds.), Changing perspectives in mental illness. New York: Holt, 1969, 702-735.

Rimoin, D. L. The medical genetics clinic and mental health. Birth Defects: Original Article Series, 1970, 6, 67-75.

Robbins, M. & Glass, G. The Doman-Delacato rationale: A critical analysis. In J. Hellmuth (Ed.), Educational Therapy, Vol. II. Seattle: Special Child Publications, 1969.

Roberts, J. A. F. An introduction to medical genetics. London: Oxford University Press, 1970.

Robson, J. R. K. Malnutrition: Its causation and control, with special reference to protein calorie malnutrition. Vol. I. New York: Gordon & Breach, 1972.

Sagor, M. Biological bases of childhood behavioral disorders.
    Ann Arbor: Institute for the Study of Mental Retardation
    and Related Disabilties, 1971.

Scrimshaw, N. S. Early malnutrition and central nervous system
    function. Merrill-Palmer Quarterly, 1969, 15, 375-388.

Seguin, E. Traitment, morale, hygiene et education des idiots.
    Paris: I. B. Bailliere, 1846.

Slater, E. T. O. Heredity of mental diseases. In F. A. Jones
    (Ed.), Clinical aspects of genetics: Proceedings of a
    conference held in London. London: Pitman Press, 1961, 23-29.

Solomons, G. Guidelines on the use and medical effects of
    psychostimulant drugs in therapy. Journal of Learning
    Disabilities, 1971, 4, 472-475.

Sprague, R. L., Barnes, K. R., & Werry, J. S. Methylphenidate and
    Thioridazine: Learning, reaction time, activity and class-
    room behavior in disturbed children. American Journal of
    Orthopsychiatry, 1970, 40, 615-628.

Springer, N. S. Nutrition and mental retardation: An annotated
    bibliography. Ann Arbor: Institute for the Study of
    Mental Retardation, 1970.

Strauss, A. Diagnosis and education of the cripple-brained,
    deficient child. Journal of Exceptional Children, 1943, 9,
    163-167.

Strauss, A. & Kephart, N. Behavior differences in mentally
    retarded children as measured by a new behavior rating
    scale. American Journal of Psychiatry, 1940, 96, 1117-1123.

Strauss, A. & Lehtinen, L. E. Psychopathology and education of
    the brain-injured child. New York: Grune & Stratton, 1947.

Strauss, A. & Werner, H. Disorders of conceptual thinking in the
    brain injured child. Journal of Nervous and Mental Disease,
    1942, 96, 153-171.

Szasz, T. The myth of mental illness. New York: Hoeber-Harper, 1961.

Thompson, T. & Schuster, C. Behavioral pharmacology. Englewood CLiffs:
    Prentice Hall, 1968.

Tourney, G. History of biological psychiatry in America. American Journal of Psychiatry, 1969, 1, 67-80.

Tourney, G. & Gottlieb, J. S. (Eds.), Lafayette Clinic studies on schizophrenia. Detroit: Wayne State University Press, 1971.

Townes, P. L. Preventive genetics and early therapeutic procedures in the control of birth defects. Birth Defects: Original Article Series, 1970, 4, 42-51.

Volpe, E. P. Human heredity and birth defects. New York: Pegasus, 1971.

Werry, J. S., Weiss, G., Duglas, V. & Martin, J. Studies on the hyperactive child: The effect of chlorpromaszine upon behavior and learning ability. The Journal of the Academy of Child Psychiatry, 1966, 5, 292-312.

Wyatt, R. J., Termini, B. A. & Davis, J. Biochemical and sleep studies of schizophrenia: A review of the literature, 1960-1970. Schizophrenia Bulletin, 1971, Issue No. 4, 9-66.

BEHAVIORAL INTERVENTIONS IN EMOTIONAL DISTURBANCE

L. I. Kameya

TABLE OF CONTENTS

1. INTRODUCTION

A. History

The philosophical precursors to the learning theorists have been clearly outlined by Ullmann and Krasner (1969), who trace the conceptual path from the Greeks and Romans to the twentieth century psychologists. For present purposes, however, we may locate the conceptual roots of the modern day learning theory and behavior modification in the works of Thorndike, Pavlov, Watson, Guthrie, Hull, and Skinner.

The systematic application of learning theory for the therapeutic modification of behavior is a relatively recent phenomenon. [Ulrich & Stachnik & Mabry (1966), Franks (1969), and Hilgard & Marquis (1961) give very complete accounts of early applications of learning theory.] Watson and Rayner (1920) demonstrated the ease with which a fear reaction could be conditioned in a child, Albert, and suggested four possible methods of deconditioning. However, because of Albert's premature departure from the hospital, none of these was attempted.

It remained for Mary Cover Jones (1924) to compare six different procedures for eliminating fears in children. The two methods that were most consistently effective were "direct conditioning" (eliciting a pleasant response in the presence of the feared object) and "social imitation" (placing the child with peers who are not afraid of the fear stimulus). Thus, behavioral therapy was born, although it did not come of age until the post-war period. Few articles described application of techniques, but conceptual models were being constructed by B. F. Skinner (1938).

The early applications of behavior modification were generally case studies within clinics, laboratories or institutions. Educational interpretations did not follow until the late fifties. The cross-fertilization which then occurred resulted in a blossoming of articles, books, and journals that devoted themselves exclusively to behavior modification, behavioral therapy or behavioral engineering.

This paper will concentrate upon the more recent applications of learning theory for the modification of behavior. Following the bifurcation generally recognized (e. g., Hilgard and Marquis, 1961), the interventions will be divided into those which are based upon reinforcement theories or operant (instrumental) conditioning, and those which flow from contiguity theories or classical (respondent) conditioning techniques. Completing the paper are separate discussions of punishment or aversive therapy (faradic techniques), modeling procedures, and the general theoretical and ethical issues that are raised by the manipulation of behavior.

B. Assumptions and Definitions

Those adhering to a learning theory model of behavior assume that all behavior (adaptive and maladaptive, in humans and infrahumans) is the result of the lawful application of principles of reinforcement and extinction; i.e., behavior is controlled by impinging stimuli. The alteration of behavior should follow the same principles that govern the acquisition of behavior. The behaviorist is not concerned with the internal state of the individual, but with observable behaviors and consequences (including social consequences).

A reinforcer is a stimulus which alters the future probability of occurrence of the behavior which immediately precedes it. A positive reinforcer increases that probability of occurrence of the behavior which immediately precedes its presentation. A negative reinforcer increases the future probability of occurrence of a behavior which immediately precedes its termination. The converse is also true: the future probability of occurrence of a behavior will decrease with the termination of a positive reinforcer and will decrease with the application of a negative reinforcer (punishment).

Extinction is the process of removing the contingent stimuli which maintain the behaviors, hence, reducing the frequency of those behaviors. Time out from positive reinforcement (stipulating a period during which positive reinforcement is not available

Table 1. Procedures for influencing strength of behavior.

	Operation	Behavioral Effects	Examples of Events	Learning Princi
I	Behavior produces positive event	Increase in strength of behavior which produces the event	Smile, money, food, approval, special privilege, affection, passing grade, promotion, pay raise, participation in game	Positive reinfo ment
II	Behavior produces removal of aversive event	Increase in strength of behavior which removes the event	Frown, poor grade, electric shock, threat of removal of play period, criticism, rejection, nonattention, penalty	Negative reinfo ment
III	Behavior does not produce the positive event associated with previous positive reinforcement	Decrease in strength of behav- which was reinforced previously by the presentation of the positive event	Same as events in Row I	Extinction
IV	Behavior does not produce the removal of the aversive event associated with previous negative reinforcement	Decrease in strength of behavior which was reinforced previously by the removal of the aversive event	Same as events in Row II	Extinction
V	Behavior produces aversive events	Decrease of strength of behavior which produces the aversive event	Same as events in Row II	Punishment
VI	Behavior produces temporary or permanent loss of positive events	Decrease of strength of behavior which produces the loss of positive events	Same as events in Row I	Punishment: Time out, resp cost

(From Gardner, W. I. Behavior Modification in Mental Retardation, Chicago: Aldine/ Atherton, 1971, p. 89.)

as a consequence of a behavior) is also a procedure which decreases
the strength of a behavior (thus, a punisher).

Primary reinforcers are those which satisfy innate needs
(e.g., food, water). Secondary reinforcers or second order reinforcers are those stimuli which are associated with primary reinforcers and in time acquire reinforcing properties of their own
(e.g., tokens).

Learning theorists find it necessary to carefully stipulate
the behavior under consideration. It must be defined in terms of
overt movements that are observable, countable, measurable and
whose occurrence or nonoccurrence can be established without
interpretation. For example, "restless behavior" is indefinite
because observers vary in their definition of restlessness, whereas "number of times subject leaves seat" is a measure on which
observers can agree since it deals with an observable behavior
that is quantifiable.

The functional analysis of behavior involves defining the
behavior under consideration (e.g., sitting in own chair) and
determining the target or terminal behavior (i.e., accelerating
or decelerating the behavior, or establishing a new behavior such
as "correctly solving 10 arithmetic problems a day") and instituting a modification procedure to secure the desired change.
To determine the effectiveness of the modification procedure
selected, an ABAB experimental design may be selected: the

frequency of the behavior under study is measured to determine the baseline, and this is compared to the frequency of the behavior during periods when the modification procedure is put into effect, removed, and reinstated.

The behaviorist utilizing a reinforcement model is interested in "contingencies of reinforcement," that is, the interrelationships between an organism's behavior and its environment. He is interested in the response, the occasion of the response, and the consequence (Skinner, 1969). It is the study of systematic contingent environmental consequences based on the empirical work of the last three decades that is important (Krasner, 1970). It is not reinforcement per se, but the contingent application of reinforcement that is the critical feature. Non-contingent reinforcement is functionally equivalent to an extinction run. That is, the rate of relevant behaviors decreases over time.

C. Principle of "Probability of Behavior"

In 1959 Premack articulated the principle which has greatly influenced behavioral engineering. Premack's principle opened an almost endless range of potential reinforcers. The principle is: given two responses, A and B, if B occurs with a greater frequency than A, it can be used as a reinforcer for A. In application, this means that if Johnny likes to play baseball and does not turn out many arithmetic problems, playing baseball could be made contingent upon arithmetic achievement (such as

"10 arithmetic problems solved correctly").

The first step in applying Premack's principle is to count behaviors in a natural setting, when a variety of behaviors can occur ad libitum; if the desirable (target) behavior is low in frequency, the other behaviors are made contingent upon its occurrence.

In determining whether an event or object is reinforcing, the experimenters' estimations and subjects' reports cannot be relied upon to provide an accurate picture, nor do they guarantee that the list of reinforcers produced are approved or legitimate. The Reinforcing Event Menu (RE Menu) (Addison & Homme, 1966) solves both problems by allowing the subject to choose from a list of approved alternatives; this insures that the response-consequence contingency is viable for each subject.

Both the Premack principle and the RE Menu can be incorporated into a program utilizing token reinforcers. Such a program (or token economy) has three requirements: (1) A specification of behaviors to be reinforced (desirable behaviors); (2) A method of making the tokens contingent upon behavior (dispensing mechanism); (3) A specification of the rules regarding the exchange of tokens for primary reinforcers, objects, or events (the "back-up" reinforcers). The tokens acquire their reinforcing qualities through association with the back-up reinforcers.

In order that the tokens be reinforcing to the subjects, they should be redeemable for a variety of stimuli (i.e., they should be generalized reinforcers). This is similar to the RE Menu since the individual selects the back-up reinforcer he wishes to "purchase" with his tokens. The back-up reinforcers should include primary reinforcers (e.g., food), objects (e.g., cigarettes, magazines), or privileges (e.g., ground passes, time to watch television, time to nap). The latter classification includes those behaviors found to occur with high frequency in normal circumstances, as with the Premack principle.

One can also include a "response cost" rule in a token economy. An errant individual loses some of the privileges previously earned. With a token economy, tokens are removed. Unfortunately, no direct comparison of the efficacy of the response cost procedure and the positive reinforcement procedure has been made, although several investigators report success with the former without any side effects noted.

Group versus individual contingencies must also be considered. Is the dispensing of reinforcers a function of group or individual behavior? For example, a group contingency would make a 10-minute recess for the class contingent upon everyone's completing their work assignment; an individual contingency would permit each child a recess if his own work was completed. The group contingency is useful in bringing group pressure to bear upon a deviant individual (especially if such behavior was previously reinforced

by the group, as in the case of an acting-out individual). However, before launching such a program, one must consider the
danger of excessive group pressure as well as the desirability
of conforming behavior in the context of long-range educational
goals.

A token system has some built-in disadvantages which should
be mentioned. It is an artificial system that does not necessar-
ly conform to the "real world," although some parallels could be
drawn to the monetary system. In most applications, however,
there is a need to "fade out" the token reinforcers and replace
them with more enduring reinforcers, such as social approval
or self-reinforcement. This type of change has been reported in
only a few programs.

For instance, the individual may function in other settings
(e.g., at home) where the token contingencies are not in effect.
Unless the tokens are "faded out," they will become discriminative
stimuli for certain behaviors, and appropriate functioning may be
dependent upon the tokens being used--that is, the behavior may
not generalize to other settings, but may become increasingly
specific to the token system environment. O'Leary and Drabman
(1971) give specific suggestions to preclude the occurrence of
this phenomenon in a school context. These suggestions are apl-
plicable to other token economy settings. To increase generalization of the appropriate behavior to other settings, they sug-

gest: (1) Be sure that "behavior disorders" are not due to academic deficiencies. The probability of inappropriate activity is minimized if the student has the appropriate academic skills in his repertoire; (2) Build the expectation that the student is capable of doing well and that he will be able to function without tokens as he grows older; (3) Have the students evaluate their own behavior. Involve them in the selection of behaviors to be reinforced and the contingencies to be used; (4) Provide reinforcement in a variety of situations to reduce the distinction between reinforced and non-reinforced situations; (5) Involve the parents to provide some continuity between school and home; (6) Gradually withdraw the tokens and back-up reinforcers and utilize the reinforcers present in the natural environment (e.g., privileges, free time).

II. REINFORCEMENT THEORIES

In this section we shall discuss past and present applications of operant technology in the clinic and classroom, as well as programs that employ behavior modification in the natural environment with parents and consultant-mediators. Some excellent collections of related articles may be found in Ullmann and Krasner (1964), Krasner and Ullmann (1965), and Franks (1964). In the thirties, conditioned reinforcers, including tokens, were used with chimpanzees (Cowles, 1937; Wolfe, 1936). The first reported use of tokens for behavior modification in a clinical or educational setting was in 1959 (Staats, 1969). The results encouraged many researchers, including Michael and Allyon who had until then relied upon social and material reinforcers.

173

A. Clinical Applications

Ayllon and Haughton. Ayllon and Haughton (1962) utilized food
as a back-up reinforcer of the early applications of tokens to a
psychiatric setting. Their goal was to control limited aspects
of the behavior of chronic schizophrenics. Fifty per cent of the
forty-five patients on the ward had a history of refusing to eat;
various measures, including spoon-feeding, tube feeding and elec-
tro-shock were ineffective in changing this pattern. At dinner
time the patients were coaxed and cajoled to eat by the nurses.
This social attention, the investigators reasoned, was reinforcing
to the patients and maintained their reluctance to eat.

A three phase program was instituted. The first phase called
for the dining room to be open only thirty minutes and no nurses
were to be in the area during the meal times; the patients were
left alone. Since twenty-four hour control was possible on the
ward, no food was made available at other times during the day.
The eating problems were eliminated; all patients began to eat un-
assisted. The meal time was then shortened to twenty minutes,
then fifteen and finally five minutes.

In phase II, a simple motor response was developed--dropping
a penny into a slot before entering the dining room. The penny
was obtained from the nurse. Although some verbal shaping was
necessary, all of the patients quickly learned the required response.

174

Again, food was sufficient reinforcement for the behavior. In phase III, a simple social response, cooperative button-pushing, was required, along with the motor task of phase II, to gain access to the food. Two buttons were placed 7.5 feet apart and had to be pressed simultaneously (by two patients) to activate a buzzer and light and dispense a penny. All but one patient learned the cooperative response required. A side benefit was an increase in verbal contact among the patients, usually centering around the task. No side effects were noted; the initial apprehensions of the staff concerning the "stressful" circumstances of the program were not supported by the results.

The token in this study, a penny, was negotiable for one event only, namely, admission to the dining room. Since food is one of the most salient of the primary reinforcers, it was a potent back-up reinforcer for all of the patients. Although both the learned responses were very simple, the study demonstrated the feasibility of utilizing tokens to control the behavior of schizophrenics. An earlier study (Ayllon and Michael, 1959) demonstrated the efficacy of using psychiatric nurses as behavioral engineers (those who dispense reinforcers, administer the program, and stipulate contingencies). Relatively untrained personnel can effectively coordinate a behavior modification program with periodic consultation with professionals. This concept (paraprofessional control) was incorporated into many of the programs which followed, solving a crucial manpower problem.

Ayllon and Azrin. Ayllon and Azrin (1968) incorporated the use of conditioned reinforcers (tokens) and the Premack principle into a complete psychotic ward program at a large state hospital (Anna State Hospital, Illinois). Their basic objective was to maximize the motivation of psychotic patients in a manner consistent with operant reinforcement theory. Because all behaviors and procedures were clearly specified, ward attendants could administer all aspects of the program. Desirable behaviors were increased and undesirable behaviors were decreased by utilizing the laws of reinforcement and extinction. Aversive stimuli and coercive procedures were eliminated from the ward through careful selection of the staff, regular supervision, and clear-cut specification of behaviors and reinforcements. The behaviors deemed desirable were those that were considered to be useful or necessary for functioning within the context of the mental hospital (e.g., grooming, mopping the floor, eating, sorting laundry, etc.). Lists of desired behaviors were posted conspicuously and read aloud by attendants. These lists described the behaviors, specified the time and place at which they were expected to occur and the number of tokens allotted for their performance. Each patient selected

176

his own jobs. Tokens collected were negotiable currency for reinforcing activities (e.g., walking through the grounds, attending religious services, admission to dining hall, musical activities, and even psychotherapy sessions). These activities were determined to be reinforcing by the probability of behavior rule (Premack principle) which states: Observe what the individual does when the opportunity exists. Those activities which are very probable at a given time will serve as reinforcers.

Ayllon and Azrin have formulated general rules which are easily adaptable to other treatment or education environments. These rules relate to the discovery, selection and definition of reinforcers and responses, and to appropriate programming (delineation of contingencies). They outline procedures for shaping and prompting of expected behavior, and for maximization of reinforcements through scheduling.

Tokens were selected as a mode of reinforcement because they effectively bridge the time gap between the desired responses and the delivery of reinforcements, permit the responses to be reinforced at any time (even when separated temporally or spatially from the reinforcement), and permit reinforcement without delay. Tokens can bear a quantitative relationship to the amount of reinforcement, may be used to operate devices which automatically deliver reinforcements, are durable and are not subject to satiation as a primary reinforcer would be. In other situations, of course, money, points, marks or similar conditional reinforcers could be employed effectively.

Ayllon and Azrin have found that, in general, the adaptive, reinforced behaviors were maintained as long as the experimental procedures were employed. Discontinuation of the experimental program reduced the frequency of desired behaviors; reinstitution of the program resulted in an immediate increase in desired behaviors.

Adaptations of the Ayllon and Azrin program have been used in such diverse settings as institutions for the mentally retarded, sheltered workshops for multiply disabled, half-way houses, correctional institutions for juveniles, preschools, classes for slow learners, and institutions for the profoundly retarded. A translation of the program for a regular classroom or a class for the emtionally disturbed is a recognized eventuality.

Schaeffer and Martin. The Patton Experiment (Schaeffer & Martin, 1969) at the Patton State Hospital, California was begun in 1964 with patients who were termed "incurable." These patients were transferred to two experimental cottages, one for men and one for women, each housing 70-75 persons. Patients had to meet these criteria: a diagnosis of chronic schizophrenia, hospital habituated (at least six months without progress), no organicity, poor prognosis, and able to function on an open ward. The patient-staff ratio was maintained at pre-experiment levels and no additional funds were sought to finance the project.

The ward personnel and auxiliary staff were included in program planning. They were trained in behavior modification techniques for 18 weeks; this included discussions and lectures on operant conditioning and simple behavior experiments. Specific behavior lists were made up for the behaviors desired on the ward. Since the ward personnel had maximum contact with the patients, they had to have the power to make immediate decisions about reinforcing emitted behaviors without first consulting with a doctor or psychologist. Doctor's orders were therefore couched in general terms and the nurses were free to operationalize them.

There were three groups in each building: an orientation group (60% patients), a therapy group (20%) and a "ready to leave group" (20%). The members of the orientation group, the lowest group, were allowed only hospital clothing, and a bare dormitory with a simple bed. They were given no bedspread and no storage space for personal items. All groups ate the same food, but the orientation group ate after the other groups at long tables, from plastic trays, and with only a large spoon as a utensil. The number of visitors was limited and no movies, parties or off-ward activities were allowed. In essence, they were accorded the minimal requirements for the preservation of human dignity.

Members of the therapy group were allowed to wear their own

clothing and slept in more comfortable beds with bedspreads.
Each had a small dresser and a rug on the floor. The dormitory was
adorned with drapes. They were permitted to entertain visitors,
attend social functions, and move about the grounds. They dined
at tables set for four, used flatware and dishes, and were served
family style.

Each individual in the ready-to-leave group had a private
room which he could decorate to suit his tastes. They were first
in the dining room, and sat at tables with tablecloths and flowers.
They could leave the hospital grounds and frequently had jobs
in nearby communities. They were expected to engage in outside
activities, use buses, attend movies, and go shopping.

In all groups, the patients had to pay for all necessities, lux-
eries and privileges (payment rates were varied from patient to
patient). The back-up reinforcers included food, beds to sleep
on, cigarettes, television, and visiting privileges.

Poker chips were initially used as tokens, but these were
replaced by brass tokens which could operate the automatic equipment eventually installed, such as turnstiles in the dining room,
a TV timer, food venders and automatic door openers. To check
on consumer practices for any patient, names were printed on tokens.

In the orientation group, the patients had to pay for privileges such as lying down, not getting up on time, not being on
time for medication, and smoking cigarettes.

180

Expected behaviors were explained to the patient and thereafter he was expected to be as independent as he would be outside
of the hospital. He was never coerced or summoned, not ordered to
dress or wash; instead, appropriate behavior was reinforced with
tokens. Over time, as an individual progressed through the groups,
there was a gradual weaning from the tokens to the social reinforcers that normally exist in any environment; that is, tokens
were faded out. Most patients found the orientation group unpleasant enough to modify their behavior appropriately within two
months; at that time they were transferred to the therapy group.

Within the therapy group, the individual was subject to intensive operant conditioning and individual attention. Once
in the therapy group he was allowed five months to attain discharge status (two of the five months must be spent in the
ready-to-leave group); therefore, if he was not ready or willing
to accept living outside the hospital at the end of the three
month period, he was returned to the orientation group. The head
nurse of the ward, in consultation with the nursing personnel,
made decisions for reassignment. As soon as a patient was assigned
to the therapy group, a social worker contacted his family, made
arrangements for half-way houses, work, etc.

Assignment to the ready-to-leave group occurred only after the
patient was willing to attempt outside living. It was the final
phase of the gradual transition from institutional life to normal
outside living. The patient usually held an outside job, handled

money and was responsible for making and meeting commitments. He learned the skills necessary for functioning in society but which are quickly lost in long-term institutionalization.

After the first 31 months of the program, the discharge rate was nine percent per month. Of the 248 discharged patients, 16 percent were readmitted; this compares with an average readmission rate of 35-40 percent for all public mental hospitals over a similar period. This statistic is all the more impressive since patients admitted to the program were those considered to be most resistant to change.

The Patton experiment is of particular interest because there is a built-in provision for a gradual transition to a discharge state. The token economy is faded out and replaced with the more "real-worldly" social reinforcement and general competence motivations. As in Ayllon and Azrin's Anna State Hospital program, ward personnel were trained in behavior modification techniques and were very effective administrators. One fringe benefit of this program, as in many others that utilize this model, was the staff's increasing awareness of the ways that behavior can be controlled. This awareness leads to a critical evaluation of their own practices that maintain or establish undesirable patient behaviors.

182

B. Educational Applications

The first reported use of operant techniques in an educational setting was by Staats in the teaching of reading concepts to children. Early work specialized in individual treatment in order to maximize control of environmental factors. Only one child's behavior in a special class or on the playground was of concern. Later the behavior of several children was monitored and manipulated simultaneously through contingent reinforcement. More sophisticated programs now utilize individual contingencies for all of the children in a group. That is, each pupil's rewards are based on his own behavior. This is typical of token economy programs in classrooms (e.g., Hewett, 1968; O'Leary and Drabman, 1971) and others which do not rely upon a total token economy (e.g., Orme and Purnell, 1970). Group contingencies may also be utilized in a classroom (or anywhere, for that matter). In that case, group privileges depend upon everyone's behavior; it's an all-or-none situation. For example, "the class may have a ten minute recess if everyone completes the first ten problems on page 148 in less than forty minutes" would be a group contingency. Problems inherent in using group contingencies include (1) having a child who cannot perform the required behavior, (2) creating undue pressure on a child, and (3) having a child who finds it reinforcing to subvert the system for the other children (O'Leary & Drabman, 1971). Presently, there is no evidence to evaluate the comparative effectiveness of group versus individual contingencies. Implications

183

of both procedures for the socialization of children could be important; present data are confined to cross-cultural comparisons (Bronfenbrenner, 1962, 1970).

Zimmerman and Zimmerman. An intervention by Zimmerman & Zimmerman (1962) illustrates the nature of early attempts in the field. The modifier was an English teacher in a residential treatment center who had three boys in class for an hour each day. A modification program was instituted for two of the three boys. In both cases the inappropriate behavior (inappropriate spelling responses for one boy and temper tantrums, baby talk for the other) was extinguished (ignored) and the appropriate behavior was reinforced (with attention, close physical proximity, etc.). For both boys, the target behavior decreased to an acceptable level and appropriate class work-oriented behavior increased. However, no pre-intervention count of the target behaviors was made and the appropriate behaviors were not specified in detail. Since there was no baseline data to begin with, the design did not include a withdrawal of the intervention to determine if there was a return to baseline. In this case, one cannot be sure that the intervention was responsible for the "change" since assessment was based on the teacher's observations and her expectations could have influenced her perceptions. But the Zimmermans' work, while methodologically weak, demonstrated an application of behavior modification techniques in a classroom, rather than in a laboratory setting.

Harris, Wolf, and Baer. One result of the applications of
the behavior modification techniques to the classroom has been the
careful delineation of those factors operating as reinforcers.
By making teachers aware of some of these factors, they can be
more effective in dispensing reinforcers. For instance, the
potency of attention as a reinforcer has been demonstrated by
Harris, Wolf, & Baer. They sought to reverse the normal in-
clinations of teachers to attend to deviant or undesirable
behavior, on the basis that this attention served to reinforce and
maintain the behavior. Baseline data on several behaviors were
obtained at a laboratory preschool. One child spent 80% of the
time crawling on the floor; another child cried or whined 8
times per morning. Understandably, the teachers spent much time
with both children to ease their adjustment. The modification
program called for teachers to ignore the problem behavior of the
children, and to give immediate attention to them for more appropriate behavior (i.e., on-feet behavior and non-crying). Within ten days, the first child spent a normal amount of time on her
feet and the second child rarely cried in the morning. To determine if the differential attention was responsible for the change
in behavior, the teachers returned to their former method of handling the crawling and whining; the frequency of both behaviors returned to pre-intervention levels. Once the appropriate behaviors

had been re-established, the excessive attention accorded to the two children was faded out (i.e., diminished) to the levels normal for any child in the class. This latter point is important since the behaviors that have been established must be maintained in a normal situation by reinforcers available naturally, or they will quickly diminish. Behaviors established through modification routines must be maintained naturally or they serve only as fruitless exercises in temporary change.

Orme and Purnell. Behavior modification techniques can also be applied to a total class. Orme & Purnell were faced with a class of eighteen, third and fourth grade youngsters who were uncontrolled: serious fighting occurred frequently and although not all of the children were aggressors, each had been struck one or more times during an observation period of two weeks. The teachers (T_1, the regular teacher and T_2, the intern) were also unable to keep the pupils in class; they would run through the halls, through other classes and offices and out of the school. Unsuccessful efforts to achieve control included selecting new curriculum material and dividing the class into two groups.

The classroom was divided into two small rooms (A & B); an attempt was made to establish control in B through conditioning and modeling. It was hypothesized that changes in behavior produced in Room B would transfer to Room A. There were four phases to the project which was run over a six week period. Videotape equipment was used both in training and in measurement of behavior (12 randomly determined five minute segments of classtime filmed each day.)

186

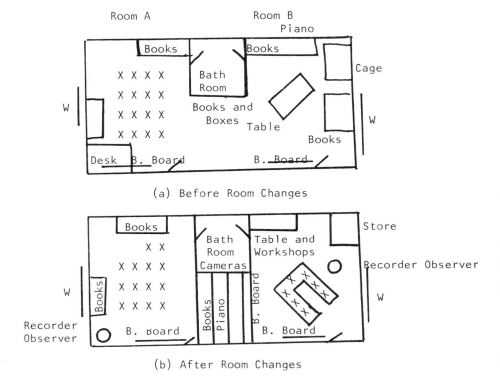

(a) Before Room Changes

(b) After Room Changes

Figure 1. Classroom plan (from Orme and Purnell, 1970).

To institute milieu control in Room B, changes were made in the room and the curriculum, the teachers were trained in new techniques and a token reinforcement program was instituted.

The room changes (see diagram) included the following re-arrangements. The room was divided in two with a piano and black-board placed in the center. All books, wall decorations and extra furniture were removed and posters appropriate to the cur-riculum were placed and changed when necessary. The desks in Room B were placed in a U-pattern and placed so that the teach-er could control the door, and was encouraged to move away from the blackboard, into the U and over to the worktable; this created a varied stimulus situation for the pupils. A store was set up in one corner of the room. All changes were designed to maximize teacher control, reduce extraneous material, make the room attractive and encourage the teacher to teach from different positions in the room.

The special training for the teachers included instruction in verbal, nonverbal, and token reinforcement procedures, basic questioning procedures (probing), and ways to vary the stimulus situation. These latter two procedures are used to elicit at-tention and curiosity; they are methods to shape pupil behavior. The teachers were also taught to engineer desirable behavior, to reinforce the desirable behavior with tokens and verbal and nonverbal reinforcement. They were told to ignore disruptive

behavior by focusing on a nearby pupil engaged in desirable behavior (modeling). They were trained to specify instructional
goals in behavioral terms and to apply differential reinforcement
techniques. Videotapes were used for analysis of each teacher's
classroom behavior.

The curriculum material was changed by the teachers involved.
Neither was given specific suggestions to follow except to use
"educational value" and "control potential" as guideposts. Both
produced changes in the curriculum that eliminated traditional
drills. For instance, choral reading and drama were used for
English literature, and role playing and student-teacher discussions were included in social studies units.

The token system utilized is novel in that the pupils shared
in the determination of behaviors receiving points, and to a
certain degree, in the selection of backup reinforcers. The
backup reinforcers included candy, gum, balloons, comics, novels,
math puzzles, the opportunity to write poetry, art lessons from
a real artist, a model airplane with a lesson on aerodynamics,
field trips to museums, etc. All items were displayed on the
table. Non-tangible reinforcements (trips, projects) were color-
fully illustrated. Most items were designed to provide further
opportunities for individual or small group study; to that extent,
the pupil determined his curriculum for part of the school day.
Prices for the backup reinforcers ranged from the candy at 15
points to projects at 450 to 1000 points. All names were listed

189

on the board and points displayed as awarded. The children were all given 25 points to use immediately as an introduction to the system and to provide an incentive. The initial rules (for receiving points) were listed on a blackboard; keep busy all the time; have good manners; don't bother your neighbor. The first few minutes of the initial class session were allotted for discussions and suggestions for specific rules that the pupils thought should receive points. There was no shortage of suggestions.

Transfer of control to Room A from Room B was achieved in the following manner: All children were exposed to the milieu control of Room B during Phase 2 of the program (Phase 1 was the pretreatment observation period). This atmosphere was designed to be highly desirable because they had a chance to earn points and exchange them at the store, among other reasons. If Room B were indeed reinforcing, then Room A contingencies could be set up to capitalize on this. The entire class was brought to Room A (after exposure to B conditions) and told that only half the class could be in Room B at any time. They were asked for suggestions regarding rules for gaining entrance to Room B. The result of the discussion that followed produced these rules: points earned in Room A would be used to gain entrance to Room B, but not to purchase store items. The two highest point earners at the end of the day in Room B would be allowed to remain there and the seven highest point earners in Room A would be allowed to transfer to Room B the following day. A constant changeover was thus maintained

throughout the study. Point earning rules for Room A were determined as in Room B through class discussion. (Unfortunately, the
authors do not indicate how much of the above structure and the
room-changing mechanism had been predetermined by the experimenters
before the discussions with the pupils.) This was the third phase
of the project.

In Phase 4 of the study, the teachers switched rooms; T_1 (the
regular teacher) went to Room B from Room A and T_2 went to Room A.
This transfer was deemed desirable for two reasons. One, it
allowed T_1 to experience the token system of Room B such that at
the end of the study he would be able to extend his skills and
implement as many of the new procedures as he desired. Two, it
was important to determine if the effects of the program were a
result of the differing contingencies of the two rooms or an
effect of the personalities or past reinforcement histories with
the two teachers; the pupils' past history with T_1 had been of an
aversive nature since he was primarily a disciplinarian during the
pretreatment state of the classroom.

The analysis of changes over the course of the study was extensive in terms of the diversity of behaviors of both the pupils
and the teachers monitored and compared. The authors' summary
includes the important points:

> In general, the data support the hypothesis of the study:
> The systematic application of teaching techniques de-
> signed to elicit and reinforce specific forms of pupil
> behavior led to relatively stable and desirable modifi-

cations in that behavior. The desirable behavior produced by the teacher was successfully transferred from
one classroom to a second room and a different teacher.
It should be clearly understood that the transfer of
desirable pupil behavior from Room B to Room A cannot
be explained solely in terms of generalization effects.
Pupils were clearly given to understand that they could
only gain entrance to Room B by behaving in certain ways
in Room A. It should also be noted that this transfer
of control stratagem produced basic changes in the nature of reinforcers operating in each room. While point-
getting behavior was the same in both rooms, it led to
different consequences....In any event, points produced
substantial increases in desirable pupil behavior under
both conditions.

(Orme & Purnell, p, 137)

Hewett. Frank M. Hewett has developed a program for emotion-

ally disturbed youngsters that stresses the resocialization of

youngsters whose behaviors are maladaptive to learning. There is

no attempt to evaluate the appropriateness of the societal goals,

the aim is merely to allow these youngsters to continue to learn

that which is considered to be important in the context of an

"engineered classroom."

The engineered classroom approach utilizes behavior modifi-

cation technology in achieving the goals of psychodynamic-inter-

personal and sensory-neurological strategies within a wholly edu-

cational context. Hewett derived his developmental strategy from

the writings of Kephart, Doll, Havighurst, Piaget, Sigmund and

Anna Freud, Erikson, and Maslow, It is a practical, educational

sequence. That is, it is couched in terms teachers know and under-

stand, and can utilize in the classroom, Hewett had determined

that teachers often could not understand the child from the var-

192

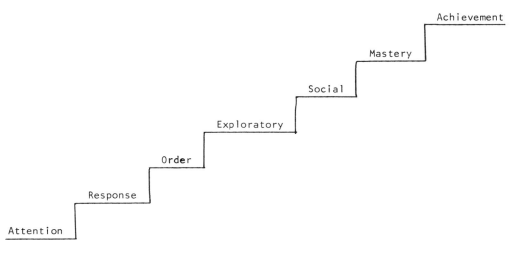

Figure 2. A developmental sequence of educational goals. (Hewett, 1968)

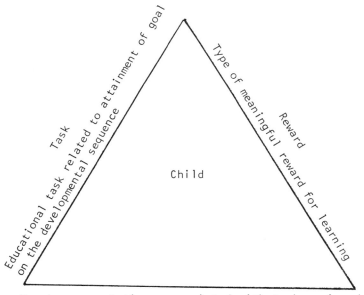

Teacher expectations associated with task assigned
child which determine conditions under which reward
will be provided.

Structure

Figure 3. The learning triangle (child). (Hewett, 1968)

ious view points espoused by psychiatrists and psychologists. Moreover, even when they were familiar with the terms and concepts. of the theorists, the teachers could not readily translate these into classroom goals or operationalize them into behaviors necessary for attainment of these goals. Hewett's schema includes behaviors he considers necessary for learning. His developmental sequence of educational goals stipulates that learning can occur if a child pays attention, makes a response, orders his behavior, engages in multisensory exploratory behavior, gains social approval, masters self care and cognitive skills and, finally, functions on a self-motivated basis with achievement providing intrinsic rewards.

A child can make progress in learning if a suitable education task provides meaningful, appropriate rewards in an environment which provides the structure necessary for efficient application of his resources and which defines the relevant task-reward contingencies. The task is defined by assessing the child's progress along the developmental sequence with instruments clearly outlined by Hewett (1968). Hewett and his collaborators have developed specific tasks for children at each of the developmental stages. They have also developed novel multi-level tasks for arithmetic and reading skills development. These provide necessary variation to otherwise traditional tasks (e.g., addition, anagrams), serve to maintain the interest of the child and simplify the teacher's preparation of individualized assignments (Hewett, 1968).

194

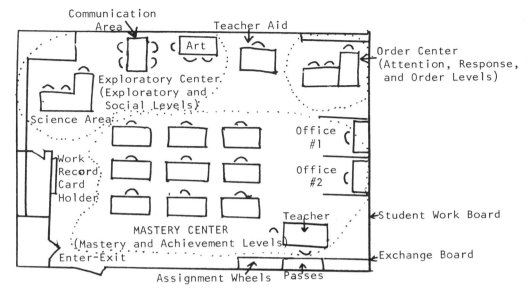

Figure 4. Floorplan of an engineered classroom. (Hewett, 1968)

The appropriate tasks, rewards and structure are incorporated into the "engineered classroom" design (Hewett, 1968 (a) (b) ; Hewett, Taylor, Artuso, 1969).

The room is divided into three areas: (a) the attention-response-order center which includes activities emphasizing participation, direction-following and task completion, (b) the exploratory-social center which includes science, art and communication tables, (c) the mastery and achievement center which includes the student's and teacher's desk and two study cubicles where assignments are given. The third area is similar to the traditional classroom. There are nine children per class and a teacher and an aide (who may be a community volunteer). The class day includes two hours for reading, writing and arithmetic, one hour for exploratory activities and one hour for recess and physical education. Each child picks up a Work Record card in the morning which he retains throughout the day; he earns a maximum of 10 check marks every fifteen minutes. These check marks are assigned for beginning and actively working on tasks and behaviors related to the developmental sequence levels appropriate for the child. These Work Record Cards may be exchanged initially for tangible rewards, eventually for self-selected activities and, finally, for graphing of total check marks earned.

The time span between exchange sessions is increased from daily to weekly within the first three weeks of the program.

196

Therefore, the child's performance is acknowledged systematically, and he learns that his behavior controls certain consequences. Children are assigned varying tasks through the day to insure that they are learning and earning marks. There is no penalty for assignment to a task of a lower level. No negative feedback is provided. If a child cannot function at an assigned task, expectations are reduced by sending him to a study booth, modifying the assignment, verbally restructuring the task, sending him to the exploratory center, sending him to the order center, taking him outside the class and agreeing on a task, tutoring individually, providing time out or exclusion. All of the interventions alter in some way one facet of the learning triangle, (or in the case of the last two, eliminate a facet).

Evaluation of the Santa Monica Project indicates that there were significant increases in task attention in the experimental group over the control group when the experimental condition followed placement in a regular (control) class. Reading achievement was not affected by the experimental condition but gains in arithmetic fundamentals were significantly correlated with the employment of the experimental condition. In two classes which had the control condition following the experimental condition, there were significant increases in level of task attention in the control condition (i,e,, after tokens withdrawn). This is in

197

contrast to most other studies that show that target behaviors decline with the withdrawal of a token reinforcement program.

Precision Teaching. Precision teaching is a system of monitoring behavioral improvement that has gained a small but ardent following among behavior modification adherents. The system grew out of the work of Lindsley (1964) with youngsters in special education classrooms. In essence, the system calls for the daily charting (on standard behavioral charts) of the frequency (number of occurrences per minute) of any specified behavior (Lindsley, 1971; Bradfield, 1970; Alper and White, 1971; Jordan and Robbins, 1972). The system also has a standardized terminology to expedite communications among project executors and to ensure that relevant variables are being isolated.

More specifically, the system uses a standard six-cycle logarithmic chart developed by Lindsley to plot the daily behavior rates. The abscissa of the chart represents the calendar days (up to 140) and the ordinate, the movements per minute (number of occurrences of a behavior divided by the number of minutes during which the count was taken). Since the numbers along the ordinate range from .001 to 1000, behavior rates ranging from one occurrence per 1000 minutes to 1000 behaviors per minute may be plotted on the same chart; this readily covers most of the behaviors amenable to modification.

In pinpointing the behavior under study, several criteria

198

must be met: the behavior must be directly observable, it must involve movement, and it must be cyclical (i,e., be repeatable); the last two specifications permit the use of the term Movement Cycle for the behavior under study. In order to determine which environmental events affect the occurrence of any movement cycle, Lindsley devised the IS-DOES formula. The IS part of the formula includes all the environmental variables which _might_ influence a movement cycle, and the DOES part of the formula includes those events which, after experimentation, have been identified as _having_ an effect upon the movement cycle (Alper & White, 1971; Bradfield, 1970). The IS part of the formula includes: the program, the antecedent event, the movement cycle, the arrangement, and the subsequent event. The _program_ is the overall environmental setting including time, location, subject taught, etc. The _antecedent events_ are those events which occur just prior to the emission of the movement and which might result in the movement cycle or affect the performance of the behavior; this includes curriculum materials, teasing from another child, etc. The _movement cycle_ is the behavior under study which meets the criteria set forth above. The _arrangement_ is the numerical ratio expressing the number of times the movement must be emitted and the number of times the subsequent event will occur. One positive comment for every 10 problems correct would be a ratio of 10:1. The _subsequent events_ are those which immediately follow the emission of the movement and which may be the result of the movement cycle and which may affect the future probability of occurrence of the cycle. The intervention phase may be an alteration in any one of the components of the IS formula (i.e., program, antecedent events, arrangement, or subsequent events). If the hypothesized relationship does exist, rate changes should occur and would be evident on the charting that is maintained from day to day. Each environmental event which when altered changed the rate of the movement cycle can be transferred to the DOES part of the formula which substitutes disposition, stimulus, response, contingency, and consequence for program, antecedent event, movement cycle, arrangement, and subsequent event, respectively. This helps to differentiate those alterations which have been attempted from those which have worked   (Bradfield, 1970 ; Alper & White, 1971).

Since a file with these DOES analyses could theoretically be of use to anyone attempting an intervention who would like access to a number of successful projects, a Behavior Bank has been set up into which one may deposit successful intervention projects for the return privilege of withdrawing others at a later date (Koenig, 1971; Bradfield, 1970).

While both behavior modification and precision teaching derive from the operant conditioning literature, some distinctions should be made. Behavior modification stresses change procedures

200

using reinforcements, while precision teaching uses measurement procedures and the more traditional change procedures such as curriculum changes which include; the child in the learning and change process. Both teachers and students can study the charts and project outcomes on the basis of a mutual sharing of data. The precision teaching process provides the teacher with a way of comparing and evaluating the daily effects of the teaching procedures they already have at their command (Lindsley, 1971). There is no requirement of adopting a behavior modification stance when using the precision teaching model; even the Behavior Bank has projects from a host of other theoretical positions, including psychotherapeutic interventions (Koenig, 1971). Because the use of a common language facilitates communication about particular projects, the precision teaching approach has proved to be readily adaptable for use with parent groups (Lindsley, 1966; Galloway and Kay, 1971) and with peer monitoring (Starlin, 1971).

Implications. These procedures and case studies are useful in calling attention to those classroom variables that operate on the behavior of both the adults and the children. This awareness should, at the lowest levels, result in more effective child management techniques. On the other hand, this knowledge could be synthesized and used as the core for different classroom programs, using reinforcers as motivators (points, praise, attention, etc.) rather than the elusive and often non-existent (within some schools) "intrinsic rewards" upon which so many first and second grade teachers depend. Indeed, in some cases, these "intrinsic rewards" may never develop.

Intrinsic rewards develop as external rewards and standards are internalized by the child. But unless appropriate feedback is provided for the child, the external standards and reward contingencies to be internalized are never clearly delineated. For example, the ability to delay gratification increases with age. We expect adults to delay gratification for at most a month (for paychecks) yet we expect six and seven year olds to work diligently for marks that are placed on their report cards four times a year. The reinforcements that are meaningful for the young child need not be the ubiquitous M & M's. They need not be tangible. They may differ from child to child, but the task of determining reinforcers is not an endless one (O'Leary & Drabman). A reinforcer could be the privilege of delivering a note for the teacher, the opportunity to go to the science center or read a treasured book, or it could be as simple as a smile or a glance from the teacher. This form of positive feedback can do much to create a healthy and stimulating and motivating learning environment. Many schools tend to concentrate on negative feed-back. A child gets attention only when he is "bad." Schools have a myriad of forms to fill out and send home when a child breaks a window, wets his pants, arrives at school ten minutes late, speaks

too loudly or too frequently, or trips a classmate on the playground. No forms exist which may be sent to the parents when
Johnny arrives in school on time for a week, or gets five more
arithmetic problems correct this week than last. Normative behavior cannot be defined by negation, especially to a child whose
behavioral repertoire is limited by experience or happenstance.

The adoption of behavior modification techniques need not
dictate a change in curriculum content. Rather, the emphasis is
on pin-pointing behavioral objectives that already exist. On the
other hand, the total environment (including the curriculum) must
be considered a legitimate object of study and evaluation. Some
experimenters choose to "create" an environment (e.g. Hewett,
Orme & Purnell) by altering aspects which they consider relevant.
Others (e.g., Tharp & Wetzel), work in the natural environment
and serve as information inputs to those who are the controllers
of the reinforcers; the information is aimed at creating an environment of systematic, contingent consequences for their target
population.

Except for work by Tharp and Wetzel and Martin (Martin,
et al, 1967) no systematic attempt has been made to integrate a
school program with home activities. This involves parental
cooperation and regular communication between home and school.
(Programs involving parents in connection with non-educational
settings will be discussed in a later section.) The task for a

teacher could become quite formidable, but it is suggested that the results would be promising.

C. Behavior Modification in the Natural Environment

Parental Involvement. Parents are "significant others" in the environment of children. Therefore, it is logical to assume that parents can mediate changes in behavior by dispensing reinforcers. Some relevant considerations are raised by Bijou and Baer (1967, p.184):

> ...to train parents...is itself an exercise in behavior modification. The fact that the parents have been living with the child whose behavior they have allowed to remain seriously deficient or deviant indicates that their everyday repertoires of behavior do not include effective instructional techniques; thus they too may well require training. The fact that they are adults and (presumably) normal does not guarantee that a simple description of new procedures will suffice to change them into successful shapers of their child's behavior. Indeed, it should be assumed that the parent's behavior, like the child's, will change only if it is connected with appropriate discriminitive stimuli (cues) and contingencies. Reliance merely on instructions will often prove ineffective. Thus attention to the reinforcers appropriate to the parent's behavior is also an essential part of the process of effective modification or development of the child's behavior. Fortunately, most parents will be reinforced by seeing their child improve as a consequence of their own efforts. However, this feedback comes about only after the program of child training has been successfully initiated. Prior reinforcement will have to be provided by the experimenter.

Since most of the child's day is spent within the home, parents are potent agents in the maintenance or modification of adaptive

204

and maladaptive behaviors. If treatment of a child is carried out within a laboratory or clinic, generalization to the home setting is not guaranteed, especially if parental behavior is not modified. It is important to involve both parents (and siblings, if any) in the treatment program.

Williams (1959) reported the earliest case in which parents were utilized to administer a behavior modification program. The child had been ill for 18 of 21 months, during which time his parents and aunt doted over him. Subsequent to the illness, tantrum behavior always occurred at bedtime unless one of the adults remained with him until he fell asleep (one-half to two hours). An extinction program was put into effect after determining that no physical problems existed. No one returned to the child's room once the door was closed at bedtime. The crying pattern was extinguished within ten days. The crying was reestablished by the aunt's returning to the room on one occasion; the second extinction period closely resembled the first. No recurrence of the behavior was evident over the next two years.

Another study by Wolf, Risley & Mees (1964) combined the application of behavior modification in an institutional setting and in the home by instructing the parents within the institution setting, allowing them to participate increasingly in ward routines, and gradually exposing the child to longer periods at home. The subject, Dicky, was a three and one-half year old male with behavioral problems which included temper tantrums, refusal to wear glasses (required due to removal of occluded eye lens), sleeping and eating difficulties. Hospital attendants and parents learned the operant conditioning procedures of shaping, extinction, time-out from positive reinforcement, and differential reinforcement; they were entirely responsible for dispensing reinforcers. By carefully specifying the environmental events and the behavioral criteria and their consequences, significant progress was made. The modification of a single behavior will be used to describe the methodology and the gradual increase in parental involvement.

Dicky, typically, would not sleep at night, requiring someone to remain with him. He was bathed at a regular hour each night, cuddled, and put to bed with the door left open. If he arose, he was told to return to bed or the door would be closed. If he did not return to bed, the door was closed and was not reopened until the ensuing tantrum had subsided. The door was left open if he stayed in bed. Bedtime was seldom a problem after the sixth night. The parents were brought in at bedtime to put him to bed and carry out the door-closing routine when necessary. Then Dicky began short home visits accompanied by the attendant. These visits were gradually lengthened. During one visit he experienced bedtime routine with his siblings, and then he was brought back to the ward for bed. The following night he spent at home. These nights at home were increased to three per week, and then five per week during the month preceeding his discharge. Other behavior modification procedures were used to eliminate food-stealing, food-throwing and glasses-throwing, and to establish proper use of eating utensils, glasses-wearing, and a wider verbal repertoire. Six months after Dicky's return home he continued to wear his glasses, sleep properly, and was becoming increasingly verbal.

Schell and Adams (1960) report on a behavior modification procedure carried out within the home by the parents. The boy Danny, had several maladaptive behavior patterns: he tugged at arms to get attention and make requests, he had frequent tantrums and engaged in repetitive behaviors. The parents were required to read several books on behavior modification and meet with the consultants regularly. A program of differential reinforcement was begun. Arm tugging was ignored, but more appropriate responses were quickly reinforced with adult attention. Tantrums were extinguished by placing Danny in an isolation room for a specified period of time. The parents made no comments before or after the periods of incarceration in the bare room. The repetitive behaviors were extinguished systematically; these tended to decrease as more appropriate behaviors were added to Danny's repertoire of responses. Secondary benefits from the program included improvement in speed, and improvement in self-care habits. Zeilberger, Sampen, & Sloan (1968) carried out hour-long training sessions five days a week with a mother and child. Problem behaviors included fighting, screaming, disobeying, and

207

bossing. A time-out from positive reinforcement procedure
(isolation following unacceptable behavior) was used to eliminate
aggressive behavior and disobedience. Differential reinforcement of acceptable behaviors, with both social and material reinforcement, was effective in increasing the percentage of instructions carried out.

Consultation with parents on a group basis is also possible,
as Lindsley (1966) has demonstrated. He met with fathers of retarded children and had discussions of accelerating and decelerating
procedures and measurement techniques. All of the nine fathers who
tried to modify behavior were successful, and three of them went
on to start their own groups the following year, hence pyramiding
the dissemination process. Some of the gimmicks or techniques that
his groups utilized are worthy of mention. One procedure is to
set up a "point store" within the home in a high traffic area. Items
or privileges are listed, as well as the number of points necessary for purchase. Points are awarded as a consequence of an increase in desirable behaviors. A "Sunday Box" can be set up to
deal with the common complaint of things being out of their place.
Anything found out of place is placed in the box and is not re-
trievable until Sunday, when all the sins of the week are pardoned.
Of course it is important for this to be a family contingency rather than one reserved for the children. Frequently, the mere act
of publicly counting the behavior to be decelerated is enough to
eliminate the behavior. Families can be shown that not all decel-

erating procedures need be painful.

Several programmed texts (Smith and Smith, 1965 ; Patterson and Guillon, 1968; Patterson, 1971) have been developed for use by anyone having regular contact with children. They clearly illustrate the influence of the environment, especially including the social environment, upon behavior. Besides explicating the parameters of behavior management, these texts provide many examples of management programs. There is an emphasis upon the management of problem behaviors (e.g., acting out behavior) but the procedures and techniques are obviously applicable with all children. The self-teaching nature of these programmed texts make them ideal for use with parent groups and many workers, including this writer, have used them in this context. Once the rudiments of the behavior technology have been learned, the parents can compare behavior change projects they have carried out, and in so doing, master the more advanced principles.

Consultant-Mediator Approach. One example of a research project which attempted to carry out behavior modification in the natural environment utilizing significant adults as mediators of reinforcement for children is The Behavior Research Project (BRP) (Tharp and Wetzel, 1970). Their procedure was to train behavior analysts (BA's) who met with those individuals (mediators) who were significant in the child's (i.e., the target's) environment. The BA's were trained by and met regularly with supervising psychologists.

209

The initial program was set up to deal with "behaviorally disordered, under-achieving, pre-drop-out, delinquent, and pre-delinquent youth." Children were referred to the BRP by principals, psychometricians, parents, social agencies, or juvenile courts. The referral criteria were: misbehavior at school or home, academic under-achievement, and evidence of an IQ of 90 or above. The children were from 6 to 16 years of age with a mean grade achievement of a D+.

A behavior analyst visited the home of the child and explained BRP's function to the family. If services were declined, no further contact was made; if services were approved, a complete assessment was made of the target's abilities and of the natural reinforcement contingencies existing in the environment. When completed, mediators were selected, criteria of appropriate behavior were selected, and roles were specified regarding the behavior of the mediator and the consultant.

Consultant	Mediator	Target
Anyone with knowledge	Anyone with reinforcers	Anyone with problems
Behavior Analyst	Person in touch with consultant for purposes of effecting changes in target. Must have reinforcers for target and must be able to place them as contingency.	Anyone whose behavior the consultant contracts to modify
Psychologist		
Social Worker		
Mother		Predelinquent
Teacher	Teacher	Patient
	Father	
	Mother	Employee
	Employer	
	Psychotherapist	Spouse

210

The training model emphasizes 'deprofessionalization.'
That is, the behavior analysts, all of whom had A.B. degrees,
were trained specifically for their role as consultants to the
mediators. They had no necessary prior experience, they did not
have to be professionals. Consequently, one professional person
could be in contact with several BA's, each of whom had a case
load. The BA's staff work was confined to contact with the mediators; they did not have direct contact with the targets, and
neither did the supervising psychologist.

The modification technique utilized contingency management.
Undesirable behaviors were weakened by non-reinforcement, and
desirable behaviors were strengthened by reinforcement. Homme
(1966) suggests that 'reinforcing event' be used as a label for
the total consequences of a behavior. A functional relationship
may exist between any act and any of the reinforcing events, each
of which may be assigned a positive or negative reinforcing value.
The combined value of these reinforcers is inferred from the succeeding behavior; if future incidence of occurrence increases, the
value is positive; if incidence decreases, the value is negative.
These patterns of reinforcement in the target's behavioral environment exercise systematic regulation of consequences. If proper
mediators are selected and if prepotent reinforcers are selected,
the probability of effecting the desired change is increased significantly.

Tharp and Wetzel report success with this model although the number of intervened cases (77 out of 227 referred) is rather small. This program has been implemented in other areas with comparable results.

This program is an example of the learning model approach to modifying variant behavior. It is different from the laboratory approach in that the significant dispensers of reinforcers are determined through assessment before implementation of the program; other programs have assumed a priori that significant others are parents and teachers without considering other role figures and have confined the intervention to predetermined locales.

III. CONTIGUITY THEORIES

A. History

The contiguity theories focus upon behaviors which are elicited by preceding stimuli, as opposed to reinforcement theories described earlier that focus on responses that are influenced by consequences. (For complete accounts see Russ, 1971; Hilgard & Marquis, 1961.) These behaviors are called reflexive, and include many emotional responses, as well as physiological responses such as salivation, perspiration, sneezing, etc. The classic picture of Pavlov's dog salivating to meat powder is, of course, the initial introduction to this form of conditioning. Watson (1920) paired the presentation of a rat, which previously elicited no fear response, with a loud noise (striking of an iron bar) behind Albert's head to produce a fear reaction. Seven such pairings were sufficient to produce the fear reaction with the presentation of the rat alone. This reaction was present after a month had passed and generalized to other animals. No therapeutic procedure was attempted with Albert, although Watson suggested possible methods.

Jones, working with seventy institutionalized children of average intelligence, was the first to systematically compare various procedures to eliminate children's fears. Several methods had no effect or limited effect. Included in this study were the methods of "elimination through disuse" (fear will disappear if

213

not aroused), "verbal appeal" (talking about the fear will break down the fear response), "negative adaptation" (repeated pre-sentation of the feared object), and "distraction" (a substitute activity). Only two methods were successful in eliminating child-ren's fears. In one method, social imitation, the child was ex-posed to the feared object in the presence of peers who were not afraid of it. (Such modeling procedures will be discussed in a later section.) The other successful method was "direct con-ditioning." In this procedure, the children were exposed to the feared object while engaged in an activity which elicited pleasant responses, such as eating. The feared object was grad-ually brought closer to the child until he could tolerate touch-ing it. This same procedure was used with a child, Peter, in another classic study by Jones (1924a). In spite of the ap-parent success of this method, not much was published in suc-ceeding years until Wolpe's book was released in 1958. The inter-vening years were largely confined to efforts to understand phenomena by producing abnormal conditions through conditioning methods rather than by reducing the severity of the condition (Pavlov, 1927; Liddell, 1944). These studies of induced neuro-sis in animals did not include attempts to restore normal be-havior until Masserman (1943) used petting, stroking and hand-feeding to re-institute normal eating in cats previously made "neurotic" by sharp blasts of air during feeding behavior.

214

The interventions based on contiguity theories have followed three major lines of development: aversion therapy, reciprocal inhibition and negative practice (Beech, 1969).

B. Negative Practice

The theory behind negative practice was first suggested by Pavlov (1927), who stated that a behavior will be weakened if made to occur many times in rapid succession (even if reinforced each time). Dunlap (1928, 1932) is usually credited with making systematic use of the method. Beech (1969) cites Wakeham (1928) as the first to use this method to eliminate an unwanted behavior. Wakeham consistently made mistakes on a certain passage of a Bach piano piece. After a fortnight of deliberately and consciously practicing the mistakes, he could give a perfect rendition of the piece. Few have adopted the procedure for neurotic complaints, since it is more suited for correcting motor errors such as typing and piano playing. The method of negative practive is distinct from experimental extinction, in that the former stipulates that a reduction in a behavior will occur even with reinforcement if the behavior is performed rapidly and at length. Extinction, on the other hand, occurs when a behavior is no longer paired with reinforcement.

C. Reciprocal Inhibition

Reciprocal inhibition is one type of counterconditioning procedure. The basic assumptions are that neurotic habits are learned, and that learning principles can be applied to effect the removal of these neurotic habits. Anxiety is the common constituent of all neurotic habits. Conditioned autonomic responses (anxiety) may be aroused in situations which pose no objective threat (e.g., standing inside an elevator). The inhibition of anxiety can be achieved by establishing a competing response. The reciprocal inhibition principle outlines the establishment of conditioned inhibition: If a response inhibitory of anxiety can be made to occur in the presence of anxiety-evoking stimuli, it will weaken the bond between these stimuli and the anxiety (Wolpe, 1958; Wolpe & Lazarus, 1966). Anxiety-inhibiting responses include a wide range of empirically successful procedures, including assertive responses and relaxation responses (systematic desensitization). Other treatments include the use of drugs, carbon dioxide, role training, "thought-stopping" and "anxiety-relief conditioning" (Wolpe, 1958; Wolpe & Lazarus, 1966). Only the first two procedures will be covered here.

Assertion training is recommended in cases of overriding anxieties in interpersonal situations. The therapist encourages and trains outward expressions of emotions on the part of the client, in situations where such actions have been previously inhibited by anxiety. Basic feelings and emotions are considered legitimate for expression. The expression itself is a counter-anxiety response and reciprocally inhibits the anxiety. This is combined

216

with operant reinforcement of the assertive response to increase its frequency and build motivation.

Systematic desensitization consists of three phases: deep muscle relaxation training, construction of anxiety hierarchies, and the contraposition of relaxation and the anxiety-evoking stimuli from the hierarchies.

To illustrate the method, an outline of the procedures used by Wolpe and Lazarus (1965) will be presented. The subject is interviewed by the therapist and presented with orienting information regarding the role of anxiety in neurosis and the process of behavior therapy. Attempts are made to minimize self-blame by the subject and to dispel any misconceptions.

In order to understand the presenting problem or problems, the antecedents of all the reactions must be known, including factors that intensify and alleviate the anxiety. The subject's past is explored in terms of the family background and attitudes, educational history, and neighborhood   occupational and sexual history and attitudes. The Willoughby Neuroticism Schedule which is composed of 25 items from the Clark-Thurstone Inventory is administered to identify situations which elicit anxiety. This is a self-rating scale in which the subject rates himself from 0 to 4 on such items as "Do you get stage fright," "Are you often lonely," and "Does criticism hurt you badly?" Eighty per cent of neurotic patients score above 30 on this schedule, although neuroticism is not contra-indicated by a lower score. Another self-rating scale, A Fear Inventory, is designed to assess the subject's reactions to various stimuli. The subject is asked to indicate the degree of disturbance to 76 items, such as noise of vacuum cleaners, open wounds, falling, worms, flying insects, crowds, journeys by car and darkness.

Following the compilation of the above data, the therapist and subject discuss their expectations regarding treatment. The delineation of benefits may include specification of positive side effects that may result from the therapy. The therapist indicates the treatment that he has deemed appropriate for the particular constellation of presenting symptoms, and the treatment program is undertaken. Although several methods may be employed, let us assume that systematic desensitization is indicated.

The deep muscle relaxation method is that of Jacobson (1938) carried out in six sessions. The ordering of muscle groups trained to relax is unimportant but the chosen sequence should be invariant. Wolpe suggest working on the arms, then the facial area including the shoulders, neck and upper back, followed by the chest, stomach and lower back and finally the hips, thighs, calves and complete body relaxation. Wolpe and Lazarus (1966) give complete details of the instruction in relaxation treatment. The process is one of alternately tensing and relaxing various muscle groups in order that discriminations be made between the contrastive sensations.

The anxiety hierarchy is a graded list of stimuli of a defined theme that elicit anxiety. The theme may be as obvious as
fear of heights, or as subtle as rejection, guilt, criticism or
disapproval. Establishing and constructing the anxiety hierarchies appropriate for a patient is a time-consuming process.
The data for the hierarchies are obtained from the subject's history, the Willoughby Questionnaire response, the Fear Inventory
response, and extensive questioning into all areas in which the
subject feels some anxiety without any objective threat. The
data are grouped into themes (such as fear of dogs, being watched),
and a progression of stimuli are constructed for each theme. The
stimuli include both endogenous as well as exogenous ones ("faint-
ing" versus "seeing someone faint").

The subject is then ready for systematic desensitization. If
relaxation is incomplete even after training, drugs (meprobamate,
chlorpromazine), carbon dioxide-oxygen mixture inhalation, or hyp-
nosis is used to induce further relaxation. Once complete relaxation is obtained, the subject is asked to imagine a neutral scene
(e.g., a street scene) to test his ability to visualize and to
determine if anxiety is aroused by features other than those contained in the scene. He is asked to raise an index finger if un-
duly disturbed.

The least anxiety-eliciting scene from the hierarchy is then
presented to the subject. Scenes are presented for about five seconds and a usual session lasts fifteen to thirty minutes. The time

between sessions does not appear to be critical; success has been reported with monthly sessions and with four sessions daily. At each session, imagined scenes are presented and represented until no anxiety is elicited. Increasingly anxiety-eliciting scenes are then introduced until relaxation is complete during presentation. The number of sessions required and the number of scene presentations necessary before therapy is complete varies with the number of hierarchies, their intensity, and the degree of generalization within each of the hierarchies. Wolpe reports a close correlation between the amount of desensitization to imagined stimuli and the degree of anxiety decrement upon exposure to real stimuli in the hierarchies.

Moreover, case records indicate no change in the patients' problematic responses between sessions although inter-session intervals were as long as five weeks and, in one case, three and one-half years. Wolpes' conclusion is that the improvement noted in all cases is due to the desensitization treatment and not processes or factors extraneous to the treatment session.

Evidence to support the potency of the desensitization treatment is not conclusive because of selection factors and high drop-out rates. Wolpe himself makes clear (1966) that the desensitization session makes up only part of the interview session and that other treatment methods were employed, but never clarifies these statements.

The procedure devised by Wolpe has been primarily applied to neurotic conditions, especially phobias. But the principle of setting up new associations to stimuli that have, over time, become associated with negative affect can be applied to other areas. For example, if patients on a ward avoid a particular attendant or nurse because he has been associated with punishment and this avoidance is interfering with ward routine; the avoided person could be assigned to the dining room during particular hours until the avoidance responses were terminated. Similarly, if low achievement children avoid school books because of a past history of failure in the school setting, the books could be temporarily removed from the room and the room could be made less school-like and more pleasurable by changing desk configurations using easy chairs in selected corners, brightening up displays and windows, and by using less traditional learning methods, such as role-playing. Once new responses in the classroom are established, more traditional learning methods and materials, including books, could be gradually re-introduced in non-threatening ways. The range of possible applications is large, but the realm of the attempted is small. More effort to explore further applications in a variety of settings should be expended.

D. Aversion Therapy

Early Attempts. The first reference to a conditioned response to an aversive stimulus was made by Pavlov (1927) regarding a study utilizing apormorphine injections into dogs. A tone paired with the onset of symptoms of nausea brought about by the apormorphine eventually was sufficient to elicit these same symptoms. Others noted that the activities of the experimenter prepatory to an apormorphine injection were also conditioned and elicited the symptoms of nausea.

Kantorovich (1935) is generally cited as the first to use aversion therapy with human subjects. In 1930 he used electric shock to treat alcoholics. The alcohol was paired with electrical shock; most of the twenty patients treated did not return to alcohol for several months. The abstracted report provided few other details.

In a convention report, Max (1935) detailed a treatment of a homosexual fixation by electric shock. Shock level was varied and differential effects noted. No follow-up work was forthcoming, however, and Max's work was largely ignored until the sixties when interest in faradic techniques applied to humans was renewed.

Interest in the use of aversive stimuli for therapy waxed and waned during the thirties, forties and fifties. The method of choice during this period was chemically-induced nausea; alcoholics were the favored treatment population.

Lemere and Voegtlin (1950), working at Shadell Sanitarium, Seattle, treated alcoholics by administering emetine to induce

nausea and vomiting at the sight, taste and smell of alcohol.
Patients poured drinks for themselves and sniffed them and looked
at them; they were allowed to taste them only at the onset of
nausea. An average of six sessions were administered to each
patient with booster sessions at six and twelve months. Follow-
up data over a period of more than ten years was obtained on over
91% of the 4468 patients treated. Fifty-one per cent were absti-
nent with one or two treatments over the thirteen year period
between 1935 and 1948. Other studies utilizing Lemere and Voegtlin's
procedures with modifications have been reviewed by Franks (1958).
Work with chemically-induced nausea in treating a variety of syndromes continued in the fifties and sixties, but never on as massive a scale as that undertaken in Seattle.

Punishment. Azrin and Holz (1966, p.381) define punishment as:

> a consequence of behavior that reduces the future
> probability of that behavior. Stated more fully,
> punishment is the reduction of the future probability
> of a specific response as a result of the immediate
> delivery of a stimulus for that response. The stimulus
> is designated as a punishing stimulus; the entire pro-
> cess is designated as punishment.

Punishment is not equivalent to a simple response decrement, since
this may be caused by extinction, satiation or drugs. The definition of punishment above is parallel to the definition of a reinforcing stimulus, since it is a response-produced stimulus consequence. It requires a change in the future probability of occurrence of the response.

223

The ideal punishing stimulus, according to Azrin and Holz, should have the following characteristics: (1) It should be capable of being specified precisely (e.g., electric shock may be specified in terms of amperes and volts). (2) The stimulus should be constant in terms of the contact it makes with the subject. (3) The subject should not be able to control the stimulus (i.e., decrease the intensity) through any unauthorized activity. (4) The stimulus should produce few skeletal reactions since these would interfere with measurement of the response to be suppressed. (5) The stimulus should be capable of being varied over a wide range. For punishment, the aversive stimulus is presented in conjunction with or as a consequence of an undesirable behavior. Hence, punishment can be utilized in a respondent or operant learning paradigm. In the former case, the aversive stimulus is used to create conditioned aversive stimuli (as with alcohol). In the latter, the punishment serves to suppress the behavior it follows.

The aversive stimulus may also be utilized within an escape or avoidance situation. That is, the stimulus could be withdrawn (escape) or withheld (avoidance) as a consequence of certain behaviors. This serves to accelerate certain behaviors. The escape situation is equivalent to a negative reinforcement sequence.

Punishment does not always utilize aversive stimuli; all aversive stimuli need not be punishing (as in negative reinforcement procedures, for example, when aversive stimuli increase a response).

The aversive stimulus of choice for most present practitioners is electric shock (faradic techniques). It meets the criteria set by Azrin and Holz for an ideal punishing stimulus and it is convenient and inexpensive to apply. Most of the contemporary punishment literature utilizes this stimulus.

Chemical aversive stimuli have been much used in the last four decades, especially in the treatment of alcoholics. Typically, the chemicals used (e.g., apormorphine, emetine) produce nausea. Unfortunately, the latency, intensity and the duration of the symptoms cannot be controlled precisely even in the same individual over repeated administrations. For some individuals, a placebo may be used on the second trial and produce the nausea; in others, ten or more trials are required before the placebo may be substituted. Moreover, the delay between the drug administration and the onset of symptoms limits the application of this method, since the target must be called to mind or presented immediately prior to or during the symptoms. Temporal contiguity is an important factor in controlling the strength of the association. Also, in order to ensure a proper association between the aversive reaction and the target thought or object, the conditions of the laboratory must be carefully controlled; however, this in turn limits the generalizability of the conditioned response to situations outside of the laboratory. Frequently, generalization to natural settings is determined by patient reports, without confirmation. It is quite possible that only verbal conditioning is occurring.

Corporal punishment is another type of aversive stimuli. Although frequent in many homes, schools and institutions, corporal punishment is rarely acknowledged publicly and hence never evaluated systematically. It has been suggested, however, that the recipients of physical punishment aggress more frequently than those who have not experienced physical punishment (Sears, Maccoby and Levin, 1957 Bandura & Walters, 1963). This argument could be levelled against the use of most forms of aversive stimulation, but the frequency of operant aggression (aggression directed at the experimenter or at the equipment applying the stimulus) and elicited (aggression directed at those unassociated with the aversive stimulus or displaced aggression) have not been carefully monitored in most studies employing any form of aversive stimuli for therapeutic purposes.

Seclusion or time-out from positive reinforcement is a form of punishment which does not utilize an aversive stimulus. The duration of the placement in the seclusion area (which should be less reinforcing than the area from which the subject was removed) should be specified in advance. Otherwise, the implementation would be subject to the whims of the administrator. The

226

actual placement in and removal from the seclusion area should be handled without fanfare, lest the attention itself provide reinforcement for the target behavior and negate the effects of the seclusion. A typical procedure would be to place a child in a bare room for two minutes each time he hits another child or has a temper tantrum (or a similar target behavior).

A response cost procedure is the removal or reinforcements earned (tokens, points, etc.) as a consequence of an undesired behavior. This procedure, as well as the time out from positive reinforcement, should be coupled with a positive reinforcement program to achieve maximum progress.

A less commonly used aversive stimulus is high intensity noise. However, the range of effective intensities is limited (Azrin, 1958) and subjects adapt to auditory stimulation. One hundred and twenty decibels is the pain threshold. Signals up to 135 decibels do not consistently produce suppression of behavior; intensities exceeding that level cannot be conveniently produced in the laboratory. Moreoever, there is a high risk of permanent damage to ear tissues subjected to such high signal intensities. Prolonged exposure to intensities above 85 decibels will result in permanent damage.

A traumatic respiratory paralysis has been produced by the injection of scoline. The drug produces temporary motor paralysis lasting up to 90 seconds or more, depending on the dosage.

Sanderson (1963) and Holzinger et al (1967), among others, have utilized this drug to treat alcoholics, but the results have been unimpressive. There is a high drop-out rate of subjects in experiments utilizing this procedure. In addition, there exists a possibility of permanent tissue damage due to a long paralysis.

Combining aversive stimuli with other modes of therapy (e.g., apormorphine used in conjunction with desensitization) has been tried, but optimum combinations cannot be determined until better evaluation techniques are employed.

Method. A few case histories from Bucher and Lovaas (1968) should suffice in demonstrating the method and a behavioral syndrome that is successfully treated with aversive stimulation. John was a seven year old boy with psychotic-like behaviors. He was diagnosed as retarded (IQ=25). Since the age of two, he had been self-destructive and, in the year of hospitalization prior to treatment by Lovaas, he was kept in complete restraints (legs, waist and arms) 24 hours each day. Without restraints he would scream, hit his head against the crib and strike his head with his fists. Scar tissue covered his head; his ears were swollen and bleeding. Two procedures were followed to extinguish the self-destructive response, an extinction procedure and a punishment procedure (although no indication is given whether the procedures were run concurrently or successively). To extinguish the behavior,

John was left alone in his crib for one and one-half hours per day for eight days without his restraints. No attention was paid to his self-destructive behavior. The rate of self-injurious actions fell from 3000 in Day 1 in one and one-half hours to 15 in Day 8. Although self-destructive behavior was nearly extinguished, over 10,000 self-injurious acts were recorded in the eight days; the reduction in self-destructive behavior did not generalize to other situations. There was damage caused by edema of his ears, although John was a relatively "careful" hitter.

The punishment procedure was carried out in a living room with one of four experimenters present. The length of these sessions was not specified. Baseline data was obtained during the first fifteen sessions; self-destructive behavior continued at a high rate during this baseline period. Twelve one-second electric shocks, contingent upon self-destructive responses, were administered over sessions 16, 19, 24, and 30. Shock was delivered with a cattle prod. Self-destructive behavior dropped immediately and was maintained at essentially zero from the 16th session to the 38th and last session. Only two of four experimenters administered the shock but the suppression effect generalized to the other experimenters. As the self-destructive behavior decreased, responses of avoiding adults and crying (which were also measured during the sessions) also decreased. Other positive behavioral side effects were noted as John was able to function without restraints. He ran, played in the tub, scratched himself and made other reinforcing discoveries as he joined in a normal ward routine.

Marilyn was a more severe case handled by Bucher and Lovaas She was a 16 year old girl who had been self-injurious since her second birthday. During the two years prior to being seen for treatment with aversive stimulation, she had been hospitalized and confined with a camisole. When without a camisole (which she sometimes removed with her teeth), Marilyn would remove her finger-nails by their roots with her teeth and bite her hands; one of her fingers had to be amputated due to the severity of her self-inflicted wounds. Marilyn's head was covered wtih scar tissue as she was also a head-banger. It was impossible to place Marilyn on an extinction schedule because she could have inflicted severe damage or even have killed herself.

The suppression data with shock administration are similar to that of John. Although there was an immediate favorable be-havior change in other respects, Marilyn's aggression towards other children on the ward increased at a later time. The experimenters concluded that she returned to a form of behavior that previously provided reinforcement (namely, attention) for her because she was not trained in acceptable behaviors. The post-treatment environment is important to the maintenance of the treatment effects. It is obviously important to include programs to build new, ap-propriate behaviors in treated individuals, along with a punishment regimen, which is effective for behavior suppression.

Evaluation. Most of the experiments or case studies reported in the literature do not employ satisfactory control groups to assess the effects of the procedure under study. Many studies do not stipulate procedures employed in detail, and important sequences and decision criteria are omitted. Temporal factors are important because they affect the strength of conditioning, and because improper delivery of the aversive stimulus could possibly decelerate desirable behaviors rather than the target behavior.

Punishment has been generally employed when the behavior is dangerous to the patient (as in self-destructive behavior), is undesirable but self-reinforcing (e.g. sexual fetishes), or is untreatable by other methods. The attempt is generally to suppress inappropriate behaviors and develop appropriate ones, although frequently the latter, and more important, concern is overlooked by experimenters in their quest to eliminate target behaviors. Without building appropriate behaviors that are subject to reinforcement in the natural environment (especially those that are incompatible with the target behavior) the probability of long-term success is diminished considerably. Other behaviors that have been demonstrated to be amenable to modification through punishment include motoric, ideational, and obsessional behavior such as conversion reactions, smoking, alcoholism, sexual perversions, tics, thumbsucking, nail-biting, and intractable sneezing.

Bijou (1971), and others have applied aversive stimuli suc-

231

cessfully and have argued persuasively that with proper controls, the use of electric shock is justified by the results, especially with otherwise intractable cases of self-destruction.

Baer (1970) also argues for carefully controlled and ethical investigations on the use of shock punishment to amass more information about the procedure. Not to do this would be "saying that we would not find out how to make therapy less socially punishing than it often is, because we object to research on shock punishment (Baer, 1970, p. 247)." "Not to rescue a person from an unhappy organization of his behavior is to punish him, in that it leaves him in a state of recurrent punishment   (Baer, p.246)." On the other hand, caution must be exercised in using punishment since experimenters are themselves subject to selective reinforcement through success. According to Baer,

> Punishment works, I submit. There is too much affirmative, careful demonstration to resist that conclusion. Consequently, punishers should succeed often in eliminating the behavior they mean to eliminate. That they reinforce them, which is to say, their rate of using punishment in the future, and in more diverse situations, will rise. Contributing to that tendency is the extreme simplicity of punishment technique and technology. Anyone with a hand to swing is equipped with a punishing device. The Sears-Roebuck farm catalog lists a number of inexpensive and reliable cattle prods. Furthermore, the punishment contingency is the essence of simplicity, compared to which positive reinforcement and its allied art of shaping looms as a formidable mystery indeed. Thus, it is possible that punishment could become the first and, woefully, the exclusive behavioral technique some carelessly trained persons might use. That would indeed be a tragic outcome.

For one thing, punishment is painful, and the essence
of my argument (and of everyone else's) is that we
should have as little pain as we can. Thus, we want to
use as little punishment as we can, not as much. To
find out how to use one form of punishment so as to
minimize other forms of punishment, and what the
exchange relationships can be, we will have to study
punishment; to study, we will have to use it. But
to use punishment successfully is to subject oneself to
an environmental event which may press one to use it
again, and more than necessary. That, we shall have
to watch with great care (Baer, 1970, p.247).

E. Modeling

Early conceptualizations of modeling processes utilized in-

stinctual interpretations. Because of scientists' reactions to the

notion of instinct, modeling, as a theoretical basis for learning,

was largely ignored. However, Bandura (1969) argues strongly that

observational learning processes must be considered to account

for many no-trial learning situations of novel responses that can-

not be accounted for by theories relying upon response-contingent

reinforcement. For instance, the learning of complex response rou-

tines (such as training a mynah to whistle a new song, driving a

car) cannot be accounted for through shaping processes alone.

For our purposes, it is also important to distinguish between

the acquisition of learning of a response through modeling, and the

performance of that response. Bandura (1965) demonstrated that

acquisition of a response was primarily due to stimulus contiguity

Performance, on the other hand, was a function of the reinforcing

consequences to the model or to the observer. In considering inter-

ventions utilizing modeling routines, we shall be most concerned with

233

variables that bear upon performance of modeled behaviors.

Exposure to modeling influences has three effects (Bandura, 1969). First the observer may acquire responses not previously in his repertoire (observational learning). Second, modeling procedures may strengthen or weaken inhibitory responses of the observer (inhibition of disinhibitory effect). This effect varies as a function of the rewarding or punishing consequences of the model. And third, the observation of a model may increase the occurrence of a previously learned response (response facilitation effect). This effect differs from the second point above in that the facilitated response is not likely to have incurred punishment and therefore the response increase is not due to a disinhibition.

Modeling is especially efficient where a desired behavior occurs rarely because of the dominance of other behaviors. In such a case, there are few opportunities to reinforce the new behavior. The frequency of the modeled behavior is likely to increase in the observer as long as the model is reinforced, irrespective of whether the observer is reinforced (Bandura, 1965). Models are more effective if they are similar to the observer, or if they are high in status. Orme & Purnell (1970) for instance, use this principle by reinforcing appropriate behavior of a student adjacent to a disruptive student.

Lovaas has incorporated modeling procedures into a program to eliminate some behavioral deficits of schizophrenic children.

234

Linguistic skills, play patterns, self-care skills, interpersonal behavior and intellectual skills are established by:

> the establishment of stimulus functions which make one amenable to social influence. This process primarily involves developing children's responsiveness to modeling cues, increasing the discriminative value of stimulus events so that children attend and respond appropriately to aspects of their environment that they have previously ignored, and endowing social approval and other symbolic stimuli with reinforcing properties (Bandura, 1969, p.152).

> The therapist first establishes control over children's attending behavior; complex response patterns are gradually elaborated by modeling activities in small steps of increasing difficulty; manual prompts are utilized if children fail to respond. The prompts are gradually withdrawn and reinforcement for prompted behavior is later withheld to counteract passive responsiveness. After imitative behavior is strongly developed, stimulus control of children's behavior is shifted from modeling cues to verbal prompts and appropriate environmental stimuli (Bandura, 1969, p.157).

The results of the modeling reinforcement method have been encouraging, especially since various lay groups have served as therapists.

Although Jones (1924) and others, utilized modeling procedures to overcome fear responses in young children, nothing systematic had been attempted until Bandura and his colleagues (Bandura & Menlove; Bandura, Grusec & Menlove, 1967b, 1968) became concerned with the factors affecting vicarious extinction of avoidance behavior. Subjects who had repeated brief exposures to a live peer model engaged in increasingly fear-provoking interactions with the feared object (dogs) in a party context or in a neutral context exhibited greater extinction of avoidance behavior than did two control groups (one viewed the dog in a positive context with no model and the other group participated in positive activities but was never exposed to either dog or model). The tests for dog avoidance were administered again, a month after the experiment, and indicated that the extinction of avoidance behavior was highly stable over that time period. Bandura, Grusec & Menlove (1968), employing single and multiple symbolic (i.e., filmed) models, also produced extinction of avoidance behavior, although symbolic modeling appeared to be less potent than live modeling in producing the desired changes. "However, the diminished efficacy of symbolic modeling can be offset by a broader sampling of models and aversive stimlus objects (Bandura, 1969)."

Bandura, Blanchard & Ritter (1968) assessed the effectiveness of modeling and desensitization procedures in producing behavioral, affective and attitudinal changes. The subjects were adolescents and adults with severe snake phobias.

The initial assessment devices included a behavioral test of strength of snake avoidance, a fear inventory (to determine if a decrement in fear of snakes is associated with changes in other areas of anxiety), and attitudinal ratings on encounters with snakes (to assess attitudinal effects of behavioral changes achieved through social learning procedures). Four conditions were incorporated into the experimental design. Subjects in the first group observed a film depicting children, adolescents and adults and a

236

large king snake in progressively threatening interactions. They were also taught relaxation procedures and asked to maintain a relaxed state throughout exposure. Furthermore, they could regulate the presentation of the film through remote control devices. When a sequence induced anxiety, they were told to reverse the film, relax, and review the film until no anxiety was evident. Subjects conducted their own treatment with no experimenter present.

The second condition combined graduated modeling and guided participation. The model would demonstrate behavior, then perform the behavior with the subject and finally allow the subject to execute the behavior alone. The sequence was graduated into small steps and rate of progression was dependent upon the degree of anxiety of the subject.

The third group received the desensitization treatment of Wolpe (1958), in which deep muscle relaxation is paired with imagined representations of snakes in a pre-established hierarchy of anxiety-provoking situations.

The control group was assessed in the initial phase with no intervention following.

Following treatment, which was carried out until all anxiety reactions had been extinguished or until the maximum time (unspecified) had elapsed, all subjects were reassessed with the instruments used initially.

The behavioral test called for approaching, looking, touching,

holding a snake with gloved and bare hands, removing it from its
cage, letting it free in a room, replacing it in the cage, holding it five inches from their faces and leaving the snake in their
laps while holding their hands at their sides. Before and after
each of the above behaviors, subjects rated their fear arousal
on a ten point scale. Live modeling with guided participation
eliminated snake phobias in ninety-two per cent of all subjects;
symbolic modeling and desensitization procedures substantially reduced avoidance behavior. The control subjects were unchanged.
Attitudes toward snakes were favorably changed as a result of the
experiences; as expected the model with guided participation produced the greatest change in attitudes. The fear inventory scores
also reflected some fear reduction of items beyond the treated
phobia. The degree of reduction was proportional to the effect of
the treatments in eliminating the phobia. Desensitization reduced
the degree of fear toward other animals only; modeling plus guided
participation produced widespread fear reductions in a variety of
threatening situations of both an interpersonal and non-social nature.

The effect of observational learning in inhibiting or disin-
hibiting responses has been studied with respect to aggressive behaviors, self reinforcement, and transgression. The degree of
influence of the model is a function of the positive or negative
consequences of the modeled behavior. Model characteristics, such
as age, sex, and social status also influence the degree to which
the modeled behaviors will be imitated.

Modeling influences in facilitating responses have been observed in volunteering one's services, performing altruistic acts,
assisting people in distress, and seeking information (Bandura, 1969).
Social phenomena are especially amenable to alteration through modeling   influences. Possessors of high status or high social power
are probably most effective as models for other group members. This
mode of influence would be much more efficient than attempting to
alter the behavior of each group member in turn.

Modeling procedures and operant conditioning procedures should
be considered as complementary methods of shaping and maintaining
response patterns rather than as mutually exclusive methods. Modeling is an effective and efficient method of instating new behaviors
into the behavioral repertoire of an individual. The maintenance
of these behaviors over time is a function of the reinforcement
consequences. Many of the token economy programs (e.g. Ayllon &
Azrin) utilize modeling procedures to shape new behaviors and to
increase the effectiveness of new reinforcers.

In any event, every intervention that requires an interaction
between the person treated and any other individual contains a
potential learning situation that could be amplified in importance
through the use of modeling procedures.

> Most conceptualizations of psychotherapy as a learning
> process depict the therapist as a source of reinforcements
> that can be manipulated in a contingent manner so as to
> develop and to maintain the client's behavioral reper-
> toires. However, little attention has been paid to the

239

importance of therapeutic agents as a <u>source of</u>
<u>behavioral repertoires</u>. (Bandura, 1965, p. 339)

The systematic use of modeling techniques, whether
singly or in conjunction with other treatment methods
is likely to accelerate substantially the successful
achievement of therapeutic outcomes.
(Bandura, 1965, p.340)

IV.   ETHICAL AND THEORETICAL ISSUES IN BEHAVIOR THERAPY

This section on the theoretical and ethical issues involved
in behavior therapy is not designed to be exhaustive; it attempts
merely to review some of the salient issues raised by advocates and
detractors of the behavioral stance. Many of these points have
been raised by consideration of Skinner's (1971) advocacy of greater
cultural control over individuals to ensure cultural survival. The
issues, however, are relevant for anyone interested in a behavior
modification program for the clinic, classroom, kitchen or crib.

Most of the theoretical issues revolve around the assumptions
that behaviorists make. One assumption, for instance, is that observable behaviors provide the only valid data. Neither the substrates of behavior (e.g., neural transmission) nor the larger
cosmos within which the behavior occurs may be considered. This
leads to disagreement with other theoretical positions regarding the
specification of the locus of the problem source and the target
of an intervention method. Subscribers to the medical model (and
the analytic model) consider the primary cause of the problem to be
distinct from the symptoms (i.e., behaviors) treated by behavior
modification programs. They contend that treatment of the symptoms,
without dealing with primary causes, results in the appearance of
new symptoms (symptom substitution). Behaviorists maintain that any
subsequent manifestation of pathological or maladaptive behaviors
can be treated in turn. However, outside of the psychodynamically-

241

oriented clinical literature, almost no cases of symptom substitution have been reported (Ullmann and Krasner, 1965). Lindsley reports one case out of three hundred treated that could possibly deserve the label of symptom substitution (Lindsley, 1966).

Theoretical and ethical considerations are involved in debates over other issues. Nonbehaviorists object to the behaviorist contention that environmental variables are the only relevant parameters of behavior. While some behaviorists have taken that stance, Skinner, in Beyond Freedom and Dignity and earlier works, acknowledges the contribution of genetic factors in delimiting behavior and in determining critical periods for conditioning (Jensen, 1972; Schwab, 1972). But these two factors, social setting and genetic endowment, detractors continue, cannot account for all of human behavior. The dismissal of concepts such as "free will" and the sense of "identity" (the experience of "me") results in a simplistic view of man. Moreover , there is the possibility that the behavior of groups of individuals is more than the summation of the individuals' behaviors. If this is so, consideration of units larger than the single organism is necessary (Schwab, 1972).

Toynbee argues that Skinner fails to demonstrate that the totality of human behavior can be accounted for by the social setting and genetic endowment.

> No one would disagree with Skinner if he had limited his counter-thesis to asserting that a human being is only partially free. We might perhaps all go so far as to agree that a major part of a human being's conduct is not self-determined. The disputable point of Skinner's

> thesis is his denial that the human being himself
> may be even a partial, if only a minor, determinant
> of his own behavior (Toynbee, 1972, p. 59).

The type of manipulation that Skinner supports is possible _if_ all

behavior could be accounted for by genetic endowment and social set-

ting and _if_ the manipulation of both of these were possible. Never-

theless, Toynbee argues, if, as Skinner posits, human freedom is

truly an illusion,

> no human being would be free to plan and carry out the
> requisite biological and social 'engineering.' The
> blind cannot lead the blind, and a camel cannot lead
> a string of camels. Experience has proved that it
> needs a donkey to do that (Toynbee, 1972, p.62).

The primary ethical problems revolve around the concept of con-

trol. In _Beyond Freedom and Dignity_, Skinner argues that the de-

gree of control to be legitimized should be increased rather than

decreased; we need more control and more precise use of this control.

Without increased control, man will not survive, unlimited access

to reinforcements have led to a population explosion and to an ex-

ponential increase in the consumption of natural resources. The

question of whether or not controls should be applied is moot, since

controls _are_ applied during the entire lifetime of the organism.

The real concerns should be the _degree_ of control to be legitimized,

condoned, sanctioned or accepted, the specification of the _controllers_,

and the intent and _goals_ of the controls that they implement: who is to

control whom and to what end? Skinner maintains that the system

designs countercontrols by controlling the consequences of the be-

haviors of the controllers (Skinner, 1971; Platt, 1972; Schwab, 1972).

243

Responsive feedback systems make these checks and balances possible. Control breeds countercontrol breeds control in a behavioral dialectic moving towards cultural survival. Others do not share
this rather sanguine view; they fear the inevitable birth of the
power-hungry individuals who remain external to the normal constraints on power acquisition, and who have historically appeared
with regularity. Empirical answers are not available for any
of these questions, but the rate of development and application
of behavioral technology makes urgent the consideration of these
issues.

If the appropriateness of controls is accepted, there still
remains the question of goals. Many present behavior modification
programs in schools instill values, such as conformity and docility.
Most clinical applications of behavior modification programs could
be criticized along similar lines; the emphasis is in adapting the
individual to the existing societal norms, rather than changing those
norms to tolerate a wider range of behavior. Moreover, given the
behaviorists' assumptions that preclude the existence of the self-
directing self-controlling individual, it is not clear exactly what
the behaviorists' ideal man is like.

It is ironic that those who are most vociferous in their ob-
jections to behavioral manipulations are also those who support and
even encourage manipulations within settings such as therapeutic sessions, educational institutions, governmental domains, and personal-
social situations. Within the psychoanalytic therapy session, for

244

example, the therapists' values enter significantly into the therapeutic goals that are espoused, and the interaction can be parsimoniously placed in a learning theory framework (Bandura, 1961). Although some therapists would argue that the eventual goal is self-directed decision-making and internalized goal-setting, that internalization is itself subject to all of the shaping forces impinging upon the person (Rogers & Skinner, 1956). It is also possible that manipulation within the traditional psychoanalytic therapy model is more palatable because the goals and procedures are nebulous and ill-defined, and hence less threatening (initially) to individual values. Moreover, the long latency from initiation of treatment to verifiable change also tends to dull any reaction on an ethical basis. On the other hand, the clearly specified goals and the relatively short time period before these goals are achieved in behavior therapy seems to pose a great threat to the idealized Free Man.

The learning theory approach provides a potent mechanism for change. The direction and the content of this change is a function of one's philosophical bent--be one a hedonist, counter-theorist, pantheist, atheist, fascist or humanist. It is to increase the knowledge of learning theories and their applications, and to foster a consideration of the important ethical issues involved, that papers such as this are directed.

Addison, R. M., & Homme, L. E. The reinforcing event (RE) menu. National Society for Programmed Instruction Journal, 1966, 5, 8-9.

Alper, T. G., & White, O. R. Precision teaching: A tool for the school psychologist and teacher. Journal of School Psychology, 1971, 9, 445-454.

Ayllon, T., & Azrin, N. H. The measurement and reinforcement of behavior of psychotics. Journal of Experimental Analysis of Behavior, 1965, 8, 359-383.

Ayllon, T., & Azrin, N. H. The token economy: A motivational system for therapy and rehabilitation. New York: Appleton, 1968.

Ayllon, T., & Haughton, E. Control of the behavior of schizophrenic patients by food. Journal of the Experimental Analysis of Behavior, 1962, 5, 343-354.

Ayllon, T., & Michael, J. Psychiatric nurse as behavioral engineer. Journal of the Experimental Analysis of Behavior, 1959, 2, 323-334.

Azrin, N. H., & Holz, W. C. Punishment. In W. K. Honig (Ed.), Operant behavior, New York: Appleton, 1966, pp.380-447.

Baer, D. M. A case for the selective reinforcement of punishment. In C. Neuringer & J. L. Michael (Eds.), Behavior modification in clinical psychology. New York: Appleton, 1970, pp.243-249.

Bandura, A. Principles of behavior modification. New York: Holt, 1969.

Bandura, A. Psychotherapy as a learning process. Psychological Bulletin, 1961, 58, 143-159.

Bandura, A. Vicarious processes: A case of no-trial learning. In L. Berkowitz (Ed.), Advances in experimental social psychology. Vol. II. New York: Academic Press, 1965.

Bandura, A., Blanchard, E. B., & Ritter, B. Relative efficacy of desensitization and modeling approaches for inducing behavioral, affective, and attitudinal changes. Journal of Personality and Social Psychology, 1969, 13, 173-199.

Bandura, A., Grusec, J. E., & Menlove, F. L. Some social determinants of self-monitoring reinforcement systems. Journal of Personality and Social Psychology, 1967, 5, 449-455. (a)

Bandura, A., Grusec, J. E., & Menlove, F. S. Vicarious extinction of avoidance behavior, Journal of Personality and Social Psychology, 1967, 5, 16-23. (b).

Bandura, A., & Menlove, F. L. Factors determining vicarious extinction of avoidance behavior through symbolic modeling. Journal of Personality and Social Psychology, 1968, 8, 99-108.

Beech, H. R. Changing man's behavior. Baltimore: Penguin Books, 1969.

Bellman, R. Pigeons on the grass, alas! Comments on "Beyond freedom and dignity" by B. F. Skinner. Paper presented at the Conference on The Social and Philosophical Implications of Behavior Modifications held at the Center for the Study of Democratic Institutions, Santa Barbara, California, January, 1972.

Bijou, S. W., & Baer, D. M. (Eds.). Child development: readings in experimental analysis. New York: Appleton, 1967.

Bradfield, R. N. Precision teaching: A useful technology for special education teachers. Education Technology, 1970, 10(8), 22-26.

Bronfenbrenner, U. Some methods of character education: Some implications for research. American Psychologist, 1962, 17, 550-564.

Bucher, B., & Lovaas, O. I. Use of aversive stimulation in behavior modification. In M. R. Jones (Ed.) Miami Symposium on the Prediction of Behavior, 1967, Coral Gables, Florida: University of Miami Press, 1968, pp.77-145.

Cowles, J. T. Food tokens as incentives for learning by chimpanzees. Comparative Psychological Monographs, 1937, 35, 267-268.

Dunlap, K. Habits: Their making and unmaking. New York: Liveright, 1932.

Dunlap, K. A revision of the fundamental law of habit formation. Science, 1928, 67, 360-362.

247

Franks, C. M. Alcohol, alcoholism and conditioning: a review of the literature and some theoretical considerations. Journal of Medical Science, 1958, 104, 14-33.

Franks, C. M. (Ed.), Behavior therapy: Appraisal and status. New York: McGraw-Hill, 1969.

Galloway, C., and Kay, C. Parent classes in precise behavior management. Teaching Exceptional Children, 1971, 3(3), 120-128.

Gardner, W. I. Behavior modification in mental retardation: The education and rehabilitation of the mentally retarded adolescent and adult. Chicago: Aldine/Atherton, 1971.

Harris, F. R., Wolf, M. M., & Baer, D. M. Effects of adult social reinforcement on child behavior. In S. W. Bijou & D. M. Baer (Eds.), Child development: Readings in experimental analysis. New York: Appleton-Century-Crofts, 1967, pp. 146-158.

Haughton, E. Great gains from small starts. Teaching Exceptional Children, 1971, 3(3), 141-146.

Hewett, F. M. Educational engineering with emotionally disturbed children. Exceptional Children, 1967, 33(7), 459-567.

Hewett, F. M. The emotionally disturbed child in the classroom. Boston: Allyn and Bacon, 1968.

Hewett, F. The Santa Monica Project: Demonstration and evaluation of an engineered classroom designed for emotionally disturbed children in the public schools. Phase 2: Primary and secondary level. U. S. Dept. of Health, Education and Welfare, Office of Education, Bureau of Research.

Hewett, F. M., Taylor, F. D., & Artuso, A. A. The Santa Monica Project. Evaluation of an engineered classroom design with emotionally disturbed children. Exceptional Children, 1969, 35, 523-529.

Hilgard, E. R., & Marquis, D. G. Conditioning and learning. 2nd edition. Revised by G. A. Kimble. New York: Appleton-Century-Drofts, 1961.

Holzinger, R., Mortimer, P., & Van Dusen, W. Aversion conditioning treatment of alcoholism. American Journal of Psychiatry, 1967, 124, 150-151.

Homme, E. Contingency management. Clinical Child Psychology Newsletter, 1966, 4.

Jensen, A. R. Skinner and human differences. Paper presented at the Conference on the Social and Philosophical Implications of Behavior Modification held at the Center for the Study of Democratic Institutions, Santa Barbara, California, January, 1972.

Johnson, E. C. Precision teaching helps children learn. Teaching Exceptional Children, 1971, 3(3), 106-110.

Jones, M. C. A laboratory study of fear: The case of Peter. Pedagogical Seminary, 1924, 31, 308-315 (a).

Jones, M. C. The elimination of children's fears. Journal of Experimental Psychology, 1924, 7, 383-390(b).

Jordan, J., & Robbins, L. S. Let's try doing something else kind of thing: Behavioral principles and the exceptional child. Arlington, Virginia: Council for Exceptional Children, 1972.

Kantovovich, N. An attempt at association reflex therapy in alcholism. Psychological Abstracts, 1935, 4, 493.

Koenig, C. Behavior bank: A system for sharing precise information. Teaching Exceptional Children, 1971, 3 (3), 157.

Krasner, L. Behavior modification, token economies, and training in clinical psychology. In C. Neuringer and J. Michael (Eds.), Behavior modification in clinical psychology. New York: Appleton-Century-Crofts, 1970, pp. 86-104.

Krasner, L., & Ullman, L. (Eds.) Research in behavior modification: New developments and implications. New York: Holt, 1965.

Lemere, F., & Voeghtlin, W. An evaluation of the aversion treatment of alcoholism. Quarterly Journal of Studies on Alcohol, 1950, 11, 199-204.

Liddell, H. Conditioned reflex method and experimental neurosis. In J. M. V. Hunt (Ed.), Personality and the behavior disorders. New York: Ronald Press, 1944.

Lindsley, O. R. Direct measurement and prosthesis of retarded behavior. Journal of Education, 1964, 147, 62-81.

Lindsley, O. R. An experiment with parents handling behavior at home. Johnstone Bulletin, 1966, 9, 27-36.

Lindsley, O. R. Precision teaching in perspective: An interview with Ogden R. Lindsley. Teaching Exceptional Children, 1971 3(3), 111-119.

Masserman, J. H. Behavior and neurosis. Chicago: University of Chicago Press, 1943.

Max, L. W. Breaking a homosexual fixation by the conditioned reflex technique. Psychological Bulletin, 1935, 32, 734.

Neal, F. W. Some questions about Professor Skinner's ideas. Dialogue discussion paper presented at the Conference on the Social and Philosophical Implications of Behavior Modification held at the Center for the Study of Democratic Institutions, Santa Barbara, California, January, 1972.

O'Leary, K. D., & Drabman, R. Token reinforcement programs in the classroom: A review. Psychological Bulletin, 1971, 75(6), 374-398.

Orme, M. E. J., & Purnell, R. F. Behavior modification and transfer in an out-of-control classroom. In G. Fargo, C. Behrns, & P. Nolen, Behavior modification in the classroom, Belmont: Wadsworth Publishing Co., 1970, pp.116-138.

Patterson, G. R. Families: Applications of social learning to family life. Champaign, Illinois: Research Press, 1971.

Patterson, G. R., & Guillion, M. E. Living with children: New methods for parents and teachers. Champaign, Illinois: Research Press, 1968.

Pavlov, I. P. Conditioned reflexes, New York: Dover, 1927.

Premack, D. Toward empirical behavior laws: I. Positive reinforcement. Psychological Review, 1959, 66(4), 219-233.

Rogers, C., & Skinner, B. F. The control of human behavior. From some issues concerning the control of human behavior: A symposium. Science, 124, 1057-1066.

Rozynko, V., Swift, J., & Boggs, L. Controlled environments for social change. Paper presented at the Conference on the Social and Philosophical Implications of Behavior Modification held at the Center for the Study of Democratic Institutions, Santa Barbara, California, January, 1972.

Sanderson, R. E., Campbell, D., & Laverty, S. G. An investigation of a new aversive conditioning treatment for alcoholism. Quarterly Journal of Studies on Alcohol, 1963, 24, 261-275.

Schaeffer, H. H., & Martin, P. L. Behavioral therapy. New York: McGraw-Hill, 1969.

Schell, R. E., & Adams, W. P. Training parents of a young girl with profound behavior deficits to be teacher therapists. Journal of Special Education, 1968, 2, 439-454.

Schwab, J. Mr. Skinner's critics and their criticisms. A paper presented at the Conference on the Social and Philosophical Implications of Behavior Modification held at the Center for the Study of Democratic Institutions, Santa Barbara, California, January, 1972.

Skinner, B. F. The behavior of organisms: An experimental analysis. New York: Appleton, 1938.

Skinner, B. F. Beyond freedom and dignity. New York: Knopf, 1971.

Skinner, B. F. Contingencies of reinforcement: A theoretical analysis. New York: Appleton, 1969.

Smith, J. M., & Smith, D. E. Child management. Ann Arbor: Ann Arbor Publishers, 1965.

Staats, A. W. Reinforcer systems in the solution of human problems. In G. A. Fargo, C. Behrns, & P. Nolen, Behavior modification in the classroom. Belmont, New York: Wadsworth, 1970, pp. 6-31.

Starlin, C. Peers and precision. Teaching Exceptional Children, 1971, 3(3), 129-132.

Tharp, R. G., & Wetzel, R. J. Behavior modification in the natural environment. New York: Academic Press, 1969.

Ullmann, L. P., & Krasner, L. (Eds.) Case studies in behavior modification. New York: Holt, 1965.

Ullmann, L. P., & Krasner, L. A psychological approach to abnormal behavior. Englewood Cliffs, New Jersey: Prentice-Hall, 1969.

Ulrich, R., Stachnik, T., & Mabry, J. (Eds.). Control of human behavior. Glenview, Illinois: Scott Foresman, 1966.

Wakeham, G. Query on a revision of the fundamental law of habit formation. Science, 1928, 68, 135-136.

Watson, J. B., & Rayner, R. Conditioned emotional reactions. Journal of Experimental Psychology, 1920, 3, 1-14.

Williams, C. D. The elimination of tantrum behavior by extinction procedures. Journal of Abnormal and Social Psychology, 1959, 59, 269.

Wolf, M. Risley, T., & Mees, H. Application of operant conditioning procedures to the behavior problems of an autistic child. Behavior Research and Therapy, 1964, 1, 305-312.

Wolfe, J. G. Effectiveness of token rewards for chimpanzees. Comparative Psychological Monographs, 1936, 12(60).

Wolpe, J. Psychotherapy by reciprocal inhibition. Stanford, California: Stanford University Press, 1958.

Wolpe, J., & Lazarus, A. A. Behavior therapy techniques: A guide to the treatment of neurosis. New York: Pergamon Press, 1966.

Zeilberger, J., Sampen, S. E., & Sloane, H. N. Modification of a child's problem behaviors with the mother as therapist. Journal of Applied Behavior Analysis, 1968, 1, 47-53.

Zimmerman, E. H., & Zimmerman, J. The alteration of behavior in a special classroom situation. Journal of the Experimental Analysis of Behavior, 1962, 5, 59-60.

PSYCHODYNAMIC INTERVENTIONS

IN EMOTIONAL DISTURBANCE

Carol Cheney

William C. Morse

253

TABLE OF CONTENTS

I. INTRODUCTION

It is popular to equate the psychodynamic approach with Freud, which would be similar to presenting Watson as the sine qua non of behaviorism. An even more restricted approach is to dwell on the nuances of difference between various theorists in the long development of the Freudian school (Fine, 1973; Ruitenbeek, 1973). Such enterprises are challenging for theoreticians. Without disparaging the significance or the stature of the leadership individuals, past or present, another approach is taken here.

The purpose of this paper is twofold. The first is to develop a synthesis of the core propositions found in the literature, which together represent a viable and challenging dynamic position related to current understanding.[1] It may be useful at this point to make note of those who have been the most important contributors to the viewpoint we will be presenting. These include both theoreticians and clinicians: Freud, Jung, Adler, Sullivan, Horney, Fromm, Anna Freud, Murray, Erikson, Maslow, Rogers, Kessler, and Redl--to name but a very few of the many.[2] The second purpose

---

1. A discussion of the historical development and diversity of the psychodynamic view is contained in Rezmierski, G., & Kotre, J. A limited literature review of the theory of the psychodynamic model. In W. Rhodes & M. Tracy, A Study of Child Variance. Univ. of Michigan Press: Ann Arbor, 1972, pp. 181-259.

2. Some basic views of certain major theoreticians are summarized in the appendix.

of this paper is to derive from these propositions a relatively
coherent set of interventions and tactics. Attention will be
focussed on work applicable to the lives of children and youth.
In this connection, while the ultimate focus is on deviant children,
deviance cannot be considered apart from the developmental process
in normal children.

It is recognized that such a truly monumental expectation
is beyond the resources of this Project. Since the dynamic position
is itself amorphous and compounded, there is always the matter of
selective judgement, synthesis and emphasis. In fantasy there is
the dream of programming every detail of every concept on a massive
deck to be stored on endless tapes. One might then command it to
the computer to create a vast unimpeachable array of the factors of
dynamic theory. But perhaps we would feel as uneasy with such precise results as we may with what follows.

While the parameters of psychodynamic theory and interventions have changed shape, amoeba-like, and defy easy codification and
neat cohesion, there are certain elements which characterize the
position as a whole. At the foundation of any comprehensive theoretical stance are both implicit and explicit assumptions about the
nature of man and the impact of experience. What are the givens
about humanness at origin and as it unfolds? How are the "givens"
altered by learning? While some theories virtually ignore one or
the other of these factors, the psychodynamic position grapples with

the substance and processes of both, albeit not always in terms which are easily comprehended.

One issue which comes up is the overlap with other positions. Since all theories attempt to explain human nature and learning, this is to be expected. It follows that observations and insights of any theory must appear, in some form, in other explanations, unless the authors choose to neglect or ignore aspects. For example, psychodynamic theory talks about the intensity of impact of traumatic events, while Guthrie (1938) describes the circumstances of one trial learning from a behavioristic view. What is really true about children is true regardless of semantics.

Further, any theory which attends to how children grow must also attend to how they should grow. This admixture of psychology and values crops up in the least expected places, hidden or overt, in all theories. Maslow (1962) is almost alone in making a bold synthesis of value and biological need, finding from what we are, a universal direction for determining where we should be going.

Since all theories must somehow accommodate both nature and learning, it becomes a matter of relative emphasis. A behavior modifier, if not utilizing tissue needs such as food, sex, and movement, has to study the pattern of contingencies which work for individuals, even if the term "motivations" is rejected as meaningless. The psychodynamicist for a long time was so preoccupied with the nuances of the internal states, that he appeared to regard the child as living in a social vacuum. The psychodynamic position

259

owes much to Freud and the analytic school, but this psychological approach is not owned or circumscribed by them; many other psychologists have been concerned with the inner life.

Thus, it is that the encyclopedic psychodynamic theory may be articulated with other positions. The level of generalization at which such articulation is made may be uncomfortable. Certain kinships often appear to be even identical until further examination shows the essential differences which underlie the issues. For example, those "perceptual" psychologists who emphasize the existential self deal extensively with how the person imposes form on his outer world. Humanistic psychologists deal with inner motivational conditions, creativity and expressiveness. In the literature, several major tenets of the psychodynamic position expand these concerns. The orienting core of the position describes the organism as a biological being. His drives and motives are discussed, as are individual differences and developmental phenomena. The diagnostic-historical interpretation of behavior stands in contrast to the existential-circumstantial approach. Recently, the power of "past determinism" has been vastly moderated by the incorporation of sociological findings and by the projection of "determinism" to the future, through examination of the individual's hopes and expectations. Thus the central theme has become the course-of-life concept. Much (perhaps overmuch) attention has been given to atypical development in the course of life. The recognition of the importance of the learning process is apparent; often the learning process is described in terms such as "identification" or "relationship." A psychodynamic position puts emphasis on the unconscious or unaware conditions which are seen in fantasy and projection. There is extensive attention to this inner life of primary emotions and feelings. The ego-come-lately aspects, expanded from defense mechanisms, now include cognitive learning and skills, products of the thinking being. But above all is the dynamic concern; the inter-relationships within and without are seldom in a homeostatic state. There is ebb and flow, tension and resolution. Thus the inter- and intra-personal conditions are seen in a dynamic state.

This brief compendium of concepts is admittedly at an abstract level and does not make a neat, coherent theory. How can we explicate such a rich, but sometimes disparate set of concerns which constitute the psychodynamic position? Since the focus is on normal and deviant children and youth, the material will be organized following this outline: biological predispositions and growth factors; the path of the child's interaction with his environment (normal and deviant): all of which lead to the interventions which follow from this theoretical position. The interventions obviously imply goals for the youngster and depend upon assessment of his status. Intervention procedures are classified as: those utilizing biological manipulations, those which rely mainly on the potential of normal growth for recovery, and those which emobdy special designs to prevent self-defeating reactions.

II. BASIC THEORETICAL CONSTRUCTS OF THE PSYCHODYNAMIC APPROACH

Two major constructs are critical to a psychodynamic explanation of the nature of the child and his development. Each construct
represents a complex network of theoretical underpinnings.

A.   The Individual Self Pattern Evolves Around
     Significant Biological Predispositions

Each individual embraces a complex set of biological predispositions, in addition to the "tissue needs" such as hunger,
thirst, and sex which themselves are found in individual degrees
of intensity. There are also individual differences in such sub-
strata as temperament, energy output, exploratory curiosity,
talents, cognitive style, and the like. The reflections of such
"biological predispositions," some of which are apparent even in
infancy, are seen in the motivational patterns which characterize
the growing child. There is little agreement concerning the degree
to which individual variation of specific attributes is genetic.
Each child has idiosyncratic givens, but it is not possible to chart
these with any precision. In some instances biological factors are
considered highly potent and determinant, as in the case of severe
organic atypicality (infantile autism, brain injury, etc.).

From the point of view of a given societal value system,
the metamorphosis of these predispositions, which one then sees in
the individual's display of creative, aggressive, affectional,
achievement-oriented, curious, etc. behavior, may be positive or
negative. Man's biological nature is not seen as comprised of

only anti-social tendencies, though those capacities are only too obvious. Just as the child can hate, so can he love, for the tendency toward altruistic and constructive behavior is also within the human potential. Man's social nature and the way in which he has learned to live with others form the substance out of which altruistic behavior grows (Campbell, 1972; Cohen, 1972). Both cognitive (such as the logic of sharing) and affective (empathy, sympathy) considerations influence the development of altruistic behavior (Berkowitz, 1970; Cohen, 1972). Its acquisition is also closely tied to the patterns of moral growth which have been observed in children and extensively described (Berkowitz, 1964; Piaget, 1932; Kay, 1968). Basic to psychodynamic theory is the power of internal motivation, that motivation recognized by the individual, and that not at an awareness level.

Three significant propositions about the nature of the child may be stated.

1. The Child is a Feeling Being

The child is a feeling being. His personal emotional world is filled with many strong feelings: anger, hurt, joy, fear, excitement, love, and so on. This world of feelings is intricately bound into the child's motivational systems. There is interaction and interdigitation on both conscious and unconscious levels. How the child feels has much to do with what he needs and wants, and his needs and desire significantly affect his feeling.

263

2. The Child Is a Thinking Being

The child is characterized not only by the irrational world of his feelings, but also by the rational world of his cognitive processes. That the child possesses cognitive functions and the ability to think has three significant implications. First, human beings make constant use, both consciously and unconsciously, of symbols and labels for the things they experience and see around them. The child is able, for example, to label things he sees or feels ("tree," "house," "soft," "hurt," etc.), to develop symbolic concepts such as number and size, and to group things into meaning-ful classes (all safe things, all dangerous things, etc.). Secondly, his ability to manipulate the symbolic world which he develops allows the child to communicate with other people. The acquisition of language, whereby the child can use word-symbols to talk (and later write) about the world within and around him, represents an important process in his development.

Finally, the child's development of cognitive skills is the basis for his gradual organization of the world within and around him and his mediation of his relationship with that world. He learns to classify things, to order them and talk about them, just as he also learns to label and communicate about his feelings and wants. His world thus takes on a structure determined by the labels and classifications he uses to organize it. Many of the most important concepts are references to himself.

The psychodynamic concept of the ego is closely related to these functions. The ego is seen as the mediator between the internal and external worlds of the child. It modulates both input and output, and thus is responsible for the development of such capacities as perception, muscle coordination and language. It is also the ego which is responsible for mediating and responding to the demands and stresses which accompany the developmental process. Among its important functions are modelling, comparison, abstraction, projection, and prediction of the future. The course of the child's growth is closely tied to the quality of ego skills and strengths which he develops.

3. The Child Experiences on Many Levels, on Some of Which He Is Not Aware

The concept of the unconscious is an important aspect of psychodynamic theory, which encompasses both the child's affective and cognitive functions. According to this view, behavior may be governed by motivations which the child does not consciously recognize, and experience--both past and present--may have impacts of which he is not aware. For the child, especially, the world of fantasy is a significant interface between the complex processes of his unconscious inner world and the concrete world of external realities (Singer, 1973).

Fantasy functions in two ways in the child's life. First, dreams and daytime fantasy provide a framework within which the child realizes some of the goals and motives which he is prevented from reaching in the real world. When the child finds himself limited by physical size or immaturity, social or economic situation, etc., he or she can envision him/herself as a famous and skillful pilot, a life-saving physician, a loving mother, a powerful athlete, etc. Or, on the other hand, the child can play out some of his more frightening motives in fantasy--he can burn down his family's house, beat up his little brother, kill his father, all in the protected (and frequently symbolic) world of fantasy.

The child also uses fantasy as a symbolic projection of processes and conflicts which are going on within him. Selma Fraiberg reports the story of "Gerald," an imaginary creation of a two-year-old boy named Stevie:

> When Daddy's pipes are broken, no one is more
> indignant than the two-year-old son who is under
> suspicion. "Gerald, did you break my daddy's
> pipes?" he demands to know. Gerald can offer
> nothing in his defense, and it's plain as the
> nose on Gerald's face that only he could have
> committed this crime. When Gerald is not the
> perpetrator of a dozen crimes a day, he is the
> sly fellow who gets other people to carry out
> his evil plans. When circumstantial evidence
> points to Stevie as the person who tossed his
> sister's dolly into the toilet, he cries out
> despairingly, "Gerald made me do it" (Fraiberg,
> 1959, p.141).

Just as the devils of some primitive men, the child's "Gerald" serves as an externalization of the forces within himself which he finds frightening or unacceptable.

These three capacities--affect, cognition, and the unconscious processes--represent the basic pool of resources for mental life, upon which the child draws as he grows and develops, and as he meets the stresses inherent in the growth process. It is important to recognize that for each child that pool of resources has some real limits. An important determinant of such limitations is physiological, but even here there is no absolute immutability. For example, grave distortions may be introduced into the growth process by inadequate diet in the prenatal period and/or the early years (Winick, 1969; Simonson & Chow, 1969), by organic brain damage, and other phenomena which directly affect cortical functions. Less directly, the child's reactions, and those of people around him, to his being sick, disabled, or deformed, may also be significant in producing limitation or distortion of the developmental process.

A limitation which is common to the experience of all children is their helplessness to deal with so many of the situations which shape their experience. For the infant this powerlessness is clear and physical; the adults around him are much bigger than he and can do many things which he cannot do, because his physical and cognitive skills are still immature. As he grows and expands his sphere of experience, important forces enter his life which the child remains powerless to influence in any significant way. The structure of the school system, the poverty of the family, prejudicial attitudes toward his color, etc., are all important influences, in the face of which the child is relatively helpless.

B. The Growing Child is Actively Involved in Interactions
with His Environment

The changes, learning and development which are the product
of the growth process do not emerge predetermined from the inner
workings of the child's psyche. A child's interactions with other
people and with his "life milieu" are very important in determining
the style and direction of his growth. The child's involvement in
the process of his own development is _active_. He is far more than
a passive responder to external stimuli, for his own strong motivational systems cause him to initiate interactions with the world
around him--to ask for things, to go out exploring his surroundings.

The complex matrix of interactions with the environment involves characteristic processes, the quality of which is important
in determining the overall outcome of the child's growth. One
such process is _identification_, whereby the child incorporates the
characteristic coping styles of the significant people around him.
A most obvious example of this process has been in sex role acquisition; girls have traditionally come to see themselves, like their
mothers, as "domestic," weak, not mechanically minded, etc., while
boys have seen themselves as more aggressive, more athletic, etc.
One identifies with age groups, race, political entities, economic
class and thereby accumulates self-referrant points.

Secondly, the child is involved in an ongoing process of
socialization, in which he gradually defines his relationship to
the social and physical world and becomes integrated as a function-

268

ing member of that larger world. As he is articulating himself with the social world defined largely by others, the child is at the same time building a growing concept of _self_. He comes to see himself as an independent entity, more than a mere extension of the adults around him.

Characteristics of Healthy Development

Although the interactional process of growth is different for each child, we can define some goals for that process by describing the psychodynamic view of mental health. An emphasis on the individual results in a certain "self"-centeredness in the psychodynamic description of mental health. The ideal situation is always seen in terms of the complete and healthy development of the individual, rather than in communal or social terms. Beyond this, the specific form of goals reflects time and culture specific values and norms. The anthropological literature is replete with examples of behaviors which are normal in one culture but considered highly pathological in another. The description of healthy development which is found in the psychodynamic literature has six basic characteristics:[3]

Attitude toward self. The healthy individual is aware of himself in a realistic way, able to recognize and deal with his thoughts, feelings, and behaviors. The development of self-esteem is important in bringing the child to a point where he both recognizes himself as an individual, and feels comfortable with what he

---

3. The substance of this section is drawn in large part from the work of Jahoda (1958) and Biber (1961).

sees and feels in himself.

Resistance to stress. Because an inability to cope successfully with the situations and crises which develop can be very destructive, the cultivation of what Bower and Kliman (Bower, 1964;
Kliman, 1968, pp.2-12) call "stress immunity" is an important goal.
The child must develop reasonable and acceptable crisis-coping mechanisms, since inadequate or inappropriate responses to stress are
characteristic of a broad range of disturbance.

Autonomy/Independence. It is important that the child develop a degree of autonomy and independence, so that he has a sense
of actively determining and regulating his own behavior. An important aspect of this goal is that the child be aware that he is
influenced by the environment and that he make "conscious discriminations...of environmental factors he wishes to accept or reject
(Jahoda, 1958, p.45)." The aim is thus to engender in the child
a strong sense of independence, tempered by a realistic recognition
of the factors which provide significant input and influence on
the behavioral decisions which are ultimately his own.

Interpersonal relations. The healthy person is able to
form meaningful relationships with other people, to share himself
with those around him. This aspect of health implies an understanding of the needs and feelings of other people, and an open-
ness to accepting people whom one sees as different from oneself.
On a broader level, the recognition and respect for the needs of
others is reflected in the process of socialization, of accepting
the behavioral patterns of the community.

270

Curiosity, creativity, expressiveness. The emphasis here is on cultivation of the individual's resources and potentials, and on the opening of channels for their expression. Although optimal situations of growth allow these to freely unfold, the experiences of many children lead them to cut off or bury these potentialities because they have been so often frustrated or rejected.

Cognitive and language skills. Finally, the heavy demands made upon the child's cognitive abilities, especially after he enters the educational system, make the support and development of these skills a significant and independent developmental goal. The child needs to understand the nature of the world about him.

This broad overview of the basic processes and implicit goals of child development will serve as a foundation for a more detailed examination of specific characteristics of the growth process, the significant variables which determine the direction and quality of growth, and the range of outcomes of the growth process.

Concepts Related to Growth

The psychodynamic view sees the growth of the child as a sequential process, which is unique for each individual. This understanding of development embodies four basic concepts:

Each individual is a unique entity. Each child is a unique individual with a unique genetic makeup and a unique history. He is endowed with and continues to develop a different constellation of capacities and interests from that of any other child. In

271

attempting to describe a child or his behavior, it is important to keep his unique nature in mind and to avoid blanket categorizations, which overlook his individuality.

Growth reflects a "continuity of experience." Dr. Jane Kessler (1971) stresses the view that the individual's experience represents a continuum, along which each experience is linked to every other. This sort of "psychological determinism" involves a constant interaction of one's history with his present experience, feelings, and motivations. Out of this interaction emerges present behavior. Wordsworth's maxim, "the Child is father of the Man," reflects the emphasis which the psychodynamic view puts on the early childhood years of this continuum. This period is seen as particularly important in the formation of the basic personality structures which inform the individual's later experience.

There are critical developmental stages. An important characteristic of the growth sequence is the existence of critical periods of vulnerability and development (Freud, 1965, pp.56-92). This concept has been approached in many ways by different psychodynamic systems; a representation of the varieties of such description is presented in the Appendix. The "staging" of growth is determined by the interaction of the on-going process of physical and intellectual maturation and growth ("readiness") and the child's experiences and motivations. Out of this interaction emerges the child's drive toward the acquisition of new skills and the conquest of new tasks. For example, the continuous maturation of the infant's

muscular strength and coordination, combined with his curiosity and
desire to explore and move about, work together as he learns, first
to crawl, and later to walk.

Gerald Caplan (1961, p.12) points out the

...importance of [these] repeated periods of individual
and social disequilibrium in human development. The
relatively smooth trajectory of individual personality
growth and eventual deterioration is interspersed by
relatively short periods of upset, during which sudden
alteration of pace and direction of personality change
may occur...[T]here is an increased susceptibility to
change during these periods, and novel methods of handling
psychologic problems may be developed by the individual
during these crises.

Another implication of the existence of significant developmental
crises is that inadequate mastery of the tasks of a given stage
will often severely jeopardize healthy development at later stages
as Erikson (1963) emphasizes.

The growth process generates new motivations. The motivational system which functions in the adult personality is certainly
not present from birth. Part of the maturational process of growth
is the emergence of new goals and interests. Here, again, there
are some tendencies which develop almost universally, such as sex-
uality which emerges as an important drive in the adolescent; but
there is also great variation in the patterns of new motivations
which develop out of childhood growth and experience. An important
implication of this premise is the view that because the child's
motivational system is not static, but changes with time and experience, there are within the child significant "psychic resources"

273

which develop over time. Among those resources which develop over time is moral judgement. Piaget's developmental theory (Piaget, 1932; Kohlberg, 1964; Kay, 1968) describes three stages of moral development--the young child's unilateral respect for authority figures, the "equality" justice based on the child's growing awareness of social realities, and the "equity" justice based on internalized moral standards.

Participants in the Growth Process

Because the child's growth is at all points an inter-active process (Wolman, 1965), it is important to examine the nature and significance of the participants in that process. The child himself with his unique set of biological givens, clearly represents a significant participant in the interactions which shape his growth. Because each child is unique, endowed with different capabilities and goals, the developmental process is different for each. There are, as well, individual differences in the conditions with which the child must cope, and in how successful he is at coping.

The young child's parents, as sources of nurturance and love, are powerful figures in his life--able to grant or deny many of his strong desires. The way in which the parental role is filled and the way in which the growing child reacts to his parents' behavior have significant (and often long-term) effects on the direction of the child's growth, and his expectations about his world.

A number of studies (Spitz, 1945; Spitz and Wolf, 1949; Davis, 1947; Bowlby, 1952) have demonstrated that "maternal deprivation" can have severe distorting consequences on personality development. Inadequate or inappropriate role models in the home, especially the absence of one parent (Wardle, 1961; Short, 1966), is also a common factor in the history of disturbed children. Similarly, a change in parent-figures through remarriage or adoption carries with it a poor prognosis (Redl and Wattenburg, 1951, pp. 132-134).

As he grows older, the child also interacts with significant adults in the social and community environment. In his early years relatives, day care staff, and friends of parents all serve as significant representatives of the community. Later, participation in church activities, Girl Scouts and Boy Scouts, etc. brings the child into wider contact with the community. The formal learning structure of the school is another sphere of significant interactions. The large amount of time which the child spends with a teacher, and his involvement with the child's acquisition of important skills, confer on the teacher a major role in the life of the child.

Siblings, as well as parents, can have important influences in the young child's life. The presence or absence of siblings, birth order and the nature of relations between sibs are all

significant parameters of the early experience of the child.
The birth of a younger sib is frequently cited as an important
event, generating feelings of hostility and rivalry in the older
child (Redl and Wattenburg, 1951, pp. 136-140).

As the child grows older, interactions with children
outside the family also take on significance. The peer group
functions as a powerful source of status, affection, acceptance,
and socialization. Its effects may be destructive, as well; a
child may gain the benefits of belonging and being accepted, at
the same time that he is socialized into a deviant subculture
which may reward fighting, stealing, and so on. Just as the
child can gain rewarding status among his peers, that group also
has the power to inflict painful rejection, accusations of in-
feriority, etc. upon the child (Ausubel, 1970, pp. 326-327).

The attitude of the society as a whole towards the child
is also an important factor in his early experience. The complex
process of socialization reflects the child's interaction with
his culture and his response to its expectations. For the
minority child, especially, cultural attitudes can have a
destructive impact. Racial slurs, discrimination, etc., all
serve as learning experiences, and generally the lesson learned
doesn't generate a positive self image. Robert Coles describes
the case of the migrant farm worker (Coles, 1970, p. 52):

> I want to emphasize how...extraordinarily cruel their
> lives are:...the need always to gird oneself for the

next slur, the next sharp rebuke, the next reminder that one is different and distinctly unwanted, except, naturally, for the work that has to be done in the fields.

The experiences of a young black girl in Roxbury are similar (Coles, 1967, p. 124):

Perhaps she is simply a sensitive human being, able to respond, like many others, to obvious, concrete situations...: the welfare lady's remarks she hears; the policeman's constant surveillance she sees; the foul and dank air she smells in one hallway after another; the rats she has felt jumping on her bed.

Finally, the quality of the child's development is determined not only by his interactions with other people but also by significant inputs from his physical environment and life milieu. First, the overall sensory stimulation level to which the child is exposed is an important variable--there is a wide range from household to household in the amount and variety of auditory, visual, and tactile stimulation with which the young child is presented. The paucity of sensory stimuli in the environment of the children studied by Spitz and Wolf (1949) and Davis (1947) was considered an important factor in the behavioral disturbances which they exhibited.

Similarly, as the cognitive skills begin to develop, the availability of stimulating games, picture books, and so on may significantly affect his interests and development. Absence of cognitive stimuli in the home--toys, games, books, may retard cognitive development. For the bilingual Spanish child, for

277

example, the cognitive content of his environment can prove very confusing.

A second important factor is the physical size of the young child's life space. How crowded the household is, how much space is available for the child to explore and how much privacy is possible, all are important characteristics of the developing child's life milieu. There will, for example, be a vast difference between the experience of a child confined largely to a crib in a boarding home and that of the middle class child who has the run of his home, and is taken with his parents to the homes of friends, to the park, to the beach, etc.

A related issue is the stability of the environment; here a sharp contrast can be made between a child who grows up living in the same house with a relatively stable set of neighbors, and the child of migrant agricultural workers, who travel from camp to camp every year, never staying in one place for more than a few months. Coles has commented on the effects of the transient life led by children of migrant agricultural workers (Coles, 1970, pp. 27-28):

> Many of the children I have studied these past years,
> in various parts of Florida and all along the
> eastern seaboard, view life as a constant series of trips
> undertaken rather desperately in a seemingly endless
> expanse of time. Those same children are both active
> and fearful, full in initiative and desperately forlorn,
> driven to a wide range of ingenious and resourceful
> deeds and terribly paralyzed by all sorts of things.

Finally, an important consideration is the physical safety of the environment--how safe it is for the child to live in and explore. Hazards in the home or streets, poor sanitation, prevalence of disease, danger to life, all produce a less healthy and supportive environment.

One cannot discuss the important influences of the social and physical milieu without noting the clear connection in this country between the quality of this environment and socio-economic class. It is clearly within the poorer communities that one finds the less stimulating, more restrictive, less safe, less stable environments. It is not surprising that there is a well demonstrated (La Pouse and Monk, 1958; Sewell and Haller, 1959; Langer and Michael, 1963) positive correlation between "mental health" and higher socio-economic status.

Interaction of Growth Factors

Within this network of interpersonal and environmental inputs and interactions, the child grows. The course of the growth process varies for each individual and may lie anywhere along a whole spectrum:

smooth and easy		stressful
success	⟵——————⟶	inability to cope
euphoria		defeat

The way in which environmental influences and internal resources and limitations work together in determining the quality of the child's growth is represented in Figure 1.

This figure is a broad adaptation (Langner and Michael, 1963, p. 11) of the concept of mental health as a dynamic interaction between the individual and the forces about him, developing over time.

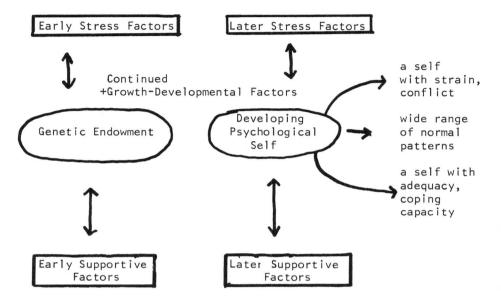

Figure 1. The interactive process of growth.

As we think of the interaction in these terms, we recognize the negative impact of low socio-economic status as discussed above, and of the variations in genetic endowment. Even the prebirth environment becomes very important (Thomas, Chess, and Birch, 1969; Pasamanik and Lilienfeld, 1955; Pasamanik et al., 1956), with mother's nutrition, drug state and well being of note. The baby/mother interactive games are an example of a supportive force. We have discussed the positive and negative input of later factors--home, peers, community, and school. As the individual develops with over-stress, a vicious cycle of detrimental input and inadequate coping mechanisms and defenses combine to make a self defeating serious mental health quandary. Since the process is interactive, there may be stress no child could meet, it may be that the coping mechanisms are defective, or both. The individual feels unworthy, has low self esteem, expects defeat, and may give up entirely or strike back to protect his life spark. It is also recognized that there may be a broad band of accepted life patterns--not one single, perfect performance. On the positive cycle, we have a self enhancing interaction which provides what Hollister has called "strens" (Hollister, 1967). The individual is able to meet life, exploit the positive aspects of the environment, and get good responses. As Peck and Havighurst (1960) have shown, in school the "good" get better while those with problems add to their grief. These individuals with strens feel loved, worthy, and purposeful, expect to meet life demands and have high self esteem.

When it comes to interventions, the significance of this process is clear. Primary prevention is the provision of adequate supportive factors for the individual child regardless of his endowment (Thomas, Chess, and Birch, 1969; Graham et al., 1973) as well as early screening for the signs which forewarn of in-cipient problems (Lambert, 1972). Secondary interventions are those which are compensatory, to counter accumulated strain. Tertiary are the very special provisions needed to help the seriously disturbed, where the vicious cycle will be self perpetuating unless we make significant and appropriate changes in the intra-and interactive conditions.

It is not only interaction which is important. As Epstein (1973) points out in a most cogent discussion, there is intraaction as well; there is a continual dynamic interaction of the individual's inner realm of cognition and affect. Epstein sees, in the evolution of self theory, the "relationship between emotions and underlying implicit cognitions (Epstein, 1973, p. 412)."

In this framework, whether the path of development is smooth and easy or rough and stressful represents the combined effect of all the internal and external factors weighing upon that process. When it goes smoothly, there has been a good fit of the child's own needs and motivations to the demands of the environment upon him. Such a child may have a favorable set of biological givens--intelligence, placidity, and so on--or a very supportive milieu. The combination of these factors creates a level of life stress with which he copes successfully.

At the other end of the spectrum, the child's internal resources and external supports are not sufficient to enable him to cope with the stress to which he is subjected. All forms of distortion of the normal developmental process represent the combined effect of stress overload--demands beyond the child's coping ability--and organismic limitations--failure to have reached a developmental level adequate to cope with a given stress. Thus a situation which might create unbearable tension for a two-year-old might be easily taken in stride by a five-year-old.

The Effect of Stress on Development

When the impact of the unbearable stress is sudden and extreme, _trauma_ results. Trauma may originate within inter-personal relationships or from the stresses and demands placed upon the child by the rest of his life milieu. Among the experiences which are commonly experienced as traumatic are physical injury and loss (or believed loss) of a parent.

An important characteristic of the traumatic incident is that it represents a significant learning experience for the child. Thus, if he later encounters an aspect of the total environmental set associated with the traumatic episode, the whole trauma and all the feelings associated with it may be vividly recalled. An example of trauma associated with feared loss of a parent, which is recalled by the experiential/environmental cues of awakening in a dark bedroom, is recounted by Selma Fraiberg (1959, pp. 79-80):

> When Carol was eight months old, she developed a sleep disturbance that was unusually severe. She wakened screaming around eleven each night and in spite of her parents' efforts to console her and reassure her, she could not be persuaded to go back to sleep for hours.

Her terror was very real and she clung to her mother desperately, in dread of her bed and of her mother's leaving her. The sleep disturbance had started when she wakened one night when her parents were out and a stranger, an unfamiliar baby sitter, came into the room. At the sight of the strange face, the baby began to scream in terror...From that night on and for several weeks to come Carol wakened regularly at night, repeated the heart-breaking cries, the tense wakefulness, even though her parents were there to give proof that they had not gone away.

As Lanner and Michaels (1963) indicate, stresses result in strain and distortion of the personality away from the ideal. Such distortions of the normal developmental processes take many forms, depending upon the unique dynamics of the child's experience. They can be roughly grouped into two categories--those distortions which primarily affect internal processes, and those which affect the way in which the child interacts with his environment.

Any of the child's internal predispositions, processes, and structures may be distorted by undue stresses during his development. There are, for example, children whose experiences fail to generate in them a <u>sense of selfness or self-worth</u> and who view themselves as inadequate to the tasks before them, unworthy of love, doomed to failure and loneliness.

The basic <u>emotional</u> and <u>cognitive</u> <u>processes</u> can also be distorted, as can the balance between them. Such an imbalance can occur at either end of the spectrum, producing at one end a submissive, thinking automatón, who is completely cut off from his emotions and feelings (Lowen, 1967) or, at the other end, a completely irrational being, a mere bundle of feelings. Finally, the child's use of fantasy may be a focus for distortion. The predictive use of imagination may be so distorted that the child bases his behavior on the wholly unrealistic world of his fantasy. For example, Eddie, one of Bettelheim's patients, had fantasies about his power to make people disappear with his frequent clawing gestures (Bettelheim, 1950, p. 232).

> The counselor asked if he really thought [the clawing made people disappear.] and Eddie said, 'Yes. It's a ray. I turn it on somebody or something and it makes him go away.'

The imaginary pursuits and creations of the fantasy world may come to dominate the child's experience until his inner world becomes his whole world. Such a case is that of seven-year-old Marie B., reported by Berkowitz and Rothman (1960, p. 17):

> Marie was a completely disoriented, confused child, who made no contact with anyone. She gesticulated wildly with her arms and her eyes darted constantly without any real perception of the environment. She seemed frightened, cried almost continuously and appeared very anxious. Marie seemed to be hallucinating, responding to inner stimuli and evidencing fear of imaginary things. She never spoke to another child nor played with any of the toys in the room. When handed a plaything, she became panic-stricken and engaged in violent destruction. She could not care for her bodily needs, soiling and wetting herself without being aware of it.

The second broad class of developmental disturbances includes those which largely affect the child's relationship to others. The child may be identification-deficient, and thus unable to empathize with the needs and feelings of others, or to form meaningful relationships with them. Inadequate socialization and failure to develop and internalize acceptable values and attitudes is another source of distortion, and accounts for many significant behavioral problems, such as delinquency. Finally, the whole area of ego controls and coping mechanisms represents an important source of distortion. When the child has failed to develop ego strengths, his ability to function is greatly compromised, since any significant stress or challenge will produce even more strain in his whole personality structure.

It is when the child's experience has produced such distortions that the medical, educational, and mental health establishments move in to provide therapeutic interventions. The rationale for this process and the range of specific interventional techniques is discussed in the second half of this paper.

III. THE PSYCHODYNAMIC APPROACH TO INTERVENTION

Since the psychodynamic position is broad and amorphous
in nature, the perspective on intervention follows suit. Regarding
development, great emphasis has been put on infancy and the early
years (Bowlby, 1952; Spitz, 1945) and on critical periods in the resolution of stages of growth (Freud as discussed in Rezmierski and
Kotre, 1972; Erikson, 1963), though the early biogenic emphasis has
come to include a more sociological approach. The attention to interventions on the interactive side has a long history--the negative
impact of institutionalization for very young children was early re-
searched by Spitz (1945) and by Anna Freud and Dorothy Burlingame
(1944) with preschoolers. The child guidance movement put strong
emphasis on working with the family, especially mothers. Aichhorn
(1935) pioneered in milieu concepts for neurotic delinquents. These
efforts, representing the interactive thesis, predicate a whole
series of interventions. It must be said that the early concept of
influence orbit included almost exclusively the intimate family relationship. It was much later that the total perspective was incorporated, though Anna Freud had early written on education (1947).

On the other side of the intervention picture, internalized
conditions have always received great attention. The development of
child analysis and play therapy, and the long involved work with
dreams and symbolic expression demonstrates the intra-focussed intervention. In fact, for some, the emphasis on sophisticated uncovering

287

and relearning of feelings in the therapeutic session was the total picture. The factors coming from within the individual and portending the unconscious, were the primary concern of the psychoanalytic strain. But it must be remembered that William James, Murray and others are also significant figures in a dynamic conceptualization of this position.

A. Categorization of Interventions

Systems for categorizing interventions range from alpha-
betical cataloging (Gioscia et al.) to those which involve a complicated conceptual system. Catterall's organization uses the following rubric:

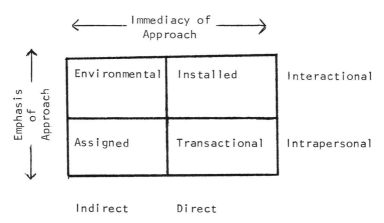

Figure 2. Categories of interventions
(adapted from Catterall, 1970).

It can be seen that Catterall is categorizing primarily on the basis
of administrative considerations, though a careful study of his lists
is most instructive to anyone interested in psychodynamic interventions. Another method is to organize interventions with regard to
where they take place. There are those which take place in the home,
the school, the neighborhood, a therapist's office or a residential
institution. Another method of making distinctions is with regard
to who the significant participants are: the therapist, the social
worker, the teacher, lay "quasi professionals," the peer group and

289

so on. It is interesting that that category of specifically what is done, by whom and to what end is often left to the term "work"--"I'm working with the child...He worked on his problem." When one examines the substance of this work, it is clear there are differences in the communications channels used. Many are strictly verbal, others emphasize non-verbal media such as touch, feeling, body language, and still others the manipulation of external cue systems. Such work can be also divided into cognitive and affective approaches. As Hersch (1968) has indicated, the whole matter of how who does what to whom, and whether you can tell if it worked, is no longer clear in the therapeutic business. In fact, almost anything goes these days.

While elements of these various systems do become part of the presentation which follows, there is an over-riding determinant. The mode of organization follows the psychodynamic theoretical position as it has been outlined. This does not imply that the set of interventions presented are unique. It can be demonstrated that there is much overlap in the actual techniques used by various schools of thought. Names and interpretations will differ even if the operation is similar. For example, some behaviorists (Bandura, 1969) would discuss role modelling, while the present description would be in terms of facilitating identification. Thus why one does something and what one conceptualizes is fully as important as any specific technique.

Another distinction about interventions concerns the

severity of the child's problem. Categorization of the child in some manner or other could be used as the determinant of the intervention. Since assessment is a factor in the psychodynamic approach, it cannot be neglected.

Following the coda of section one, interventions will be grouped around the following headings: assessment process, which sets the stage for selective intervention; interventions with a biological emphasis; interventions which depend upon regenerative growth factors, given reasonable interactive conditions; and interventions which clearly require the imposition of various specialized regimes, because of the diminished (or limited) capacity to learn. Obviously these divisions are neither theoretically exclusive nor discrete. They accommodate to the concepts presented in section one.

The structure for looking at interventions, which will be used here, focuses on the fundamental processes which serve as both the media and the target for change. The psychodynamic view of normal development assumes the necessity of interactions with the environment and with other people. The goals for mental health similarly focus on interactions and on the processes that facilitate them. In dealing with methods for reconstructing healthy patterns of interaction and behavior, it is thus appropriate to focus on those processes which are emphasized and manipulated by various interventions.

B. Goals of Interventions

The overall goals behind the interventions for the disturbed child are those already stated as the goals of the interactive system for normal growth. These are the values which reflect
a psychodynamic interpretation and have been stated in detail by
Jahoda (1958). As was pointed out, they include social relationships
(empathy, concern for others, social skills), self feelings (awareness, autonomy, and a sense of well being), expressive qualities,
use of one's talents, ability to love, and above all, an integration
and balance of the "parts" so that the individual can cope without
excessive defense.

But the level of self actualization possible for many children, even with appropriate interventions, falls far short of the
ideal. Because of biological limitations and/or severe interactive
damage, there are children who have a limited prognosis. There
will be autistic children who make minimal gains even with extensive intervention. But the gains they do make may make a
critical difference, though they may still need to live a sheltered
life, unable to meet certain responsibilities of an independent
youth or adult. The goal for a schizophrenic child is to peel
off any secondary overlay which may have been added by poor
handling and minimize the basic limitations which remain. Likewise
for a brain injured child or a sociopath, one maximizes what the
child can do, but does not expect that underlying difficulty to

292

disappear.   The work of Thomas, Chess and Birch (1969) and others
depicts this point of view most appropriately.   While there are
broad goals and subgoals for particular interventions, the determining goal matrix for any specific youngster is a complex of
assessment and the pragmatic test.

c. Clinical Assessment

Diagnosis connotes assignment to a category in the psychiatric nomenclature. A number of sophisticated diagnostic systems and classification schemes have been developed, of which those by McConville and Purohit (1973), Prugh (unpublished manuscript), and Rutter et al. (1969) represent the most complete efforts. Categorical systems often cannot describe specific children; in particular, the problems of minority children do not fit most schemes. But assessment is a broader concept than diagnosis. Assessment involves describing various dimensions of the child's development, as well as codifying the conditions of the interaction of the environment with the child (Engel, 1969).

Three criticisms can be leveled at the psychodynamic position in the area of assessment. One is the preoccupation with historical factors--even to the point, at times, of reading backwards from current conditions and implying antecedents which fit theoretical constructs, in the absence of any verifying information; i.e., the mother must have been such and so because the child is now such and so. While this is still a problem, the dynamic position has incorporated certain non-historical elements and also utilizes status assessment through psychological tests and interviewing. A child's functioning level, and his potential are judged. His hopes and worries about the future are also important. The second criticism of traditional assessment may be directed towards the concentration on the child's unconscious world, as interpreted through projections. It has been as if there were nothing directly understandable of any importance. Again, such an approach tends to be theory-bound rather than evidence-bound. For instance, if the child is believed to be in the midst of the Oedipal struggle, it isn't too hard to find possible evidence. But the ability to talk meaningfully with youngsters and to assist in the direct recognition of feelings is certainly a major contribution to assessment. The third criticism has been that, in interpretation, not only did the individual's fantasy life loom over-large, but it was assumed that all behavior was a consequence of internalized pathogenic features. In truth much of the behavior of even a very deviant child is situation specific. Psychodynamics applies to external as well as internal interventions. Redl (1959; Redl and Wineman, 1952) has been a pioneer in clarifying this principle; some deviant children carry their pathology to every circumstance, but most disturbed children are highly responsive to external conditions. In fact, it is their misreading of certain environmental conditions which can set them off. When one visits a good school program for disturbed children, the pupils may, at first glance and most of the time, behave like normal children. This is because the environment has been manipulated to fit their coping capacity, and every effort has been made to modulate provocative cues.

The main difficulty with the traditional assessment process

has been the high reliance on the single case study approach which, incidentally, is a common method in behavior modification as well (Long, Morse, and Newman, 1971, Ch.2). The single case is often presented unsystematically, open to idiosyncratic interpretation, and subject to every known bias. Even when a case conference is held to collate diverse sets of historical evidence, there is no assurance of objectivity. Since the psychodynamic position emphasizes the uniqueness of the individual, group studies of children often mask the reality.

Two things have happened to move the case approach to assessment to firmer ground. One is the development of dimensions for assessment, with anchor points, when possible. The other development is the "N of 1" technology (Morse, Schwertfeger, and Goldin, 1973). This enables objective experimental research on the single case, which is a more useful process than group studies. The corrolary is pattern search to reveal similar "single cases" from the profile of characteristics, related interventions, and outcome. It is possible to have research on a life stream basis (Allport, 1962; White, 1964) which follows the psychodynamic position.

But selection of interventions and study of change requires assessment. Moving from diagnosis to assessment, there are many patterns which have been proposed to organize data collection. Relating the previous discussions to the concepts of Rabinovitch (1968), assessment should include the following dimensions:

Neurological integration
Intellectual potential
Intellectual functioning
Clarity of ego boundaries
Reality testing
Capacity for depth relationships
Acculturation
Anxiety (endogenous)
Anxiety (exogenous)
Motivation
Self-esteem

The sources of information to scale such dimensions should be multidisciplinary-neurology, psychology, child psychiatry, education, social work, and so on. The sources should be test data, clinical examination, various interviews, visits, observations, and trial placements. (Medical examination, psychological tests, psychiatric interviews, and social histories have always been a major source of information. School history and performance have received more emphasis of late.) Whoever can supply past or present relevant information should be included. While many dimensions can be scaled, and subscaled, when there is no normative comparison information, the consensus of judgements based upon divergent observations is important. Assessment is neither simple nor mechanical.

The history of psychodynamic assessment of interactive factors has not been a glorious one. External conditions were often viewed with bias. Teacher and parent input were seen as explanations, whether they were or not. While this aspect is receiving more careful attention, the codification of information remains vague. Two things

297

should be said: since a great deal depends upon the child's perception of the environment, the reality is only one part of the
study. Second, to test how specific behaviors represent responses
to situations, especially with young children, observational nur-
series have been used, where the input can be controlled and results
studied.

The purpose of assessment is not to collect status knowledge, though this is a vital step. The real purpose is to discover
the best possible intervention for the child. But the prescriptive
teaching rubric in current vogue lacks the comprehensiveness needed
for in-depth work. One must examine carefully both internal and
external variables. Consideration of the child's internal capacities and limitations must always reflect an awareness of his
overall developmental status. As Anna Freud (A. Freud, 1965,
pp. 25-54) points out, interventional techniques must be tailored
to the developmental level of the individual. The young child,
for example, deals much more confidently with the concrete world of
play than he does with words; traditional verbal approaches to
intervention are only appropriate when the child has reasonably
well developed cognitive and language skills. Thus for the younger
child, concrete techniques such as those of play therapy are more
appropriate. Special care must be taken in dealing with the child
whose cognitive development has lagged behind his chronological age
or with the child who has severe language problems.

Determination and assessment of significant external
variables is fully as important as the examination of the child's
internal dynamics and resources. The quality of the child's interpersonal, societal, and physical environments must be determined,
and the accessibility of these factors to therapeutic change must
be assessed. The ascertainment of accessibility and feasibility
is crucial, for theory is of little use if it can't be put to work.

Closely related to the process of pre-intervention evaluation and assessment is that of continual monitoring and follow-
up study. The poor record of so many therapeutic approaches when
reviewed upon follow-up (Cromwell,1971) can be attributed to two
factors. First, rigidly prescriptive approaches are often used and
the resulting process fails to match intervention to the unique
dynamic of the youngster's problem. Matching superficial symptom
with treatment could hardly be expected to be very effective.
Secondly, many interventions fail to foster the development of
"stress immunity." The intervention may have been appropriate
to reduce malfunction but the total therapeutic environment may
have been so protective that the strength for unprotected life
has not evolved. Or the environment to which the child is returned
remains so stressful, that the child cannot function when he returns.
Conversely, some so-called therapeutic institutions are themselves
highly stressful and cultivate deviance (Rosenhan, 1973) in such a
way that the child may learn to cope within the context of those

expectations, but remains unready to return to his native environment.

The specific interventional techniques which are chosen
and defined as a result of the assessment process all share certain
basic characteristics. The aim of any therapeutic program is to
maximize, redesign, and restructure the relevant components of the
child's interactional system to facilitate growth, provide for unlearning and relearning, and mobilize needed internal resources.
To this end the biomedical, mental health, and educational institutions interact with one another in providing significant therapeutic input to the whole range of children classed as "disturbed,"
"socially maladjusted," etc. (Michigan Association for Emotionally
Disturbed Children, 1973).

300

IV.   TECHNIQUES OF INTERVENTION

A. Biological Interventions

A correlate to the theoretical emphasis which the psychodynamic school places upon biological predispositions and development is the use of medical interventions and other approaches which
affect constitutional and physiological variables. There is concern for perinatal health and diet, for the physical care which
the child receives, and for other parameters which facilitate optimal growth and development. Where physiological deficits or abnormalities contribute to the child's problem, a broad range of
biomedical intervention may be indicated.[4] These include special
compensatory diets (such as those for phenylketonuria), drugs which
facilitate recovery (such as the major tranquilizers used for some
schizophrenics), and drugs which regulate and minimize pathological
processes (such as the amphetamines used in hyperactivity).

Fully as important as the fact that biomedical interventions are used by the psychodynamicist, is the way in which they
are used. This, in fact, is the keystone of biomedical intervention from the psychodynamic view. Because one is always concerned
with the total child and the complex dynamics of his problem, biological interventions are never used without also employing paral-

4.   This group of interventions is discussed in detail in L.I.
     Kameya's paper, "Biophysical Interventions in Emotional
     Disturbance," which appears in this volume.

lel interventions which speak to the child's psychological needs. The individual and his intimate participation in therapy must never be overlooked. From this viewpoint, to prescribe drugs for a child without discussing with the child that decision and his feelings and fears about it may do more harm than good. Such isolated use of biological tools may undermine a child's already precarious feelings about the intent of others, foster dependency, etc. Thus, although biological approaches are necessary and important, they are appropriate only as an integral part of a comprehensive dynamically oriented program for intervention.

B. Interventions Which Depend Upon the Normal Growth Process

Some psychodynamic interventions focus on the mobilization of normal growth assertions to facilitate corrective changes. Another set of interventions is indicated for more severe deviance where carefully designed specialized programs are required to restore health. The overlap of the same process in these two categories is obvious in many instances. The same psychological support function becomes intensified at the second level because of the difficulty of penetrating the child's consolidated deviant system. Yet, while he carries within himself certain pre-set patterns of behavior, his repertoire is still, in varying degrees, always in responsive interaction with a given set of external conditions.

It would be difficult to argue that there is an "instinct to grow up healthy and relatively conflict free." Yet we see so many examples of youngsters wanting to join the normals, be like others, and find a reasonable solution to their stress. As indicated, the psychodynamic position sees a life sequence in Eriksonian terms, with the modulator of growth being the interactive processes, both within and without. Also, as stated, the pattern of growth is qualified by biological limitations. The evolution of the life sequence is always highly individualistic. If we can reduce the stress and provide the interactive substance needed by children, the growth process will bend toward assuming the normal developmental sequence. This requires two things: getting an environment suited to the child's level and coping ability, and providing an environment which has the psychological nutrients necessary to foster growth. Given a reasonable interactive environment, there are many children who would respond and mobilize their resources (in an erratic up-and-down course, to be sure) toward eventual normal behavior. We turn first, then, to interventions which are designed to give the distraught youngster what he should have had all along, cut to his individual measure. These include restoring the family function, compensatory schooling (breaking the transference bind, specific curricular programming), and broader community interventions. It will be evident at once that this material does not add up to a systematic and integrated taxonomy of interventions. It is held together only as a reflection of the basic psychodynamic position as presented. Growth is an interactive process with an hygienic environment: can we suggest interventions that would rest at the level of restoring this environment?

Processes Which Aim to Restore the Family to a Reasonably Function-ing Interactive System

The long history of the child guidance movement is evidence of the concern to help the family become an adequate "child-upbring-ing" institution. There have been several approaches to working with the various significant persons in the child's life. Perhaps the most widely practiced is that of family therapy (Ackerman, 1961a, 1961b; Loehner, 1971). This technique is based on the belief that "the family group can make or break mental health

304

(Ackerman, 1961a, p.231)." The interactions of the primary target child with the other members of his intimate family are instrumental in the development and support of disturbance (Henry, 1965). Family therapy rests on the assumption that the identified patient is not necessarily the only deviant member of the family system. Those who have interacted with him in destructive ways may need help and sometimes formal treatment.

Although the therapist may or may not also see family members individually, the emphasis is on interviews with the entire family group, excluding no one in the family counseling or therapy sessions. Such a situation gives the therapist a firsthand view of the stressful or even pathological dynamics of the family, in a far more reliable way than reconstruction of those dynamics from an individual patient's narrative, interviews with the family members, or case history records. The techniques employed by the therapist include observation and verbal interpretation, pointing out the processes, fostering insight and honesty, and examining the alliances and behaviors that he observes. He may bring in reality factors, occasionally support family members against alliances of others, suggest or ask for alternative solutions to problems, give interpretations, and so on. At all times the emphasis is on family process and dynamics. The assumption is that some families can make that degree of change necessary to allow the child normal growth. The concepts used are those of the psychodynamic persuasion, with the same concern for assessment of the system as for assessment of the individual.

The interpretative base includes both conscious and unconscious behavior considerations. It is important to consider major differences between family styles. There are inadequate families, who
cannot cope and need advice and help and often are willing (at their
level) to take direct suggestion. Then there are neurotic (psychotic) families who are so intertwined that to unravel the child's
problem is to unravel the family.

An extension of the principles of family therapy is embodied
in the technique of network therapy. This approach is designed to
include in the therapeutic intervention those extra-familial persons
who have significant influences over some or all of the family members. Speck (1967) reports the case of a twenty-year-old autistic
man and his mother. He treated them first by making them the
"children" in an artificial family for which they chose the "parents,"
and then meeting weekly with this "family" and all of their friends.
This group of about thirty people met for six months; at the end of
this time the son broke many of his strong maternal ties, moved
into his own apartment, and soon started a job, which he had never
held before. Among the other group members, Speck also was able to
identify improvements in a number of dyadic relationships.

The analysis of the family dynamics may identify specific
problems, such as the child being the scapegoat (Vogel and Bell,
1960) or being given double messages (Bateson **et** al., 1956) about prope
behavior. Johnson (1972) describes the phenomenon of "superego
lacunae" as a mechanism underlying antisocial behavior in certain

306

adolescents. There are strong secondary rewards in disturbance for
these children whose

> parents <u>unconscious condoning of the acting out of
> asocial impulses</u> by the child may serve the two-fold
> purpose of allowing the parent vicarious gratification
> of forbidden impulses as well as the expression of
> hostile destructive impulses felt toward the child
> (Johnson, 1972, p.525, underlining ours).

When such dynamics underly the child's behavior, it is clearly necessary to work with both the parents and the child, either separately or in family therapy.

When the child is a family scapegoat (Vogel and Bell, 1960)
or finds pseudo-stupidity his route to survival, the total family
interpersonal environment must be altered. Such alterations are
particularly difficult with families that cannot face the loss of
their diversion. When changes cannot be fostered, it may be necessary to insulate the child from the family through compensating
school life, which enriches the opportunity for normal growth.

In brief, the major supporting (or diverting) agency in the
child's life is still his family--his parents, siblings, and extended
family members. Relying on the interactive process, the psychodynamic therapist seeks to restore health-giving potentials in the
family when possible. What should it provide? Love, security,
concern, models, care and systematic training. Of course, few
families approach the ideal. Sometimes mitigating the stress, far
short of perfection, will allow the child survival. There are
distorted families and inadequate families, doing their best, but

overwhelmed. The psychodynamic approach stresses the need for adults with strength as well as love, who can limit as well as give to children.

In discussing the child's learning of sanctions for misbehavior, Rudolf Dreikurs (1960) suggests that the "natural consequences" of a child's behavior are most effective, and Ferster (1967) indicates that natural reinforcers are to be preferred over arbitrary rewards or punishments. If, for example, coming home late for dinner means eating a cold dinner (Holt, 1972, p.106), the child will come to learn that his behaviors have clear and inherent consequences, above and beyond whatever punishments he may attribute to fickle or mean adults. Conversely, the child can learn the pleasureable benefits of his own behavior when a consistent environment responds to the child's progress and successes. Love has been so much discussed that it is easy to overlook the importance of the "reality" principle which Freud himself delineated. There are so many children with fantasies of omnipotence and with exaggerated notions of their place in the world, that reality must be emphasized.

Intervention, then, aims to provide restorative assistance through giving the child a reasonable family in which he can grow "well." But it is not always possible to orient families and seldom is it easy even at best. Some of the most normal appearing families are the most difficult to alter. The intertwining relationships have solidified and any alteration of one disturbs them

all. The naive interviewers frequently underestimate the complexi-
ties, expecting too much from advice-giving or contracts which might
be suggested for certain inadequate families but seldom change
neurotic ones with unobtrusive problems.

Providing a Restorative-Supportive School Environment

There are those children who have personal problems of various
types but demonstrate neither academic nor school adjustment difficulties. There are other youngsters who are exposed to severe
stress outside the school but they "transfer" their acting out to
the school setting--especially if they are fearful of the consequences in the home. A teacher is less threatening. Developmental
and crisis difficulties may be accessible because the school is
used as the arena for the acting out. Then there are those pupils
with academic and/or behavioral reactive responses to a poor school
environment. Because of the holistic nature of the child's development, the problems in one stress area tend to flood into other
previously conflict-free areas as well; conversely, there may be
complete segmentation of contaminated and free spheres in some
children.

The modern analytic literature contains extensive discussion
of the range of causes of learning difficulties (Buxbaum, 1964;
Liss, 1955; Pearson, 1952; Klein, 1949; English and Pearson, 1972;
Grunebaum, 1962) and school phobias (Sperling, 1967; Klein, 1945;
Sperry et al., 1958). As with any other specific symptom, there are
many dynamic situations which may result in school-related problems.

Among these are trauma, withdrawal from school to avoid hurt, with-drawal from school to stay close to mother and home, and the dis-placement of problems from other sectors to the school learning sit-uation, even to specific subjects or skills.

Just as in any other situation, careful assessment of the severity and dynamics of the problem must precede the institution of any intervention. In the present upsurge of so-called school phobic problems, close collation of school and mental health efforts is suggested, with a plan for early and strong pressure to maintain the pupil in school. Elective mutism is seen as a strong manipula-tive negativism rather than a speech problem per se, calling for both individual therapy and situational inducements.

Since the school is a mini-culture, its psychological poten-tials as a resource for disturbed children are almost endless. But there must be flexibility to meet particular pupil needs. The need for aides, tutors, and conjoint work of teachers and therapists is indicated. The assessment process avoids surface, self-defeating efforts. For example, there are pupils who are described as pre-occupied with attention getting when in reality they may need the substantiation of love and caring to feel worthwhile. The psycho-dynamic approach would not recommend modification of surface behav-ior without humanizing care. School procedures for the mildly and seriously disturbed obviously overlap, and the rectification of the school environment is a matter of degree, the same basic human needs being present for the normal child, mildly disturbed, and the seri-ously disturbed.

Minimization of stress in the school environment. What is the possible psychological substance of school? The range is from the impact of a total tone or stance which promotes certain values and expectations to the impact of specifically designed interventions for an anxious learning-disability pupil. Sarason has described how the "constitution of the classroom (Sarason, 1971)," which embodies the rules of behavior, is usually set early and arbitrarily by the teacher. From the psychodynamic point of view, the participation of pupils in the evolution of the code and working through issues is therapeutic.

The school can regulate the degree of comfort vs. stress in many ways. According to the reality principle, conformity can generate rewards and survival. On the other hand, the pleasure principle is also significant. Gratifications can be intensified. Ego growth through skills and accomplishments can increase both personal competency and self esteem to cope with life as well. There are ways to reduce anxiety and fear of failure through the careful selection of material, through gradation of steps to assure success, and through ending demands for "perfection." School is a place of work and creativity and of fun and play. The social context of school provides a laboratory for peer and authority corrective role learning for the scapegoat or bully. There are so many reality factors, that direct interpretation is a natural expectation. There are peer and adult models available. Competition can be mitigated, cooperation enhanced through educational methodology, if one so chooses. There

311

is bibliotherapy and a vast array of cognitive-curricular approaches described elsewhere. A unique blend of cognitive-affective synthesis can be undertaken systematically. Any environment with such potentials has at once the power to be corrective or destructive. A youngster can find a new target for hate and fear, or new and useful things to do and people to care about. The capacity for utilizing the potential of the school resources for mental health ends requires special education insight as well as flexibility to do what is needed.

The school, from this viewpoint, provides special people who do therapeutic teaching (dealing with the affective-cognitive mix) rather than remedial teaching. The individualization can include peer and lay parent surrogates, such as proposed in the Teaching Moms concept (Donahue and Nichtern, 1965; Fenichel, 1966). Therapeutic personnel, however, lay or professional, do not become so because assigned a role. One's concern would be with the identification image provided by the person. There should be people available who can help when you are in crisis, or to speak to when you need special help with your "internal curriculum." Crisis intervention as a mental health teaching process has been described by Caplan (1964). Such school resources are especially important for disturbed youngsters (Newman, 1967).

School can even provide help for the child's life in many ways which have long-term implications. We can see in the school normal activities which are similar to established therapies:

312

recreation, work, relationship, group, identification, achievement, music, art, dance, and even Slavson's activity group (Slavson, 1943). If they can become special therapies, the school can use them as therapeutic tools.

The therapeutic consequences of active involvement and participation are facilitated by experiences which are intrinsically appealing to the child's normal interests and curiosity. A study by Kounin et al., (1966) has demonstrated that in the classroom a high level of "seatwork variety change" produces an increase in appropriate behavior in both normal and disturbed children. Thus a situation which minimizes boredom and maximizes involvement can improve overall pupil behavior. The open classroom, when it is guided by a perceptive teacher, can embody a high therapeutic potential (Knoblock, 1973; Dennison, 1969). Since the psychodynamic position anticipates interaction, this is not a proposal for laissez faire or for converting the class into a classical clinic type setting (Berkowitz and Rothman, 1960).

One cannot discuss the school situation without touching on the issue of stress, particularly the almost universally experienced test-anxiety (Sarason, et al., 1960). One hopes, of course, for the temporary and eventual total elimination of tests, with the substitution of better methods of feedback and evaluation. Many alienated delinquents and deprived children find it impossible to cope with failure induced by present practices. As Kohl (1969) points out, however, nearly all children must deal at some point with batteries of standardized tests, often with baffling coded answer sheets and unfamiliar types of questions. As Glasser (1969) says, schools should be without failure. But until test taking is not a survival skill, special education hopes to gradually, over a period, acclimate the pupil to the harsh reality, starting with possible tasks and no failure. Since mainstreaming is a goal, and since school success is critical to that goal, the matter cannot be ignored. Kohl thus undertook to teach his Harlem youngsters how to take the tests that determined such important things as their class placement, their IQ ratings, etc. As students took practice tests and discussed how tests were structured, "their anxiety decreased to a manageable level, and therefore they were able to apply things they had discovered in their own thinking, reading, and writing to situations that arose in the test (Kohl, 1969, p. 340)." After their short introduction to test-taking, students' reading scores jumped one to three years over scores they had achieved a few months earlier.

Breaking the transference: minimizing undesirable interactional gains. One of the major problems in the school programs from the psychodynamic view is the lack of recognition of the disturbed child's motivational structure, conscious and unconscious. Relevant here is the concept of transference. To some extent the child responds to even purified situations as if they were like those of the past, on

314

the basis of incorporated response patterns. An accepting teacher
is "as if" he were a rejecting authority figure encountered in the
past. As the perceptual psychologists put it, the pupil makes over
the external world according to his past experiences, many of which
may have been traumatic. He has a set of expectations which he
seeks to replicate, even though they may be painful. This "behaving as if" may be easy to dispell by a corrective influence or
it may require extensive, long-term repeated relearning experiences,
and even then linger. It should be faced with a combination of
insight-awareness and external conditions which rectify the cause.

Often the problem is that unwittingly we reinforce the very
behavior patterns we wish to eradicate, because we ignore the
environmental responses we are producing. Random or inappropriate
"reinforcement overkill" may encourage the child to do what we
would like to eliminate (Forness and MacMillan, 1972, Becker, et al.,
1967). The behaviorists, with their emphasis on acute, careful
observation of events, have moved this from a vague general concept
to a concrete data-base, though with different resolutions. As
suggested in a prior section, a pupil craves love and relationship
and behaves to demand attention. His real need is often very hard
to meet, and he forces attention from the teacher by obverse
behavior. The more the appetite for being wanted and cared for
is whetted but not met by attention, the more the pupil behaves to
maintain second-best, which is increasing attention at all costs.

Or, another pupil may expect hostility from adults or peers, and persist in provocation until his expected view of the world comes true. We give in and get angry. This also may permit the child the license for guilt-free counter-hostility. If a child feels he can't do the work and continually demonstrates "I can't," he is sometimes consciously or unconsciously substantiated by his teachers who virtually do his work for him. When one has learned to feel he is an unworthy person, his quest is to continually explore the truths of his fear. You are what you think you are, and so behave to prove it.

Since it is obvious that not all past experience remains equally potent in the present configuration of the youngster, the danger of the psychodynamic approach is in making false linkages with history, or in neglecting the fact that habitual behaviors often come to have a sequence of their own; a habitual response may be based upon arousal cues connected to historical events, but which occur even in the absence of the original psychological condition. We all persist in many behaviors even though the situations no longer produce the original deep generating motivations. There are those still expecting tokens of love on birthdays long after we have substantiated our "lovability." The youngster approaches a new task with "I can't" when it is clear he realizes he can. For those behaviors which have outlasted their useful personal dynamic and which no longer are deeply invested in an active motivational matrix, the analysis-of-cause approach is unwarranted. In most instances we could find something if we looked hard enough. However, environmental manipulation, with awareness of what is going on, is sufficient.

Thus, it is important not only to generate positive motives for change but also to reduce the attractiveness of being disturbed. Redl and Wineman's (1952) tactic of "planned ignoring" is an example of such a technique. If the interest and attention that bizarre behavior usually generates is withheld, the behavior is less likely to be attractive to the child. There are examples of patients "learning" to give what their therapist wants, rather than what is real.

Or, in another context, where a child's relationship with his teacher is felt to be overly dependent, Hansen (1971) suggests the use of the tape recorder as a means of presenting the student with pre-recorded individualized lessons, without monopolizing the teacher's time and attention.

Curricular approaches as interventions. Among the basic considerations for curricular approaches to emotional disturbances which Rhodes (1963) outlines are:

1. The child should have new experiences in relation to his old problems.

2. The child should be surrounded with new opportunities which will call up such positive motives as adventure, achievement, exploration, and discovery.

317

3. Learning should be active and involve sensory input through as many channels as possible.

4. Activities should center on those goals which the child values most.

5. The child should be encouraged to reflect back on experiences and consider what meaning they hold for him.

In addition to such specific educational interventions as indicated above, there have been suggestions for a restorative curriculum which capitalizes on the latent self-corrective capacities of the disturbed child to enhance emotional growth and mental health. Insight and understanding of emotional problems do not always have to be gained within the highly individualized learning context of counseling or individual psychotherapy. Personal discovery can be made through the curricular context as well. The curricular approaches to mental health vary greatly in their focus, from establishment of basic learning skills to fostering awareness of the child's feelings and needs.

In their experimental study Minuchin et al. (1967) used ten sequential lessons to develop basic skills needed for learning and communication. The subjects of their lessons included:

> listening
> implications of noise
> staying on the topic
> taking turns, sharing in communication
> telling a simple story
> building up a longer story
> asking cogent and relevent questions
> categorizing and classifying information
> role-playing

Several curricular approaches focus more specifically on the child as an emotional being. Such curricula reflect several basic beliefs:

1. It is both unrealistic and undesirable to try to eliminate the child's emotional involvements from the classroom.

2. Children learn best when the subject matter is relevant to their experiences and interests.

3. As Weinstein and Fantini write, "unless knowledge is related to an affective state in the learner, the likelihood that it will influence behavior is limited (Weinstein and Fantini, 1970, p. 28)."

Although these curricula were not specifically designed for use with emotionally disturbed children, these basic concerns (as well as many of the specific techniques within each curriculum) conform closely to Rhodes' criteria for work with the disturbed. The point here is, the psychodynamic approach does not favor an antiseptic, exclusively cognitive or skill-oriented educational experience, for either normal or disturbed children. The fact is that most classrooms for the disturbed already have a surplus of unexploited emotional experiences. The curricular programs which have been developed to exploit experiences are thus very relevant to teaching the disturbed child.

Several curricula and textbooks reflect these concerns explicitly. Jones (1968) discusses "Man, A Course of Study," a curriculum developed from the ideas of Jerome Bruner. The subject matter of this social studies curriculum is man's nature--his universal characteristics and his differences from culture to

319

culture. Much use is made of realistic films and stories depicting important aspects of the lives of men in other cultures. Attention is paid to the cognitive content which they contain. Jones suggests equal time for the affective responses aroused. Materials include allusions to such emotion-laden subjects as the selenecide and infanticide practiced by the Netsilik, the relative values of being male or female, and pictures of the bloody killing of a seal. The subjects presented in the program have been chosen for their relevance to the developmental tasks of childhood, and the relationship between emotions and subject matter is reciprocal. Subject matter should be chosen for its relevance to the child's emotional concerns, and the child's emotional involvement facilitates his work with the subject matter. An example of the interrelation is presented in the discussion of family life in Iraq presented below:

> Student: "We don't have the whole family living with us like they do."
> Student: "The girls there can't get married until the grandfather dies. Thats different from us."
> Student: "I agree with Sylvia. My whole family doesn't live together."
> Student: "Here it's different about the boys and girls. Here girls learn faster and are smarter, and the mother enjoys having girls around because the boys are just rough."
> Student: "I disagree. Boys do just as much around the house as girls."
> Student: "Sometimes men can sew better than women. Also the chefs in restaurants are usually men."
> Student: "Boys and men are built more rugged."
> Teacher: "Therefore?"
> Student: "I read a book about the frontier days. When the mother and father died the son worked all his life

320

to help the sisters and brothers grow up and get educated."
Student: "Boys don't change the baby's diapers."
Student: "In Puerto Rico I had to work in the fields and
the girls could stay home."
Student: "Mrs. Jackson, I want to defend my statement.
Because it is less work to hunt and fish than it is to
prepare the food, so the woman works harder."
Student: "Men have stronger constitutions than ladies."
Teacher: "Therefore?"
Student: "If it weren't for ladies, men wouldn't even be
born."
Student: "How come they say 'It's a woman's world?'"
Student: "I disagree with the girls who say that girls
are better, because if you put a girl in a cage with
a bear, she would just cry." (Jones, 1968, pp. 167-168)

In the course of the discussion such important concepts as bio-

logical and individual differences, division of labor, and the human life

cycle are elicited; identity problems and the loaded issue of sex

roles are discussed. Such an encounter reflects the usefulness

of incorporating the child's emotional involvements into the

process of his education.

The approach of Weinstein and Fantini (1970), whose curri-

culum of affect was originally developed to address the needs of

the underprivileged child, is very similar. They place a strong

emphasis on identification of the child's personal concerns, which

they group into three broad classes: self image, disconnectedness,

and control over one's life. To the psychodynamic psychologist,

these are the very things which confound the child with problems,

"the intrinsic drives that motivate behavior (Weinstein and Fantini,

1970, p. 24)." Education must speak effectively to these concerns

in order to function. Among the techniques which have integrated the affective and the cognitive realms are:

1. Creating situations which arouse the pupil's emotional
   involvement.
   A new unit on revolution, for example, was begun by a new
   teacher who immediately began to forcefully order all
   blue-eyed children out of the room. The anger aroused
   prompted a lively discussion of justice, protest, etc.
   (Weinstein and Fantini, 1970, p. 60).

2. "One-way glasses".
   Pupils practice "seeing specific persons through "glasses"
   which are colored "curious," "things-aren't-really-that-bad,"
   "suspicious," "gloomy," and so on   (Weinstein and Fantini,
   1970, pp. 70-90).

3. Procedures to identify pupil concerns.
   The Faraway Island.
      Students are asked to describe the six people they would
      choose to accompany them to a secluded island.
   Ten Years from Now.
      Children are asked to speculate about what they will be
      doing in ten years. This situation often provides an
      excellent opportunity for clarification of reality factors.
   Time Capsule.
      The class selects pictures and songs and makes a tape
      recording to depict what they think is significant about
      their lives.

4. Games
   Games were devised by the Western Behavioral Science Institute
   to help students develop their view of self and increase their
   self-esteem. Examples are presented below:
   "Complain, Gripe and Moan".
      Each child gets coupons labelled "home," "school,"
      and "block." There are booths of the same names
      where the children "spend" their coupons to complain
      about each of these aspects of their lives.
   "Spies from Xenon".
      Children are designated spies from "Xenon" and directed
      to report back what makes earth children mad, afraid,
      strong or happy.
   "Amnesia".
      An adult appears, dazed. He reports being hit and
      losing his memory. Through an elaborate earphone
      arrangement, the children tell him what has been
      happening and help him reconstruct his memory.
   "Mirror".
      The child is directed to "stand up in front of that
      mirror, look right at yourself, and say something nice
      to yourself (Weinstein and Fantini, 1970, p. 191)."

322

The goals of the curriculum developed by Raths, Harmin, and Simon (1966) are closely related to those we have discussed. Their approach has grown out of the feeling

> that the pace and complexity of modern life has so exacerbated the problem of deciding what is good and what is right and what is worthy and what is desirable that large numbers of children are finding it increasingly bewildering, even overwhelming, to decide what is worth valuing, what is worth one's time and energy (Raths et al., 1966, p. 7).

Their curriculum thus focusses on the problem of value formulation and clarification. Their emphasis is on the child's own exploration of alternatives, on consideration of goals, and on behavior consistent with his choices; no one tells him what is best.

The mechanisms which Raths et al. have developed to achieve these goals include:

1. Value clarification responses.
   This technique consists of responding to statements made by the child in such a way that he must clarify his feelings or attitudes to himself and his teacher. Raths et al. (1966, pp. 56-67) enumerate thirty "clarifying responses" such as "How did you feel when that happened?" "Did you have to choose that; was it a free choice?""What other possibilities are there?" "Do you do anything about that idea?" and "What do you have to assume for things to work out that way?" Appropriate use of such value clarifications requires sensitivity to those situations and statements which suggest unstated values. Raths et al. (1966, pp. 65-72) list five statement topics which lend themselves to value clarification: attitudes, aspirations, purposes, interests, and activities.

2. Value sheets.
   These are lists of value-related questions which are prompted by a provocative statement or reading.

3. Role-playing.

4. Contrived incident.
    The teacher contrives a situation to "shock [his] students
    into an awareness of what they are for and against
    (Raths et al., 1966, p. 123)."

5. Open-ended questions.

6. Public interviews.
    The teacher interviews one of the pupils "publicly"
    on some emotionally-charged question such as "What do you
    hate about your sister?" (Raths et al., 1966, p. 143)."

7. Action projects.
    Students participate in projects which actualize the values
    and goals they have been discussing.

In addition to these proposals, there have also been

textbooks developed to strengthen the child's emotional health,

self-concept, etc. Limbacher's (1969) Dimensions of Personality

series is designed to help the child learn to "accept himself,

others, and their society (Limbacher, 1969, p. v)." The texts

contain lessons focussing on self-awareness (Getting to Know

Myself," "Knowing I'm Alive," "My Mirrors"), feelings ("When

I Cried for Help," "My Feelings are Real"), and other people ("How

Different are We?").

Bruck's "Guidance" series (Bruck, 1968-1970) shares a

similar emphasis. The series consists of "workbooks" (sic!)

each of which presents the child with provocative reading material,

specific questions raised by its content, and suggestions for

discussion topics. The child is presented with suggestions for

action related to the lesson, and asked to choose one of those

presented or develop his own plan. Later, he returns to the

lesson to reflect on how effectively he has fulfilled his plan. The hope is that the teacher will use these as stimulants rather than as workbooks.

Jones' point was that regular curricular experiences have enough emotional stuff, and these can be approached naturally as part of the total cognitive-affective binding together of ideas. With disturbed youngsters there is the life of the class itself, which is laden with emotionally charged "curriculum." These matters should not be handled with repression, authoritarianism, or rule fixation. Here is where the class converts to a social-emotional laboratory, giving the time needed to penetrate events. It may take additional personnel to help, and the Reality Interview or Life Space Interview is the technique (this is discussed elsewhere). It is mentioned here to point out that curriculum is life, as well as "books."

The implications of this section of intervention techniques are clear. One deals with the affective aspects in the educational context, which of course means that teachers must be as well trained in these procedures as in other mental health techniques. Mental health implies the proper bonding, synthesis and integration of the thinking and the feeling components of the individual. The school, being a microcosm of life, offers a wide variety of opportunities for unwinding tangled lives, and for providing new images to be integrated into troubled personalities.

325

Providing a Supportive Community Environment

The psychodynamic approach stresses the importance of providing restorative growth potentials through not only family surrogates, but through the broader community systems. There has been an imbalance in the amount of intra-psychic work with children, implying the omnipotent belief that a therapeutic hour can counteract the other twenty-three-hour-a-day experiences of a child; it is easy to forget the attention given, by social work in particular, to foster homes, and the emphasis of many writers, such as Redl, to the hygienic life space needs of disturbed children.

When the family support system cannot be made adequate through interventions, a substitute must be provided. When this is not done, we can see what happens (e.g., the use of the gang as family). Various programs have used non-professional personnel working with emotionally disturbed children to facilitate the identification process. The foster grandparent program, sponsored by the Office of Economic Opportunity, has used selected low-income grandparents who meet for several hours daily with children institutionalized because of parental loss or neglect. A follow-up study of one such program reported that:

> for many of our children the relationship with their
> foster grandparent is the first positive relationship
> they have had with an adult...The foster grandparents
> have helped children establish a sense of identity
> by each transmitting to the child his feelings that
> the child is special, through helping him know what he
> can do, and through helping him accept control (Johnston,
> 1957, pp.50-52).

The foster parent plan is well known. The Big Brother and Big Sister movements are an extension of this approach. The common basis is to provide desirable identification figures for each child.

Extra-family socialization opportunities are provided by recreational, religious, play, and work experiences, and by group programs in the community. Many of these are manned by volunteers. Most disturbed children and youth, however, are characteristically deprived of these extensions into the extra-familial community life. Their behavior does not fit well. The leadership is seldom prepared. The "boss" on the job for work experience can't be bothered. From the psychodynamic point of view, the mediation of regular services to aid disturbed children requires consultation supervision and careful planning. There are work stations where bosses do care enough to try to help an adolescent. Here is where the infusion of mental health concepts in the community is important. The community leaders need consultation and support by the mental health professions when they are confronted with youngsters who "need our program but they spoil it." While proper placement in stable groups or settings in itself may be enough for some youngsters, others will still respond atypically. The role of community mental health interventions is to expand the parameters of the community services to take in more children through consultative functions.

327

Particularly with adolescents, at this impulse-serving time of life, the broad cultural environment demands special attention. Mass media, the screen and music business are "choreographed" to present a confused value picture to youth, which exceeds the extent of viable life style variation. Crime in high places, fraud and dishonesty in all walks of life, exaggerated materialism--these every normal delinquent knows about. They provide him license for personal value distortion. The psychodynamic position sees these images as critical in the struggle to grow up with proper values. There is a great necessity to intervene in these matters. The tactics are several. Much more open discussion and frank exchange on the raw reality of the society is required, not avoidance or demand. This must be done with adults who live reasonable lives--not perfect but reasonable. Opportunities must be provided to sort out the values, and to see the fact that many adults do try and succeed in evolving a set of acceptable behaviors. One of the saddest aspects of the present emphasis on new styles of help is the conduct of enterprises by people who themselves model by clearly communicated signs, their identification with, if not actual performance of, the behavior which is a problem for the adolescent they seek to help. Thus they condone such things as "justified" aggression, impulse satisfaction without empathic feelings for others, the view that "it's no use so let's give up," inhuman behavior because "that's the way institutions are," and on and on. Here lies the significance of the psychodynamic preoccupation with the identification process and the provision of adequate models. Professional "rites" are no substitutes for the living model of behavior. Clearly, from the psychodynamic point of view, green thumb operations have their limitations, and mental health workers need training and self awareness.

C. Specially Designed "Therapeutic" Interventions

It has been indicated that the division between the good supportive growth environment interventions and those of more special design is a matter of descriptive convenience. This section discusses the extension and intensification of therapeutic techniques through special arrangements, rather than a separate set of concepts of how the more seriously disturbed child can be helped. The issue is this: from the psychodynamic point of view many seriously disturbed children are seen as not having the resources to restore or develop balance in their lives, even with adequate environmental conditions. The external conditions must be much more than just reasonable, because the seriously disturbed child has internalized and habituated certain behaviors. There is a huge unlearning, as well as new learning, to accomplish. The ensuing conflicts which accompany the restoration may be both inter-active and intra-active, and they are of such depth as to resist simple mediation.

The following sub-headings are used to group these interventions: the "classical" therapeutic approaches (individual, group, and family therapy); interventions through specially designed environments (schools, day schools, and life space mediation); expressive "therapies;" and finally, special designs to facilitate identification. These divisions are not theoretically logical, nor do they comprise a systematic sequence. In speaking of both designs and processes in a single series, the purpose is to explicate the major emphases of the psychodynamic approach rather than to attempt an integrated connection. Also, since classical interventions are well known, less space is devoted to these in contrast to some other approaches.

The Classical Therapies

Just as there is a theoretical core to the psychodynamic view, which is derived from the work of the Freudian school and other dynamic psychologists, so there is a group of classical therapies. All of these techniques embody a strong focus on the inner life of the child. Cognitive processes (e.g., insight and awareness) and affective processes (e.g., identification and transference) are interfaced in an effort to facilitate externalization of feelings, awareness of repressed conflicts and attitudes, and the development of new patterns of behavior. Traditional therapies take place both in individual and group settings.

The classical individual therapies emphasize the role of the therapist as a model for identification and transference as well as a facilitator of self-understanding. Albert (1963, p. 175) describes the importance of the identification processes in her corrective object relations therapy, in which the therapist

> strives to make good the phase-specific deprivations
> suffered by the child in its earlier experiences
> with its mother....She [the therapist] systematically
> builds up a dependent relationship of trust to which
> the child responds with increasing receptivity.

331

With older patients, the cognitive processes, directed toward development of insight, come also to play a significant role. With the young child, communication is through play. Special approaches are indicated for adolescents because of their emotional lability.

The therapeutic interview process has received much emphasis in the analytic and dynamic literature. Books are written (Lippman, 1962; Witmer, 1946; Pearson, 1968) and every nuance discussed and rediscussed (for example, the place of interpretation and explanation). For many, the office interview has been the beginning and the end. This, in spite of the problems of taking what was learned there out to the real world. It should be noted that while most adults talk a lot "at" children, often moralizing, repressing, and admonishing, the special type of communication needed to relate to a child or adolescent is of the understanding variety. We must listen, for a major goal is to understand and deal with the child's experience of himself and his world.

The classical group therapies (Slavson, 1943; Slavson, 1950; Speers and Lansing, 1965; Kraft, 1971) capitalize on the strong "social hunger"(Slavson, 1943, p. 15) which conditions the effectiveness of group processes and on the powerful role which peers can play in influencing one another. A therapy group, in which each child is unconditionally accepted by the therapist, provides a situation in which the child need not prove himself or conform to a role which is pre-determined by his peers, for the process of group definition is one in which all members can take part. As they do so, they may become aware of the roles that they play both within the group and outside it. The free atmosphere of the group allows the child to "try on" new patterns of behavior and to discover how they feel to him. Finally, the open atmosphere which is cultivated within the group facilitates each child's getting direct feedback about how his behavior makes other people feel. Again, this is a much discussed intervention. The group can be used as a place where children bring their problems to discuss, or where the interaction of the members provides the material for discussion. Basic in any case is the understanding of the dynamics of the manifest behavior.

Lastly, the family therapies described elsewhere in this report, represent another "classical" approach. Here focus is on the unique dynamics which produce the child's problem, and input is directed towards the whole family complex, which is seen as responsible for the problem. Again, the work may be done with individual family members or with family interaction as displayed in a group session.

Special Supportive Environments

Considerable material has been presented relative to normal development and restorative help. The more intensive efforts, for the more seriously disturbed youngster, to be discussed in this

333

section, should be seen as an extension of the same techniques.[5]

The degree to which environmental situations should be abstracted or "therapized" is a continual question. The psycho-dynamic viewpoint, with its historical and implicit tendency toward ritualistic professionalism and its vulnerability to over-selling esoteric aspects, has cause to be most reflective when it comes to such matters. The belief in the powerful magic of the pressurized cabin world of the individualized interview (Redl, 1959b) versus the broader based child need-support systems can lead to sorry results. The other twenty-three hours (Trieschman, et al., 1969) is the child's total life space input. It is not either/or, but a balance of intra and inter efforts which must be maintained.

Another problem is the belief that specially created, sep-arated environments (run by professionals) will solve all the dis-turbed child's problems. He will get "well" there and subsequently be immune to a distorted support system when he returns to regular living. The success of an intervention is evaluated on the basis of the psychological experience the child actually has during ther-apy; the structuring of this experience is related to information obtained in the assessment procedure. The complications of pro-viding corrective development--given the concept of human nature

---

5 Many of the environmental mediations discussed in this section
are treated in Melinda Wagner, "Environmental Interventions in
Emotional Disturbance," in this volume.

and learning held in this paper, suggest no facile solutions are likely to be found.

The areas to be considered are several. The family is the first. (Family therapy has already been discussed.) It should be added that foster family care for seriously disturbed children cannot be done without providing a great deal of support and interpretation. Green thumb expertise does happen, but most frequently the patience, control of counter transference, and ability to both accept and structure the surrogate family do not come automatically. The twenty-four-hour-a-day abrasiveness, regressive periods, and testing which take place are not easy for any foster care personnel to handle. There will be, even in the most well trained personnel, the need for careful examination of interactive processes which develop between adult and child. As Jules Henry (1965) has proposed, the interaction of what seem on the surface to be normal families can generate pathological environments for children. Thus, it would be necessary to continually monitor and support the up-bringers in foster family situations. It is well known that disturbed youngsters have a great deal to work through in even the most benign foster placement, because of the significance of the "other than real parents" for identity formation. Treatment of the disturbed child by foster family must be attuned to the psychological components and underlying motivations. This requires participation of mental health personnel.

The extra-familial community life, a source of much nor-
malizing potential, also requires a great deal of mental health
input to function as a resource for the seriously disturbed.
The range here is from astute utilization of the community group
life, to the development of therapeutically operated substitutes.
Leaders and the peer groups themselves must be helped to integrate
even the very hard-to-accept atypical child. It should be remembered that the first labelling of the disturbed child takes place
with peers who find the child's behavior a source of threat to
their own integration: there is no automatic osmosis which produces automatic dividends. It must be worked out in detail.

The concrete issue implied is this: do we integrate the
schizophrenic child into a regular scout troop or do we establish
special groups for them? Do we have work therapy where a mental
health worker cushions the adolescent's regular employment or do
we have sheltered workshops? The simple reality is that the sheltered condition may be necessary for some as they learn to maximize their potentials, and for others as a lifetime protection.
But, with medication and psychotherapy, the number who need a lifetime of custodial, nullifying, degrading (even if benign) total
isolation is infinitessimal. The purpose of intensive psychotherapy
(whatever the limitations) is to help the child so that he will be
able to live in the least specialized environment possible. To be
toilet trained, to be able to dress and feed oneself, to find one's

way, to function in a "work" station--these expand the potentials for a normalized life. The idea of a protective therapeutic sub-community which enhances the individual's maximum normal partici-pation, but provides necessary protection, responds both to the limitations for development found in certain individuals and to their resources.

The specialized school intervention. Highly specialized school is one of the essential restorative-supportive interventions, with a vast range of programs and styles (Wolman, 1972). It may be a therapeutic nursery (Furman and Katan, 1969) or a parent training program as developed by Fenichel's League School. It may be a "kindergarten" level program for adolescents who need it, or a curriculum of learning self-care survival skills which enable one to live outside a back ward. On the other hand, school may be a modified typical school program. The cultivation of particular artistic or mathematical talents may be the core for some young-sters. A therapeutic school responds to "academic" problems and "life problems" as they become evident in the school environment. School for the seriously disturbed contains a more astute combi-nation of the components described in the prior educational sec-tion.

It has been pointed out that the psychodynamic position has been less specific when it comes to cognitive processes and learning than in dealing with the affective area. There was even

337

a time when school interventions for disturbed children were but
an extension of a permissive, let-the-poison-out, catharsis-will-
heal view of psychotherapy which was then in vogue. Contrary to
such a simplistic notion, the school is really a micro-world, a
life space where, since many things happen, there are many possible
avenues for subinterventions. The attention to neurotic uses of
learning (Sperling, 1967; Pearson, 1952; Grunebaum, et al., 1962;
Sperry et al., 1958; Liss, 1955; Klein, 1949; English and Pearson,
1972) is one phase of this position. Learning problems can be a
displacement to cover the real source of the tension, which is too
difficult to face. Failure to learn is a consequence of some outside problems--resistance, anger, fear, role expectations--which
are displaced to the school arena. Just as such neurotic uses of
schooling should not be ignored, neither should they be applied to
all school problems as a universal explanation. For most children,
learning skills of reading, computation, and comprehending their
world is the core of development. While they will always be pre-
occupied with their life problem, for these children not to achieve
is destructive to self esteem. This is true of learning to read
as well as learning to behave reasonably with peers and authority.
The benefits of academic learning are thus seen as direct--self
accomplishment necessary to self esteem--and indirect, or instrumental to pleasing important others and thereby gaining recognition.

Since the selection of the methodology employed to

338

stimulate any kind of learning is indicated by the assessment process, no methodology is of and in itself good or bad. The question
at hand is, what procedures will facilitate school learning in a
given child? There is both a developmental (Hewett, 1964) and a
characterological component of what will motivate a youngster at
a given point in his psychological life. For this reason, the use
of natural rewards, points, privileges and the like have their
places; our goal is to help him learn and this may be the procedure
of choice as indicated by the assessment. Severe punishment as a
contingency would be seen as a violation of the individual, but
there is no question, as Redl has said, that pain in some degree
enters into the learning complex. Again, the avoidance of over-
loads of punishment or traumatizing "unrewards" is essential.
Punishment, after all, is in the perception of the receiver and
not in the act alone. The only way one can utilize contingencies
is to know what they are. The only one who can tell us is the
individual. His needs and drives are what make the contingencies
operate.

Expanded though the parameters are, school always contains
an element of reality which requires flexible though established
limits on what the child may and may not do. Minimally, considerations of the child's own safety and that of those around him requires that there be some things he simply is not allowed to do.
The purpose of limits is more than adult convenience. As has been

stated, "disturbed children fear their own loss of control and
need protection against their own impulses; what they need are
teachers who know how to limit as well as accept them (Fenichel,
1971, p. 339)." The establishment of such limits serves to provide help with a whole range of decisions about behaviors. The
child is provided with established guidelines for what actions
will hurt others or himself, as well as with what should be goals
for his life patterns.

For the child who violates such limitations, even brief
non-punitive physical restraint may be required at times. When
he breaks the rules because he cannot control himself, restraint
is applied so that the child will hurt neither himself nor others;
the restrainer takes over and provides an external control temporarily until the child has regained his own. The basic message
of the adult's responding with physical restraint must come across,
and the situation is used for discussion and talk with the youngster:

> We like you. There is nothing to fear, but there
> is also nothing to gain by such behavior. You
> didn't get us mad by it, for we know you can't
> help it right now. But we sure hope this will
> reduce as time goes on. We aren't holding it
> against you, either. You can't "make up for
> it." You needn't; the behavior is too crazy and
> unreasonable for any such thought. We want only
> one thing; get it over with, snap back into
> your more reasonable self, so we can communi-
> cate with you again. Right now you don't even
> see who is with you doing what. Remember?
> This is not an ogre out of the past or a figment

340

of your delusions. This is me, the guy who
likes you and is here to help. Right now he
is helping in only one way, by taking over...
No hard feelings...Don't think of it even.
It's all water over the dam. You will soon
be able to do without this...(Redl and Wineman, 1952, p. 212).

When a child has committed an act which clearly violates

the established limits, punishment may be an appropriate interven-

tion. Redl comments that punishment is only a constructive inter-

vention when it represents a "planful attempt by the adult to in-

fluence either the behavior or the long-range development of a

child or a group of children, for their own benefit, by exposing

them to an unpleasant experience (Redl, 1971a, p. 435)." To this

end, the punishment experience must fulfill the following seven

criteria (Redl, 1971a, pp. 435-6):

(1) The child experiences the displeasure to
    which the adult exposes him.
(2) The experience makes the child angry.
(3) The child perceives that his situation
    is the result of his previous behavior.
(4) The child gets angry with himself for
    getting into this predicament.
(5) The energy of his anger gets transformed
    so that it can be used for his benefit.
(6) He uses this energy to:
    (a) regret what he did.
    (b) resolve not to repeat the incident.
(7) Future incidents call up the punishment
    experience and are met with increased ego
    control so that his misbehavior is not
    repeated.

Another approach to maximizing a reasonable reality is to

limit the behavioral options open to the child to those which are

acceptable and in which he is sure to succeed. Since choice-making

341

and the development of autonomy are vital developmental goals, it
is crucial that the child's initial ventures in this direction do
not meet with failure. Thus careful structuring of situations,
with increasing options over time, but with all options promising
success, is an important tactic. This discussion has embodied a
reflection of Freud himself, who was attentive to the reality
principle as well as to the id.

The hope is that the child will receive personal dividends
in self esteem and life coping by what he has learned. The psychodynamic position emphasizes the human aspects: the response of a
respected teacher, the fulfillment of buried or overt hopes and
aspirations of the individual. The technique is of and in itself
always subservient to the meaning of the intervention with a given
youngster in a given condition. Applications are dependent upon
assessment and clinical awareness. Lovitt (1973) has described
the use of charting and behavior management to facilitate the
development of independence. While it would seem more appropriate
to approach such problems in terms of their dynamics, the essential use of the learning process is certainly a reasonable intervention. It has been the observation of many using behavior modification that other human and self rewards are often sufficient
to motivate learning when the pupil discovers he can learn. On
the other hand, diagnostically speaking, there are children, youth,
and adults who respond only to external contingencies. The psycho-

342

dynamic assessment would guard against ignoring these conditions, and would also include techniques appropriate to those with inner conflict.

Therapeutic education implies specific design of the educational situation to limit stress at any time to that level with which the child can cope. Jacobson and Faegre's (1959) technique of <u>neutralization</u> is one method of limitation of stressful stimuli. It is based on the view that curricular materials which touch in some way on the child's own problems can "arouse multiple associations and distracting fantasies (Jacobson and Faegre, 1959, p. 244)," and thus serve as a serious block to mastering the intended cognitive skills or subject matter. Types of materials which may carry such emotional loading include "happy-family" stories depicting middle-class life styles, scenes involving bodily damage, and object lessons. Conversely, topics which are generally neutral are those which take place far away or long ago, struggles against nature, or scientific facts. Basic to this concept is that many tasks may signal failure. One then approaches the task in an entirely new way to avoid the arousal of defeating reactions. Or one uses small doses of the experience to avoid build-up. But one does not always avoid such issues. The teacher may discuss and counsel around the reaction, so that the youngster begins to consciously deal with his behavior.

Since schools are group work agencies for the most part,

there are realities to the conduct of the operation. Pupils with a low frustration tolerance need an escape. They may need to leave entirely at times as Chapman (1962) suggests. Under this plan, student and teacher mutually agree upon conditions under which the child will be unobtrusively requested to leave the school because of his inability to conform to necessary behavioral standards. When a school situation becomes so stressful that the child cannot control himself, systems like this, or Redl and Wineman's "antiseptic removal" (1952), provide a mechanism (which the pupil has had a part in constructing) whereby he can be removed from the stressful situation without any punitive connotations. But the act of removal should be utilized in crisis intervention or with a crisis teacher to help the child learn to understand and cope with school.

Failure, and the child's fear of it, constitutes a very significant source of stress, especially within the school situation. Glasser (1969) sees school without failure as mandatory. As Bettelheim comments, "the most important therapeutic contribution the teacher can make is in giving the children a real chance to succeed in their work (Bettelheim, 1959, p. 140)." Thus, whatever arrangements and environmental manipulations can be made to minimize or eliminate failure experiences will be highly therapeutic. Temporary grouping with specially moderated expectation systems is often helpful, as is tutorial assistance where only

344

one trusted person sees the failure to perform.

Frequently a particular task or concept may be the source of a great deal of frustration and may result in disruptive behavior. Thus a teacher's "hurdle help"--giving the child directed tutorial guidance--may, by heading off incipient failure, result in behavioral as well as intellectual benefits (Redl and Wineman, 1952, p. 176).

In addition to the appeals to the child's overall cognitive apparatus which we have discussed, there are also techniques which address themselves to the more specific skills of reading and language. The keeping of calendars and diaries provides a focus for reflection of feelings, experiences, and expectations. Indirect benefits are accrued to any adults with whom these might be shared, as they present a focussed view of events which are most important to the child. This can be very helpful to those who are trying to understand and help him. The writing of auto-biographies as a classroom assignment serves a similar function.

From the psychodynamic position, the teacher always plays an important role in pupils' school life, and thus it is logical to have that person deal with affective issues. The important role which the teacher plays in the restorative identification process shall be discussed in a later section. It is sufficient to note here that the teacher can embody a powerful force in her/his students' lives. For this reason, the degree of self

345

understanding and interactive control needed by a special teacher is parallel to the theoretical knowledge. The persistent, formative patience needed to promote learning by a group of autistic youngsters is rare indeed in the mental health profession. The fact is, it is a rare combination in mental health workers: there are few who are able to spend long periods of time in intensive, goal-oriented activities with very disturbed children. It is to be noted that the original high priority accorded the interview hour is now shared by school and living time in the milieu as Redl (1959b) has indicated.

To provide the chance for maximum adult transference reactions, a male and female teacher have been employed in some settings. In addition to being the teacher, the adult is a model for identification, a counselor, a group worker, a worker with parents, an advocate, mediator, and much more. The role is most complex. There is reason to believe that limited accomplishments of many very disturbed youngsters is a consequence of not getting enough intensified, personalized education. The results of one child and one teacher working a long time together with a precise and consistently executed education plan are depicted in Tommy (Steucher, 1972), which reflects the unique combination of pressure and giving necessary with most difficult children.

The three dimensions of the educational environment which contain the potentials for specialization are the adult-child

346

reaction, the peer group phenomenon, and the learning substance-method complex. We are speaking here of the utmost sophistication in the adjustment of these three elements in relationship to the individual child's needs (Morse, 1971a; Long, Morse, and Newman, 1971; Hewett, 1964). The teacher as an adult figure, and the group aspects have been mentioned elsewhere. The type of substance taught and the method are responsive to need structures, pupil relevance, and individual learning style. These were discussed in the prior school section.

The provision of extended day or total day programs is considered necessary when more of the interactions must be controlled, and more of the child's life must be under protective planning short of total residential care.

Specially planned and controlled milieu interventions. From the psychodynamic position, it is clear from the start that all children live and learn in a milieu. Sometimes this life space needs alteration. When the needed changes cannot be accomplished in situ, largely because the child has high needs and/or has internalized aberrant responses, a very special milieu is required. In contrast to putting a child away, this is seen as putting him in the place with the highest investment to help. The choice, for those very few who need such intensive support, is not whether to provide institutionalization. It is what care we are going to provide. Should it be a mental health saturated

347

controlled mileu, (Brunstetter, 1973) or a purely custodial placement; or as has been amply documented-an actually punitive, negative learning environment which constitutes the milieu in many
institutions? In dealing with delinquents, it is evident that
most institutionalizations increase the chances of a delinquent
career (Robins, 1966).

Redl (1959a) has described in detail what a therapeutic
milieu means for children. It is a setting which maximizes the
many resources the child needs on a twenty-four-hour-a-day basis,
until he can utilize a less specially maximized environment. It
goes without saying that there is never a child who needs to be
cut off one hundred per cent from the outer world, and even with
institutionalization one separates from the total community only
where it is functionally necessary. If resources are not adequate--
no transportation, one worker to ten children, and the like--it may
not be possible to take children out of the confines. But this is
an artifact of the design, not a feature of a child's problem. All
good institutional work is very, very expensive. Large institutions increase the mechanistic, dehumanizing aspects. After all,
the purpose of institutional care is to provide a surrogate family
experience, with acceptance, care and identification. That it can
be done has been demonstrated (Guindon, 1970).

Within the planned microcosm, the total tone, identification figures, adequate and pleasant life care (food, shelter,

348

clothing), a rich activity program, appropriate schooling, recreational life, monitored group life, free time, community contact with hygienic management and care rules are blended with special individual and group therapies as well as medical care. It must be a rich environment, an economy of abundance. Bettelheim's (1950) descriptions and films indicate the treatment potential for psychotic children.

From the dynamic viewpoint, multidisciplinary focus is critical. There must be a homogeneous character to all actions in the milieu, with a mental health viewpoint. It is interesting to note that many exemplary institutions are an extension of the image of an outstanding mental health leader. The over-reliance on architecture (which is important and contributes, of course) and the willingness to forget that the Gestalt is more than the sum of the separate disciplines have contributed to the sad state of children's institutional care. The need for personnel supervision and total integration of services is seldom met, though again it can be done (Guindon, 1969, 1972).

Intervention through Reality Interpretation and Mitigation

Whatever the milieu and whatever the reality, there will be, with discordant children, abrasive times which can be used to therapeutic ends. Since we have postulated the essential place of the interactive process in helping children, it is necessary to reinforce the fact that the psychodynamic approach has moved from over-reliance on the classical therapeutic interview for change in the child. The idea was that the child will then transfer growth to the outside world. It is now recognized that learning demands the exploitation of the real life interactive difficulties themselves. While it took those who dealt with delinquents to develop and sharpen this idea, the same attention occurred whenever therapists had to deal with milieu behavior. Caplan (1964) called this concept crisis intervention.

The intervention technique designed to resolve reality conflicts is called by Redl (1959b) "Life Space Interviewing" and by Glasser (1964) "Reality Interviewing." While it starts with the outside conflict, it combines this with an awareness of the motivational aspects of the individual. Nor is this the province of the mental experts alone: it is an "on the line" intervention which can be learned by teachers and others (Morse, 1963). Whatever the reality, there are most likely (though not always) periods of conflict. The attention to mitigating conflict and learning around conflict is just as crucial as the attention devoted to internal conflict. In fact, one without the other shortchanges the psychodynamic approach. A comprehensive theory which permeates the many realms of life is required to help disturbed children.

Another procedure considered important is to reduce the competing stimuli in an environment when necessary. Redl talks about the seductive nature of props. The external world is filled with

cues which may be too suggestive. Twelve cans of paint and a lot
of big brushes invite disaster. There are always figure and
ground in the outer world, and the teacher tries to arrange
these in a pattern which will be within the child's coping
capacities for the goals at hand.

"Expressive" Therapeutic Interventions

From the psychodynamic point of view, the synthesis of
the affective and cognitive life is essential for mental health,
since individuals are both thinking and feeling beings. Too often
descriptions are used as explanations in such matters as catharsis,
sublimation, projection, symbolization, externalization, "handling"
one's problems and the like. However, regardless of the difficulty
of understanding how these processes work, one is on accepted ground
in setting up interventions which depend upon such well recognized
processes. There is, in addition to the conscious aspect of these
devices, much of which reflects the unconscious. Youngsters dream,
symbolize, act out, fantasize, and project. The supposition is
that emotional aspects and conflicts are often expressed in indirect
ways. After the King assassination, ghetto children drew their fear
pictures. The inner angry child draws aggressive pictures, etc.
Externalization through various means reduces the tension, and even
though there is no conscious interpretation of the content, the expression enables the individual to reduce the debilitating force
of the problem. We have grouped the techniques with this aim under

the overall rubric of expressive therapy. Since they can be conducted on a non-interpretive basis (though there are advocates of interpretation) it is obvious what important significance these interventions have for the special school. The same processes are used by normal as well as disturbed children. Play has been called the natural therapy of children. It is interesting that seriously disturbed children often cannot utilize play without help.

This group of interventions supports and develops the child's expressive abilities. Such techniques serve to mobilize the child's internal resources in a number of ways: they facilitate involvement through activity rather than retreat and withdrawal; they provide acceptable channels for cathartic release; they serve as means of both externalizing the child's conflicts and communicating his feelings about them to others (though both the signal and response may be nonverbal, and nonconscious and not discussed); and many of the expressive media seem to embody inherent "therapeutic" qualities. For children with verbal inhibitions, the whole "language" may be nonverbal.

The sequence and dynamics of such processes have been found to take place even with youngsters who have been written off as having no inner life or potential for positive goal generation. There are ways to get to youth who would resist any psychotherapy, or "shrinks". Slack (1960) paid juvenile delinquent boys to be subjects for an experimental study. In a very nurturant atmosphere, the subjects met with the therapist, took psychological tests, and spent hours alone talking into a tape recorder while being paid. Slack reports that this format proved very successful in introducing unwilling subjects to the realities of psychotherapy. Over time they came to recognize needs and problems within themselves and to accept help to deal with them. There was a sequence which followed a pattern. First came hostility, blaming and anger. This was followed by depression. Then the intolerable realization of how bad things were began to be replaced with the search for hope and a rationale. This produced goals, the start of hope and the readiness to get help. Then help had to be provided to prevent deterioration. If this be true of hard core cases, we should certainly recognize the importance of the potential inner life of all children.

The view that <u>catharsis</u> is an inherently therapeutic process underlies a number of therapeutic approaches. The idea that the expression, acting out, or "release" of strong feelings is therapeutic in itself has generated the development of techniques for facilitating such release.

Various forms of play therapy serve this function. Levy's (1938) <u>release therapy</u> utilizes the child's play with toys provided in the treatment setting to reconstruct traumatic situations associated with the onset of the child's symptoms. Levy presents case studies of patients who, after only a few sessions, were completely free of symptoms, after having achieved expression of their trauma-associated anxieties in the play situation.

In the life of the normal child games and play serve a cathartic function. Children play out fears and hates with the "make world" game; they role play and pretend much of their play time. They impose form and structure on the objects about them, thus revealing and externalizing their inner life. Games, such as "Red Rover" or punching a punching bag, which ritualize and provide structured opportunities for aggression and other strong emotions serve an important "defusing" function. In fact all games have an overt form and a covert psychological function. Various roles are created, limitations enforced, contracts embodied, emotions generated. Some games are of high role visibility (baseball), others low identity (tug of war). Games of all sorts have become adult pastimes as well as childhood occupations.

Interventions which strengthen ego controls do not have to rely on crises or stressful situations to be effective. Participation in games, for example, can provide a low-pressure, high-reward structure for learning the concept of rules. The idea that there are "rules of the game," once learned, may be transferred to less structured situations (Bower, 1964).

Verbal catharsis may also be therapeutic for the child. The creation of situations which accept and foster the expression of strong feelings of anger, hate, fear, etc. is thus an important therapeutic approach. The phenomenon of transference frequently results in those feelings being expressed toward the therapist rather than the parent, sibling, or teacher who may originally have elicited them. Although the situation which generated strong feelings may remain unchanged, the process of "getting it all out" is therapeutic in itself. Baruch (1944) has used the expression "let the poison out."

Externalizing and communicating feelings and conflicts proves useful in both direct and indirect ways. For the child, the therapeutic effect of such expression is closely tied to the phenomenon of sublimation, which Kramer defines as

> any process in which a primitive asocial impulse
> is transformed into a socially productive act, so
> that the pleasure in the achievement of the social
> act replaces the pleasure which gratification of
> the original urge would have afforded (Kramer, 1958,
> pp. 11-12).

All of the creative arts--music, art, dance, drama, poetry, and creative writing--represent forms for symbolization and sublimation whereby the impulses get translated into products which are socially tolerable, useful or even rewarded. Play represents a similar phenomenon in children. The externalization process also has indirect benefits, for those working with the child can learn much about his feelings, conflicts, and needs from the way he expresses himself in such communicative activities.

The expressive medium which has been most extensively

exploited by those who work with children is that of <u>play</u>. Play

forms an important and integral part of the growing child's exper-

ience. It is a medium by which he first imitates those around him,

and then gradually comes to explore his surroundings, test out new

behaviors, and form physical and conceptual models of his world

(Sutton-Smith, 1971). Play thus occupies an important part in the

normal and deviant child's physical, emotional, and cognitive de-

velopment.

In the course of their play (and especially in that which

is spontaneous rather than ritualized) children "from three on up

project...the basic time-space patterns of their lives (Murphy,

1972, p. 119)" as well as how they see themselves and others, what

they feel, etc. It is this expressive component of play which

has been extensively used in the development of the play therapies.

Erikson comments on the range of expressive capacities inherent in

play:

> True, the themes presented betray some repetitive-
> ness such as we recognize as the "working through"
> of a <u>traumatic</u> experience: but they also express
> playful <u>renewal</u>. If they seem to be governed by
> some need to communicate, or even to <u>confess</u>,
> they certainly also seem to serve the joy of
> <u>self-expression</u> (Erikson, 1972, p. 131).

The technique of <u>non-directive play therapy</u> (Axline, 1947;

Moustakas, 1952) is designed to utilize the expressive components

of spontaneous play. It is conducted, either individually or in

a group, in a playroom setting which is equipped with a variety of

356

toys and dolls, finger paints, puppets, clay, paints, nursing bottles, and often a large sandbox. The child is invited to use any of these materials as he wishes, within established limits of safety. The function of the therapist is to create an atmosphere of faith, acceptance, and respect for the child (Moustakas, 1953, p.2). Within the play situation, Moustakas, Axline, and many others use the Rogerian technique of reflection of those feelings that are expressed by the child in his play. As the child comes to see that, despite the strong feelings he expresses, he is still accepted and respected, he often gains in security. At the same time, the therapist's reflection of the child's feelings helps the child to focus his generally negative feelings on specific persons or things, and to deal with them more effectively. Generally, as the negative feelings become more defined, the child begins to express positive feelings as well. The success of this technique is seen as dependent, in large part, on the ability of the therapist to communicate his acceptance to the child and to accurately reflect the child's feelings without being judgmental.

Another expressive medium which has proved very useful in therapy is <u>art</u> (Kramer, 1971). Children, far more than older persons, are open to free artistic expression, for "defenses and repressions are not yet firmly established, and the reality principle has not gained complete ascendance over the pleasure principle (Kramer, 1958, p.18)." Art is thus seen as "a method of linking the conscious and unconscious (Lyddiatt, 1970, p.3)." Because it replaces the acting out of fantasies with the creation of visual images, art clearly represents an important channel for sublimation of unacceptable impulses. But, Kramer contends, "works of art always remain emotionally charged...Art differs here from most other forms of sublimation (Kramer, 1958, p.16)." This emotional loading of artistic creations is one reason that it is a useful therapeutic tool.

Art therapy programs generally focus on the therapeutic effect of artistic production--the "fusion between reality and fantasy, between the unconscious and the conscious (Kramer, 1958, p.23)." In some cases they may also use the communicative aspects of the child's creations to help understand his feelings and conflicts.

The art therapist's function is primarily to support and facilitate the child's artistic expression. There are advocates of interpretation but many therapists let the matter rest with an uninterpreted creative production. For the severely disturbed child, who is afraid both of failure and of his feelings, to begin with pencil or paints and a blank paper may be very threatening; in such situations, first tracing and then copying are "safe" ways of gradually introducing the child to the experience of artistic creation (Berkowitz and Rothman, 1951). The availability of a range of materials for art and related craft activities makes it possible

for each child to choose media appropriate to his needs. As
Slavson writes, "some youngsters require materials that can be
easily molded, flexed or changed. The aggressive and strong, on
the other hand, can work with materials that challenge their powers
(1954, p.191)."

Because each creation is valued for itself, as a complete
and expressive product of the child, art work can be an important
source of self esteem and success experiences. Display of the
children's works (without choosing them for technical quality) in
a common area of the school or center can provide an important
boost for the child's self-image.

Finally, for those who also use the child's art as a
projective tool, it reveals much about his conflicts and feelings.
What he draws (real events or fantasies, people or things) and how
he draws it (distortions of body image, use of color, etc.) show
a great deal about how the child feels and how he views himself and
the world around him (Kellogg, 1967).

Music has been used as both a stimulus and a medium for
expression. Heimlich (1965) describes an extensive therapeutic
program using music as a means of communication. The therapist may
sing or play music which she feels speaks to the child's conflicts;
this is then used as a stimulus for responses which may include verbal comments, finger painting, singing along, moving to the music,
etc. These communications provide useful insights into the feelings

aroused by specific musical content. Frequently, when cognitive skills are not sufficiently developed to permit the child to comment verbally on a given song, he may indicate his involvement with its content by asking to have it repeated. For example, a boy who had been mute for eight months repeatedly asked for "Do, Do Pity My Case," "Sleep, My Little One," and "Mama, Gimme, Gimme."

The child's participation in the making of music can also be used therapeutically. Since rhythm is an important determinant of the emotional content of music (Altshuler, 1954) and rhythm instruments are the simplest to use, much music therapy with children centers on this aspect of music. Heimlich uses small-group improvisations, with therapist back-up, as the opening activity in her therapy sessions. In individual sessions, the child may provide a story and basic rhythm, upon which he and the therapist build a song. Like any story-telling process, the creation of such songs reveals much about the issues which are important to the child. The addition of the rhythmic component provides a medium for emphasizing the words or phrases that are most important to the child.

In addition, music alone has long been known to have therapeutic effects, especially on mood. Music has been used as therapy for anxiety (Girard, 1954), depression (Herman, 1954a), fatigue (Herman, 1954b), grief (Brown, 1954b), headache (Brown, 1954a) and psychosomatic gastric disorders (Sugarman, 1954).

Group singing is a universal social experience. With

adolescents, learning to play the guitar has been popular recently, and there are those who find much release and self esteem in mastering musical performance. The power of music can be seen in the rock-drug culture and in the explosive emotional experiences in mass gatherings, to say nothing of the symbolic lyrics. Should such a medium be left to commercial exploitation?

The therapeutic use of _dance_ as an expressive medium reflects the recognition that

> children are in the period of transition from nonverbal communication to communication using verbal symbols. They have not yet given up the use of their bodies in direct action in response to emotion (Chace, 1959, p.119).

Dance, either "free-form" or inspired by music, represents a basic medium of expression for the child. Its ritualism facilitates externalization of feelings and conflicts. At the same time, dance also fosters new awareness of the physical organism and encourages the development of improved motor coordination. As the child becomes more sure of his ability to move and to be rhythmic in his movements, Chace comments, "he often develops a feeling of greater security and confidence in himself (1959, p.120)." The stilted and rigid movement of disturbed children is well recognized.

That the content of _dreams_ reflects the emotional content of the unconscious has long been observed by psychodynamic therapists. Thus, when an intervening adult has gained the child's trust sufficiently that the child will share his dreams, those dreams may

361

serve as a useful vehicle for communicating what is important to him. The therapeutic use of dream material need not be restricted to the analyst's couch, as Jones' report of the use of "dream time" in a first grade class demonstrates (Jones, 1968, pp.246-252). Class time was set aside for children to fantasize--to stories, to music, or without external stimuli. These "dreams," as well as remembered nighttime dreams, were shared with the class. Examples of dreams the children reported are:

> This isn't a dream, but it didn't happen either. My bed turned into a horse.

> I dreamt that a snake was chasing Joe. I was up in an airplane, and I came down and killed the snake before it killed Joe.

> I dreamt there was a fight in school. Mrs. Werlin [the teacher] was clubbing everybody and they were clubbing her back with their heads. Their heads fell off. A big bird picked you [the teacher] up and me up and dropped us in the sea. I sank to the bottom. Under the water I was looking for you (Jones, 1968, pp.246-250).

A related use of the child's fantasies, which has been extensively developed as a therapeutic technique, is that of writing or telling stories. Storytelling as a projective technique is a well-established part of the psychologist's repertoire. Such tests as the Picture Story Test and the Children's Apperception Test present ambiguous situations about which the child is asked to tell a story. These standardized tests have grown out of the observations that children's stories closely reflect what is going on in their own emotional world.

362

Story-telling alone serves the dual functions of externalization and communication. In his _mutual story-telling_ technique Gardner (1971) has extended the use of story-telling to make it a medium for therapeutic input as well. The child is invited to participate in a "TV program" which will involve taping stories told by both himself and the therapist. He is then directed to tell a story and to explain the moral of the story. The therapist then re-tells a similar story which

> involves the same characters, settings, and initial
> situation as the child's story, but...has a more
> appropriate or salutary resolution of the most
> important conflicts...[The therapist] attempts to
> provide the child with more _alternatives_. The com-
> munication that the child need not be enslaved by his
> neurotic behavior patterns is vital. [The therapist's
> moral] is an attempt to emphasize further the healthier
> adaptations included in [the therapist's] story (Gardner,
> 1971, pp.29-30).

After both stories have been taped, about one-third of Gardner's patients choose to hear a replay of the whole "show," which provides a second exposure to the message which the therapist is conveying through his story.

As Hansen (1971) points out, the lure which machines hold for the child makes the _tape recorder_ itself a strong motivator for such expressive activities as story-telling, making "radio-plays," etc.

Drama represents another important therapeutic medium which can be used in a number of ways. Role playing is one facet. Drama facilitates the clarification of the feelings associated with and

363

the realities of situations about which the child feels strong

conflict. Among the ways in which this is achieved include:

(1) Focus on real occurrences
re-enacting an incident, with directions to attend
to the feelings that it arouses
re-enacting an incident, but with the participants
reversing roles and focussing on what their new
position feels like
soliloquy--(Moreno, p.190)--recreating a loaded
event with an emphasis on expression of feelings
which were hidden or held back when it first occurred.

(2) Focus on significant persons
portrayal by the child of a significant person in his
life, about whom the therapist suspects he feels
a good deal of conflict.

(3) Focus on process and feelings, using new situations--
directions may vary in specificity from:
Bill, you play a counter man at a lunch counter in
the South that has never served Negroes. You be
behind the counter attending to some washing. Chuck
and Mary, you be Negro teenagers who have come to
demand service. [After they have proceeded a bit.]
Fred, you be a white person who enters the lunch
room and helps with the argument on the side that
seems to be getting the worst of it; to merely "Who
will be three friends arguing on a street corner?"
(Ratho, et al., 1966, p.121)

This last structure is especially well suited to classroom

use and can serve to provide a "safe" situation for trying out new

behaviors (Gray, 1969) and generating material for reflecting on

feelings, realities of conflicts, and so on.

Bibliotherapy (Schultheis, 1973), started as a method of

helping delinquents externalize. They were asked to participate

in a continuing contract to read certain material and then write

follow up letters to the court. The choice of reading materials appropriate to the child's needs and disturbance is an opportunity to provide an individualized stimulus to thinking about reasonable solutions to personal problems. Stories may be chosen which reflect many of the circumstances of the child's life but within which, for example, the main character chooses more appropriate and rewarding patterns of behavior (La Benne, 1967). The introduction of reading material and/or films which speak to issues which are important to the child may generate new insights and understandings on his part.

Although the specialized way in which many of the expressive forms have been adapted to psychotherapy may not be directly employed in the classroom, the basic principles which underlie the therapeutic use of the expressive process are essential for any special classroom. The importance of involvement in captivating activity should certainly be considered in planning classroom programs. Physical education programs can be structured to include games and activities which facilitate cathartic release. The "therapies" based on play and the arts are feasible in the school: the inclusion of art, music, dance, drama, writing, and play in the educational program for the disturbed child creates a therapeutic channel, by virtue of the sublimation and cathartic expression that the arts provide. The psychodynamic position eschews basket weaving and ritualistic occupational therapy. It is not a cooking class but an experience with food, an oral involvement.

The life of school can incorporate many important processes

which occur outside of school. The expressive therapies are but an extension of the significant processes of the culture, and should not be alien to the classroom. Dance ceremonials are present in most cultures; art, music, painting--all are the essence of culture. They can generate or modulate feelings and are the most natural, abiding experiences of mankind. They are, in the ultimate sense of the term, schooling. When they are recognized as such, special schools need no longer hesitate to offer these therapies as "curriculum."

Of course teachers need training in such media. Collaborative multidisciplinary efforts are anticipated. The pity is, so often these therapeutic channels are so "educationalized" in classrooms that they become dull, drill-like, perfunctory time-spacers, or are neglected altogether.

Recognition of the benefits of arousing interest and involvement in constructive activities has generated programs specifically designed to foster such involvement. For younger children the small activity group discussed above represents such a program. As children get older, work experiences, if carefully planned, can fulfill a similar function. A sheltered workshop may be the most vital therapy for adolescents. As with any intervention, the work must be designed to meet the needs and resources of the specific child. Bond (1962) points out that a choice of a progressive series of tasks for the child provides an opportunity for the gradual acquisition of new skills, and for repeated success experiences as new jobs are mastered. It is vital, for work to be therapeutic, that the child be paid for his services and that the tasks be meaningful, more than routine housework or maintenance chores.

Particular programs have been devised which focus on making employment a viable and attractive alternative to the delinquent boy. Work must become work therapy. Events in a high valence situation with significant rewards (work), can be a channel for understanding and coping with reality, if the therapeutic aspect is included. Massimo and Shore (1967) worked with boys aged fifteen to seventeen who had just withdrawn or been suspended from school. A program of psychotherapy and remedial education was instituted, with the central focus always on preparation for and acquisition of a job. The therapeutic focus was job-oriented; the attempt was to foster attitudes which would facilitate successful relationships with the boss and other employees. Although most of the youths experienced failures on their first jobs, at the end of the program the overall employment record of the group was significantly better than that of controls. One joins the mainstream and starts a sequence of interrelationships of a supportive type.

Interventions Designed to Facilitate the Identification Processes

As indicated earlier, a large group of disturbances are characterized by deficiencies in identification. With such children it is appropriate to institute interventions which are designed to remediate and facilitate the identification process. One

367

approach is to work with those persons who already play important roles in the child's life in order to create more appropriate role models. One such approach is that of <u>filial therapy</u> (Andronico and Guerney, 1967; Guerney, 1964; Stover and Guerney, 1967). This technique has evolved out of two considerations: (1) the lack of adequate traditional therapeutic resources to conduct long-term therapy with all disturbed children, and (2) the recognition that "<u>given the skill</u>, parents, who are the most important figures in a child's life, have more opportunity to make significant improvements in their child's mental health than anyone else (Andronico and Guerney, 1967, p.5)."

The technique essentially consists of teaching parents, in small groups, to conduct non-directive play sessions with their children. The parents are taught to observe their children and reflect back to them the feelings which the child expresses during the play sessions. A controlled study has demonstrated that this parental training results in more reflective and less directive statements on the parents' part, and a more "positive" attitude in the child (Stover and Guerney, 1967). Contrary to initial expectations, parental participation in the play sessions seems to stimulate, rather than inhibit, the expression of threatening, family-related material (Guerney, 1964). A report from the mother of a seven-year-boy who was very passive and nervous before play sessions began is presented below:

He punched the "bob bag" on the head and said
"That's Sally [his eight-year-old sister]...
I have to kill her. Look how the blood rushes out
her head." I said, "Yes, it is really messy."...
He said, "Look at her cute belly button." He was
almost imitating people who admire Sally's looks.
I run into this constantly; people always admiring Sally
and nobody saying "Boo" about him...[In the next ses-
sion] he said to me "I will call out the spiders and
tell them to put you in a web; the spiders are my mean
friends...better yet, I'll get the ghosts to hang you!
They will close your eyes and shut your mouth!" I
said, "You want my mouth shut, you think I talk too
much." He said, "Yes, you boss too much!" (Guerney,
1964, pp.309-310)

It appears that the mother has become quite skillful at observing

and reflecting the son's feelings and that he has begun to express

some aggressions that he had previously held inside him.

The child's teacher always plays an important role in his

life and thus is a logical vehicle for such an effort to create

adequate role models. Jones comments on the powerful influence

which the teacher can have over the young child;

All the submissiveness, the readiness to be led,
the eagerness to be shown, which has developed out
of the particularly human condition of being relatively weak and ineffective in the proprietary hands
of comparative strength and competence, is transferred
to the teacher, with--for a while at least--almost none
of the ambivalent wariness which is a consequence of
these same conditions. Add to this the pull of the
future, the new worlds which the teacher symbolizes,
and you have an awesome potential for influence (Jones,
1168, p.264).

The teacher may represent for some disturbed children the first

adult whom the child can trust and identify with, who seems to have

the child's interests at heart, and who offers paths to new skills

369

and strengths. Clearly, a teacher who presents himself as punitive, interested only in how much the child can learn and how fast, and without concern for the child's feelings and fears can be just as destructive as the skillful teacher is constructive.

A second approach which is useful with the identification-deficient child is the provision of new objects for identification from outside his existing interactional sphere. A number of programs have been designed to meet this end. Because they are young, college students serve as particularly useful models for identification (Reinherz, 1964). Programs involving college students vary widely, from working with children within an institution (Reinherz, 1964), to work in the school setting (Cowen, et al., 1969), or to work outside of any structured setting (Goodman, 1967). The activities of the student volunteers range from conducting non-directive play therapy sessions (Stollak, 1969) to "[doing] what they please (Goodman, 1967, p.1773)." In general, the children come to anticipate and value their contacts with the student volunteers, and reports on behavioral adjustments show improvement (Cowen, et al., 1969; Reinherz, 1964).

A second program which embodies this aim is the Big Brother/ Big Sister movement. It represents a directed effort to provide a supportive relationship with a mature adult of the same sex as the child, in order to "enable the [child] to form more adequate identifications, to have an opportunity to imitate a mature adult, and to develop an association that can broaden his activity horizons (Lichtenberg, 1956, p.396)." The adult volunteers are oriented to the needs and problems of the children with whom they will be dealing and are given supportive help, especially in the early period of the relationship. What the Big Brother/Sister and the child do together they alone decide--it may be anything from playing ball, to going to a concert, to cooking a meal together.

Besides the approaches we have discussed which are designed to facilitate the identification process, there are others which use that very process in therapeutic ways. One such example is that of role playing or "trying on roles." By playing the role of someone who behaves very differently from himself, the child gets some sense of what that person "feels" like. Such role-playing may facilitate the development of new behavior patterns or may help the child to both understand and empathize with those around him who act differently, are a different color, a different religion, etc.

Another approach to the therapeutic exploitation of identification phenomena is embodied in programs which involve children observing and reporting on the behavior of other children. One paradigm is that described by Bower (1964) in which pubescent junior high school students, as part of the "social studies" experience, spend time at the child care center. Each student is assigned one younger child to observe and report on. Such a program

371

has potential for generating significant insights about relation-ships, aggressive versus passive behavior, growth and development, and so on.

Minuchin, et al. (1967) report on their trial of a peer-observation situation with disturbed delinquent children. Members of a small classroom group alternated between participation in curricular activities and observation of classmates from behind a one-way mirror. While observing, each student rated those he was watching on a zero-to-five scale, emphasizing learning performance rather than "good behavior." At the end of the session the raters discussed with the other students their observations and why they awarded the scores they did. Such a program put the children in the position of observing and passing judgment on the effects which certain kinds of behavior have in impeding or facilitating learning. To the extent that the observers were able to recognize in themselves the same behavior that they rated destructive in others, the observational protocol played an important part in the improved behavior they demonstrated.

Finally, another therapeutic use of the identification process is that of role reversal-instead of being identified as the "problem" who needs help, the child is put in the position of "helper." This is especially useful for children with learning difficulties, for the goals are much more clearly defined than those implicit in work with behavioral problems. As Bettelheim writes:

372

> children who have just successfully outgrown
> one emotional or learning difficulty are some-
> times the best persons to help others with theirs.
> In this way they can test their own newly acquired
> gains and also fight the temptation to submit to
> their former behavior in the way it is easiest to
> do that--namely by fighting it in others, instead
> of themselves (Bettelheim, 1950, p.163).

Benefits accrue to both parties. When sixth grade students with

reading problems were assigned to tutor fourth graders with similar

problems, both groups showed marked improvement in their reading

skills (Reissman, 1965). Just as important, the "helper" role can

boost self-esteem and provide important success experiences. There

are also unique advantages for the child being helped, for he may

be far more open to accepting direction and help from a peer than

from any representative of the adult world.

Appeals to the processes of identification are especially

appropriate for work with the value-deficient child. His failure

to internalize or even conform to an acceptable code of behavior

frequently reflects the lack of adequate models for identification

and/or his failure to form satisfactory relationships with such

models as exist in his interactional sphere. Such youths generally

do not see themselves as candidates for therapy and are very sus-

picious of those who offer it. Hoffer (1949) describes Aichhorn's

success in dealing with such cases by "deceiving the deceiver"--

essentially beating the sociopath at his own game. By capitalizing

on the weaknesses which his patient reveals and "outdoing the im-

postor's tricks in cleverly conducted fantasies a deux (Hoffer, 1949, describes Aichhorn's success in dealing with such cases by "deceiving the deceiver"--essentially beating the sociopath at his own game. By capitalizing on the weaknesses which his patient reveals and "outdoing the impostor's tricks in cleverly conducted fantasies a deux (Hoffer, 1949, p. 152)," the therapist establishes a "narcissistic transference" by virtue of which the patient comes to feel himself in the position of those he has tricked or cheated. He comes to feel awe toward the person who plays his games even better than he. Once such a powerful lever on the child's ego ideal has been established, his attitudes become amenable to input and change through the vehicle of the now-awesome therapist.

V. SUMMARY

In this paper we have summarized the current psychodynamic understanding of normal childhood and growth. This view emphasizes both the inner (affective, cognitive, and unconscious) life of the child, and the significant interactions in which he is involved. Biological, developmental, and interactional factors which combine to produce pathology are defined, and the implications of the psychodynamic view for treatment of the deviant child are discussed. Biological interventions are important--always in conjunction with attention to the child's psychological needs. For many children, a set of interventions designed to restore his environment to adequacy is sufficient. For the more severely disturbed child, a more specialized group of interventions (always tailored to specific needs and problems) is required. These special techniques can be grouped into four broad classes: the "classical" therapies (individual, group, and family), special supportive environments, the expressive therapies, and interventions designed to facilitate the process of identification.

At all levels, the concern must be with the child's unique constellation of resources and limitations, and with the special dynamics of his situation. One's aim is to maximize his resources and minimize the external stresses and limitations in order to permit the child to live in the least specialized environment possible.

From the psychodynamic view, the role of the educator in dealing with the deviant child is a major one. Positive school experiences with the teacher, peers, and curricular programs can play a major restorative role for the mildly disturbed child. Similarly, many of the special interventions are well integrated into the child's school experience. In addition to special curricular programs, all of the expressive media are well suited to the school, and the child's intimate interaction with his teacher and his peers lends itself to therapeutic exploitation of identification phenomena.

THEORIST	CRITICAL STAGES IN DEVELOPMENT
FREUD	1. oral 2. anal 3. phallic 4. latency 5. genital
ADLER	first 5 years are crucial in personality development; doesn't delineate specific stages
JUNG	1. birth to 5 years nutrition & growth self-protection 2. 5-------➤ adult sexuality
SULLIVAN	1. infancy 2. childhood 3. juvenile 4. preadolescent 5. early adolescent 6. late adolescent
MURRAY	5 Important "Complexes": claustral oral associated with anal 5 sequentially urethral developing castration pleasurable experiences
ERIKSON	1. infancy--mutual recognition 2. early childhood--will to be oneself 3. childhood--anticipation of roles 4. school age--task identification 5. adolescence

REFERENCES

Ackerman, N. W. Emergence of family psychotherapy on the present scene. In M. I. Stein (Ed.), Contemporary psychotherapies. Glencoe, Illinois: The Free Press, 1961a.

Ackerman, N. W. Further comments on family psychotherapy. In M. I. Stein (Ed.), Contemporary psychotherapies. Glencoe, Illinois: The Free Press, 1961b.

Aichhorn, A. Wayward youth. New York: Viking Press, 1935.

Albert, A. A special therapeutic technique for prelatency children with a history of deficiency in maternal care. American Journal of Orthopsychiatry, 1963, 33, 161-182.

Allport, G. W. The general and the unique in psychological science. Journal of Personality, 1962, 30, 405-422.

Altshuler, I. M. The past, present, and future of music therapy. In E. Podolsky, Music therapy. New York: Philosophical Library, 1954.

Andronico, M. P., & Guerney, B. G. The potential application of filial therapy to the school situation. Journal of School Psychology, 1967, 6, 2-7.

Ashlock, P., & Stephen, A. Educational therapy in the elementary school. Springfield, Illinois: Charles C. Thomas, 1966.

Ausubel, D. P., & Sullivan, E. V. Theory and problems of child development. New York: Grune and Stratton, 1970.

Axline, V. M. Play therapy: The inner dynamics of childhood. Chicago: Houghton Mifflin, 1947.

Bandura, A. Principles of behavior modification. New York: Holt, Rinehart, and Winston, Inc., 1969.

Baruch, D. W. Parents can be people. New York: Appleton-Century-Crofts, Inc., 1944.

Bateson, G., Jackson, D., Haley, J., & Weakland, J. Toward a theory of schizophrenia. Behavior Science, 1956, 1, 251-264.

Becker, W., Madsen, C., Arnold, C., & Thomas, D. The contingent use of teacher attention and praise in reducing classroom behavior problems. Journal of Special Education, 1967, 1, 287-307.

Berkowitz, L. The development of motives and values in the child. New York: Basic Books, Inc., 1964.

Berkowitz, L. The self, selfishness, and altruism. In J. Macauley & L. Berkowitz, Altruism and helping behavior. New York: Academic Press, 1970.

Berkowitz, P., & Rothman, E. Art work for the emotionally disturbed. Clearinghouse, 1951, 26, 232-234.

Berkowitz, P., & Rothman, E. The disturbed child: Recognition and psychoeducational therapy in the classroom. New York: New York University Press, 1960.

Bettelheim, B. Love is not enough. Glencoe, Illinois: The Free Press, 1950.

Bettelheim, B. Truants from life: The rehabilitation of emotionally disturbed children. Glencoe, Illinois: The Free Press, 1955.

Biber, B. Integration of mental health principles in the school setting. In G. Caplan (Ed.), Prevention of mental disorders in childhood. New York: Basic Books, 1961.

Bond, R. J. Work as a therapeutic medium in the treatment of delinquents. American Journal of Orthopsychiatry, 1962, 32, 846-850.

Bower, E. M. The modification, mediation, and utilization of stress during the school years. American Journal of Orthopsychiatry, 1964, 34, 667-674.

Bowlby, J. Maternal care and mental health. Geneva: World Health Organization, 1952.

Brown, L. M. Music and the tension headache. In E. Podolsky, Music Therapy. New York: Philosophical Library, 1954a.

Brown, L. M. Music therapy for acute grief. In E. Podolsky, Music Therapy. New York: Philosophical Library, 1954.

Bruck, C. M. Guidance series for the elementary school: Focus--Grade 8, Search--Grade 6. New York: The Bruce Publishing Company, 1968-1970.

379

Brunstetter, R. W. A milieu treatment program for psychotic children. In S. A. Szurek, & I. N. Berlin, Clinical studies in childhood psychoses. New York: Brunner/Mazel, 1973.

Buxbaum, E. The parents' role in the etiology of learning difficulties. Psychoanalytic Study of the Child, 1964, 19, 421-447.

Campbell, D. T. On the genetics of altruism and the counter-hedonic components in human culture. Journal of Social Issues, 1972, 28(3), 21-38.

Caplan, G. General introduction and overview. In G. Caplan (Ed.), Prevention of mental disorders in childhood. New York: Basic Books, 1961.

Caplan, G. Principles of preventive psychiatry. New York: Basic Books, 1964.

Catterall, C. D. Taxonomy of prescriptive interventions. Journal of School Psychology, 1970, 8, 5-12.

Chace, M. Dance in growth or treatment settings. Music Therapy, 1958, 1, 119-122.

Chapman, R. W. School suspension as therapy. Personnel and Guidance Journal, 1962, 40, 731-732.

Chess, S. An introduction to child psychiatry. New York: Grune & Stratton, 1969.

Cohen, R. Altruism: Human, cultural, or what? Journal of Social Issues, 1972, 28(3), 39-58.

Coles, R. The south goes north. Boston: Little, Brown, & Company, 1967.

Coles, R. Uprooted children. New York: Harper and Row, 1970.

Cowen, E. L., Zax, M., & Laird, J. D. A college student volunteer program in the elementary school setting. In B. G. Guerney Jr., Psychotherapeutic agents: New roles for nonprofessionals, parents, and teachers. New York: Holt, Reinhart, & Winston, 1969.

Cromwell, R. Videotape made in conjunction with the Conceptual Project, Institute for the Study of Mental Retardation and Related Disabilities, The University of Michigan, Ann Arbor, Michigan, November 8, 1971.

ruickshank, W. M., Bentzen, F. A., Ratzeburg, F. H., & Tannhauser, M. T. A teaching method for brain-injured and hyperactive children: A demonstration-pilot study. Syracuse, New York: Syracuse University Press, 1961.

ulley, M. Essential characteristics of a therapeutic program for emotionally disturbed preschool children. In N. Long, W. Morse, & R. Newman, Conflict in the classroom. Belmont, California: Wadsworth Publishing Company, 1971.

avis, K. Final notes on a case of extreme isolation. American Journal of Sociology, 1947, 52, 432-437.

ennison, G. The lives of children: The story of the First Street School. New York: Vintage Books, 1969.

ttman, A. T., & Kitchener, H. L. Life space interviewing and individual play therapy: A comparison of techniques. American Journal of Orthopsychiatry, 1959, 29, 19-26.

nahue, G. T., & Nichtern, S. Teaching the troubled child. New York: The Free Press, 1965.

eikurs, R. Psychology in the classroom. New York: Harper & Bros., 1957.

stein, R. The acquisition of learning readiness--task or conflict? In From learning for love to love of learning. New York: Brunner/Mazel, 1969.

stein, R., & Motto, R. From learning for love to love of learning. New York: Brunner/Mazel, 1969.

gel, M. Dilemmas of classification and diagnosis. Journal of Special Education, 1969, 3, 231-239.

glish, O. S., & Pearson, G. Difficulties in learning. In S. I. Harrison, & J. F. McDermott, Childhood psychopathology. New York: International Universities Press, 1972.

stein, S. The self-concept revisited. American Psychologist, 1973, 28(5), 404-416.

ikson, E. Eight stages of man. In Childhood and society. New York: W. W. Norton, 1963.

ikson, E. Identity: youth and crisis. New York: W. W. Norton, 1968.

381

Erikson, E. Play and actuality. In M. W. Piers (Ed.), Play and
development. New York: W. W. Norton, 1972.

Fenichel, C. Mama or M. A.? The "teacher-mom" program evaluated.
Journal of Special Education, 1966, 1, 45-51.

Fenichel, C. Psychoeducational approaches for seriously disturbed
children in the classroom. In N. Long, W. Morse, & R. Newman,
Conflict in the classroom. Belmont, Ca., Wadsworth Publishing
Company, 1971.

Ferster, C. B. Arbitrary and natural reinforcement. The Psychological Record, 1967, 17, 341-347.

Fine, R. The development of Freud's thought. Reviewed in Psychotherapy and Social Science Review, 1973, 7.

Forness, S. R., & MacMillan, D. L. Reinforcement overkill: Implications for education of the retarded. Journal of Special Education, 1972, 6, 221-230.

Fraiberg, S. H. The magic years. New York: Charles Scribner's
Sons, 1959.

Freud, A. Normality and pathology in childhood: assessments of
development. New York: International Universities Press, 1965.

Freud, A. Psychoanalysis for teachers and parents. New York:
Emerson Books, 1947.

Freud, A., & Burlingame, D. Infants without families. New York:
International Universities Press, 1944.

Furman, R. A., & Katan, A. The therapeutic nursery school. New
York: International Universities Press, 1969.

Gabrielson, J. B. Small activity groups aid children who are emotionally disturbed. Clearinghouse, 1962, 58(6), 32-34.

Gardner, R. A. Therapeutic communication with children: The mutual
storytelling technique. New York: Science House, 1971.

Gioscia, V., Rabkin, R., Speck, R., Rabkin, J., Beckett, T., &
Werner, H. Dimensions and innovations in the therapy of
children. Report to Task Force IV. International Commission
on the Mental Health of Children.

irard, J. Music therapy in the anxiety states. In E. Podosky, Music therapy. New York: Philosophical Library, 1954.

lasser, W. Reality therapy. New York: Harper & Row, 1965.

lasser, W. Schools without failure. New York: Harper & Row, 1969.

oodman, G. An experiment with companionship therapy: College students and troubled boys--assumptions, selection, and design. American Journal of Public Health, 1967, 57, 1772-1777.

raham, P., Rutter, M., & George, S. Temperamental characteristics as predictors of behavior disorders in children. American Journal of Orthopsychiatry, 1973, 43, 328-339.

ray, F. The Philadelphia advancement school. In B. Gross & R. Gross (Eds.), Radical school reform. New York: Simon & Schuster, 1969.

runebaum, M. G., Hurwitz, I., Prentice, N. M., & Sperry, B. M. Fathers of sons with primary neurotic learning inhibitions. American Journal of Orthopsychiatry, 1962, 32, 462-472.

uerney, B. J. Filial therapy: Description and rationale. Journal of consulting psychology, 1964, 28, 304-310.

uindon, J. Les étapes de la rééducation. Paris: Editions Fleurus, 1970.

uindon, J. The reeducation process. Lecture given at the 47th Annual International Convention of the Council for Exceptional Children, April 12, 1969.

uthrie, E. R. Psychology of human conflict: The clash of motives within the individual. New York: Harper and Bros., 1938.

amblin, R. L., Buckholdt, D., Bushell, D., Ellis, D., & Ferritor, D. Changing the game from "Get the Teacher" to "Learn." Trans-Action, 1969, 6, 20-31.

ansen, E. The use of educational technology in teaching emotionally disturbed children: How can we use the tape recorder? In N. J. Long, W. C. Morse, R. G. Newman, Conflict in the classroom. Belmont, California: Wadsworth Publishing Company, 1971.

arrison, S. I., & McDermott, J. F. Childhood psychopathology. New York: International Universities Press, 1972.

Heimlich, E. P. The specialized use of music as a mode of communication in the treatment of disturbed children. Journal of American Academy of Child Psychiatry, 1965, 4, 86-122.

Henry, J. Pathways to madness. New York: Random House, 1965.

Herman, E. P. Music therapy in depression. In E. Podolsky, Music therapy. New York: Philosophical Library, 1954a.

Herman, E. P. Relaxing music for emotional fatigue. In E. Podolsky, Music therapy. New York: Philosophical Library, 1954b.

Hersch, C. The discontent explosion in mental health. The American Psychologist, 1968, 23, 497-507.

Hewett, F. M. A hierarchy of educational tasks for children with learning disorders. The Exceptional Child, 1964, 31, 207-214.

Hewett, F. M. Teaching speech to an autistic child through operant conditioning. American Journal of Orthopsychiatry, 1965, 35, 927-936.

Hirschberg, J. C. The role of education in the treatment of disturbed children through planned ego development. American Journal of Orthopsychiatry, 1953, 23, 684-690.

Hoffer, W. Deceiving the deceiver. In K. R. Eissler (Ed.), Searchlights on delinquency. New York: International Universities Press, Inc., 1949.

Hollister, W. G. Concept of strens in education: A challenge to curriculum development. In E. M. Bower & W. G. Hollister (Eds.), Behavioral science frontiers in education. New York: ·John Wiley & Sons, 1967.

Holt, J. Freedom and beyond. New York: E. P. Dutton, 1972.

Jacobson, S., & Faegre, C. Neutralization: A tool for the teacher of disturbed children. Exceptional Children, 1959, 25, 243-256.

Jahoda, M. Current concepts of positive mental health. New York: Basic Books, 1958.

Johnson, A. M. Sanctions for superego lacunae of adolescents. In S. I. Harrison, & J. F. McDermott, Childhood psychopathology. New York: International Universities Press, 1972.

Johnston, R. Some casework aspects of using foster grandparents for emotionally disturbed children. Children, 1967, 14, 46-52.

Jones, R. M. Fantasy and feeling in education. New York: New York University Press, 1968.

Kay, W. The development of moral judgment--Piaget. Moral development. London: George Allen & Unwin, 1968.

Kellogg, R. The psychology of children's art. San Diego: CRM, 1967.

Kessler, J. W. Psychopathology of childhood. Englewood Cliffs, New Jersey: Prentice-Hall, 1966.

Kessler, J. Videotape made in conjunction with the Conceptual Project. Institute for the Study of Mental Retardation and Related Disabilities, The University of Michigan, Ann Arbor, Michigan, May, 1971.

Klein, E. Psychoanalytic aspects of school problems. Psychoanalytic Study of the Child, 1949, 3-4, 369-391.

Klein, E. The reluctance to go to school. Psychoanalytic Study of the Child, 1945, 1, 263-273.

Kliman, G. Psychological emergencies of childhood. New York: Grune & Stratton, 1968.

Knoblock, P. Open education for emotionally disturbed children. Exceptional Children, 1973, 39, 358-366.

Kohl, H. A Harlem class writes. In B. Gross & R. Gross (Eds.), Radical school reform. New York: Simon & Schuster, 1969.

Kohlberg, L. Development of moral character and moral ideology. In M. L. Hoffman & L. W. Hoffman, Review of child development research: Volume I. New York: Russell Sage Foundation, 1964.

Kounin, J. S., Friesen, W. V., & Norton, A. E. Managing emotionally disturbed children in regular classroom. Journal of Educational Psychology, 1966, 57, 1-13.

Kraft, I. A. Child and adolescent group therapy. In H. I. Kaplan and B. J. Sadock, Comprehensive group psychotherapy. Baltimore: The Williams & Wilkins Company, 1971.

Kramer, E. Art as therapy. New York: Schocken Books, 1971.

Kramer, E. Art therapy in a children's community. Springfield, Illinois: Charles C. Thomas, 1958.

La Benne, W. Differential diagnosis and psycho-educational treatment for the emotionally disturbed. Psychology in the Schools, 1967, 4, 366-370.

Lambert, N. M. Intellectual and nonintellectual predictors of high school status. Journal of Special Education, 1972, 6, 247-259.

Langner, T. S., & Michael, S. T. Life stress and mental health. Glencoe, Illinois: The Free Press of Glencoe, 1963.

La Pouse, R., & Monk, M. A. An epidemiological study of behavior characteristics in children. American Journal of Public Health, 1958, 48, 1134-1144.

Lazarus, R. S. Personality. Englewood Cliffs, New Jersey: Prentice-Hall, 1971.

Levy, D. M. "Release therapy" in young children. Psychiatry, 1938, 1, 387-390.

Lichtenberg, B. On the selection and preparation of the big brother volunteer. Social Casework, 1956, 137, 396-400.

Limbacher, W. J. Dimensions of personality: Here I am. Dayton, Ohio: George A. Pflaum, 1969.

Lindzey, G., Hall, C. S. Theories of personality: Primary sources and research. New York: John Wiley & Sons, 1965.

Lippman, H. S. Treatment of the child in emotional conflict. New York: McGraw-Hill, 1962.

Liss, E. Motivations in learning. Psychoanalytic Study of the Child, 1955, 10, 100-116.

Loehner, C. A. The sick-thinking family and its treatment. Upland, California: Phalarope Publishing Company, 1971.

Long, N. J., Morse, W. C., & Newman, R. G. Conflict in the classroom: The education of children with problems. Belmont, California: Wadsworth Publishing Company, 1971.

Long, N. J., & Newman, R. G. Managing surface behavior of children in
    school. In N. J. Long, W. C. Morse, & R. G. Newman, Conflict in
    the classroom. Belmont, California: Wadsworth Publishing Company,
    1971.

Long, N. J., Alpher, R., Butt, F., & Cully, M. Helping children cope
    with feelings. Childhood Education, 1969, 45 , 367-372.

Lovitt, T. C. Self-management projects with children with behavioral
    disabilities. Journal of Learning Disabilities, 1973, 6, 138-150.

Lowen, A. Betrayal of the body. New York: Collier Books, 1967.

Lyddiatt, E. M. Spontaneous painting and modelling: A practical
    approach to therapy. London: Constable & Company, 1970.

Maddi, S. R. Personality theories: A comparative analysis. Home-
    wood, Illinois: The Dorsey Press, 1968.

Maslow, A. H. Toward a psychology of being. Princeton, New Jersey:
    Van Nostrand, 1962.

Massimo, J. L., & Shore, M. F. Comprehensive vocationally oriented
    psychotherapy: A new treatment technique for lower-class adolescent
    delinquent boys. Psychiatry, 1967, 30, 229-236.

McConville, B. J., & Purohit, A. P. Classifying confusion: A study
    of results on inpatient treatment in a multidisciplinary children's
    center. American Journal of Orthopsychiatry, 1973, 43, 411-417.

Michigan Association for Emotionally Disturbed Children. Educating
    emotionally disturbed children (Chart), 1973.

Minuchin, S., Chamberlain, P., & Graubard, P. A project to teach
    learning skills to disturbed delinquent children. American
    Journal of Orthopsychiatry, 1967, 37, 558-567.

Mischel, W. Introduction to personality. Chicago: Holt, Rinehart
    & Winston, 1971.

Moreno, J. L. Psychodrama. New York: Beacon House, 1946.

Morse, W. C. Crisis intervention in school mental health and special
    classes for the disturbed. In N. J. Long, W. C. Morse, &
    R. G. Newman, Conflict in the classroom. Belmont, California:
    Wadsworth Publishing Company, 1971a.

387

Morse, W. C. The crisis or helping teacher. In N. J. Long, W. C. Morse, & R. G. Newman, Conflict in the classroom. Belmont, California: Wadsworth Publishing Company, 1971b.

Morse, W. C. Intervention techniques for the classroom teacher of the emotionally disturbed. Presented to the First Annual Conference on the Education of Emotionally Disturbed Children, 1965.

Morse, W. C. Working paper: Training teachers in life space interviewing. American Journal of Orthopsychiatry, 1963, 33, 727-730.

Morse, W. C. Worksheet on life space interviewing for teachers. In N. J. Long, W. C. Morse, & R. G. Newman, Conflict in the classroom. Belmont, California: Wadsworth Publishing Company, 1971c.

Morse, W. C., Schwertfeger, J., & Goldin, D. An evaluative approach to the training of teachers of disturbed preschool children. Ann Arbor, Michigan: School of Education, University of Michigan, 1973.

Moustakas, C. E. Children in play therapy. New York: McGraw-Hill, 195

Moustakas, C. E. Psychotherapy with children: The living relationship. New York: Harper & Brothers Publishers, 1959.

Munroe, R. L. Schools of psychoanalytic thought. New York: Holt, 1955

Murdock, H. M., & Eaton, M. T. Music as an adjunct to electroshock therapy. In E. Podolsky, Music therapy. New York: Philosophical Library, 1954.

Murphy, L. B. Infants' play and cognitive development. In M. W. Piers (Ed.), Play and development. New York: W. W. Norton, 1972.

Newman, R. G. Psychological consultation in the schools. New York: Basic Books, 1967.

Newman, R. G. The school-centered life space interview as illustrated by extreme threat of school issues. American Journal of Orthopsychiatry, 1963, 33, 730-733.

Norbeck, E., Price-Williams, D., & McCord, W. M. The study of personality: An interdisciplinary appraisal. Chicago: Holt, Rinehart & Winston, 1968.

Pasamanick, B., & Lilienfeld, A. M. Association of maternal and fetal factors with the development of mental deficiency: I. Abnormalities in the prenatal and paranatal periods. Journal of the American Medical Association, 1955, 159, 155-160.

Pasamanick, B., Rogers, M. E., & Lilienfeld, A. M. Pregnancy experience and the development of childhood behavior disorders. *American Journal of Psychiatry*, 1956, 112, 613-618.

Patterson, G. R., Jones, R., Whittier, J., & Wright, M. A. A behavior modification technique for the hyperactive child. *Behavior Research and Therapy*, 1965, 2, 217-226.

Paul, R., & Stand, V. M. Music therapy for the mentally ill: A historical sketch and a brief review of the literature on the physiological effects and on analysis of the elements of music. *Journal of General Psychology*, 1958, 59, 167-176.

Pearson, G. H. (Ed.). *A handbook of child psychoanalysis*. New York: Basic Books, 1968.

Pearson, G. H. A survey of learning difficulties in children. *Psychoanalytic Study of the Child*, 1952, 7, 322-386.

Peck, R. F., & Havighurst, R. J. *Psychology of character education*. New York: John Wiley & Sons. 1960.

Piaget, J. *The moral judgment of the child*. Glencoe, Illinois: The Free Press, 1948.

Price, H. G., Mountney, V., & Knouss, R. Selection of music to accompany electroshock therapy. In E. Podolsky, *Music Therapy*. New York: Philosophical Library, 1954.

Prugh, D. G. Psychosocial disorders in childhood and adolescence: Theoretical considerations and an attempt at classification. Appendix A to the Report of the Committee on Clinical Issues, Joint Commission on Mental Health of Children. To be published by Harper & Row.

Quay, H. C. Some basic considerations in the education of emotionally disturbed children. *Exceptional Children*, 1963, 30, 27-32.

Rabinovitch, R. D. Reading problems in children: Definitions and classifications. In Keeney & Keeney (Eds.), *Dyslexia: Diagnosis and treatment of reading disorders*. St. Louis: Mosby, 1968.

Raths, L. E., Harmin, M., & Simon, S. B. *Values and teaching*. Columbus, Ohio: Charles E. Merrill, 1966.

Redl, F. The concept of a "therapeutic milieu." *American Journal of Orthopsychiatry*, 1959a, 29, 721-736.

Redl, F. The concept of punishment. In N. J. Long, W. C. Morse, & R. G. Newman, Conflict in the classroom. Belmont, California: Wadsworth Publishing Company, 1971.

Redl, F. Strategy and techniques of the life space interview. American Journal of Orthopsychiatry, 1959b, 29, 1-18.

Redl, F. When we deal with children. New York: The Free Press, 1966.

Redl, F., & Wattenberg, W. Mental hygiene in teaching. New York: Harcourt, Brace & Company, 1951.

Redl, F., & Wineman, D. Controls from within: Techniques for the treatment of the aggressive child. Glencoe, Illinois: The Free Press, 1952.

Reinherz, H. The therapeutic use of student volunteers. Children, 1964, 11, 137-142.

Rezmierski, V., & Kotre, J. A limited literature review of the theory of the psychodynamic model. In W. C. Rhodes, & M. L. Tracy (Eds.), A study of child variance. Ann Arbor, Michigan: University of Michigan, 1972.

Rhodes, W. C. Curriculum and disordered behavior. Exceptional Children, 1963, 30, 61-66.

Riessman, F. The "helper" therapy principle. Social Work, 1965, 10, 27-32.

Robins, L. Deviant children grown up. Baltimore: The Williams & Wilkins Company, 1966.

Rogers, C. R. Significant learning: In therapy and in education. In On becoming a person: A therapist's view of psychotherapy. Boston: Houghton Mifflin, 1961.

Rosenhan, D. L. On being sane in insane places. Science, 1973, 179, 250-258.

Ruitenbeek, H. The first Freudians. Reviewed in Psychotherapy and Social Science Review, 1973, 7, 7.

Rutter, M., Lebovich, S., Eisenberg, L., Sneznevskij, A., Sadoun, R., Brooke, E., & Yi Lin, T. A tri-axial classification of mental disorders in childhood. Journal of Child Psychology and Psychiatry, 1969, 10, 41-61.

390

Sahakian, W. S. Psychology of personality: Readings in theory. Chicago: Rand McNally, 1965.

Sarason, S. B., Davidson, K. S., Lighthall, F. F., Waite, R. R., & Ruebush, B. K. Anxiety in elementary school children. New York: Wiley & Sons, 1960.

Sarason, S. B. The culture of the school and the problem of change. Boston: Allyn & Bacon, 1971.

Schultheis, M. A guidebook for bibliotherapy. Glenview, Illinois: Psychotechnics, 1973.

Sewell, W. H., & Haller, A. O. Factors in the relationship between social status and the personality adjustment of the child. American Sociological Review, 1959, 24, 511-520.

Short, J. F. Juvenile delinquency: the socio-cultural context. In L. W. Hoffman, & M. L. Hoffman (Eds.), Review of child development research. Volume II. New York: Russell Sage, 1966.

Simonson, M., & Chow, B. F. Maternal diet, growth, and behavior. In S. Sunderlin (Ed.), Nutrition and intellectual development in children. Washington, D. C.: Association for Childhood Education, International, 1969.

Singer, J. L. The child's world of make-believe. New York: Academic Press, 1973.

Slack, C. W. Experimenter-subject psychotherapy: A new method of introducing intensive office treatment for unreachable cases. Mental Hygiene, 1960, 44, 238-256.

Slavson, S. R. Analytic group psychotherapy. New York: Columbia University Press, 1950.

Slavson, S. R. An introduction to group therapy. New York: International Press, 1943.

Slavson, S. R. Re-educating the delinquent through group and community participation. New York: Harper & Brothers, 1954.

Smith, C. C. Using films in group guidance with emotionally disturbed socially maladjusted boys. Exceptional Children, 1958, 24, 205-209.

Speck, R. V. Psychotherapy of the social network of a schizophrenic family. Family Process, 1967, 6, 208-214.

Speers, R. W., & Lansing, C. Group therapy in childhood psychosis. Chapel Hill, North Carolina: The University of North Carolina Press, 1965.

Sperling, M. School problems: Classification dynamics and treatment. Psychoanalytic Study of the Child, 1967, 21, 375-401.

Sperry, B., Staver, N., Reiner, B. S., & Ulrich, D. Renunciation and denial in learning difficulties. American Journal of Orthopsychiatry, 1958, 28, 98-111.

Spitz, R. A. Hospitalism. The Psychoanalytic Study of the Child, 1945, 1, 53-74.

Spitz, R. A., & Wolf, K. Autoeroticism. The Psychoanalytic Study of the Child, 1949, 3-4, 85-120.

Staats, A. W., & Butterfied, W. H. Treatment of non-reading in a culturally deprived juvenile delinquent: An application of reinforcement principles. Child Development, 1965, 36, 925-942.

Steucher, U. Tommy: A treatment study of an autistic child. Arlington, Virginia: The Council for Exceptional Children, 1972.

Stollak, G. E. The experimental effects of training college students as play therapists. In B. Guerney, Psychotherapeutic agents: New roles for nonprofessionals, parents, and teachers. New York: Holt, Rinehart, & Winston, 1969.

Stover, L., & Guerney, B. G. The efficacy of training procedures for mothers in filial therapy. Psychotherapy: Theory, Research and Practice, 1967, 4, 110-115.

Sugarman, P. Music therapy in psychosomatic gastric disorders. In E. Podolsky, Music therapy. New York: Philosophical Library, 1954.

Sutton-Smith, B. Children at play. Natural History, 1971, 80, 54-59.

Thomas, A., Chess, S., & Birch, H. Temperament and the behavior disorders in children. New York: New York University Press, 1969.

Trieschman, A. E., Whittaker, J. K., & Brendtro, L. K. The other 23 hours. Chicago: Aldine Publishing Company, 1969.

Vogel, E. F., & Bell, N. W. The emotionally disturbed child as the family scapegoat. In N. W. Bell, & E. F. Vogel (Eds.), A modern introduction to the family. Glencoe, Illinois: The Free Press, 1960.

392

Wardle, C. J. Two generations of broken homes in the genesis of conduct and behavior disorders in childhood. <u>British Medical Journal</u>, 1961, <u>2</u>, 349-354.

Weinstein, G., & Fantini, M. D. <u>Toward humanistic education: A curriculum of affect</u>. New York: Praeger Publishers, 1970.

Wepman, J., & Heine, R. W. <u>Concepts of personality</u>. Chicago: Aldine, 1963.

White, R. W. (Ed.) <u>The study of lives</u>. New York: Atherton Press, 1964.

Winick, M. Nutrition and intellectual development in children. In S. Sunderlin (Ed.), <u>Nutrition and intellectual growth in children</u>. Washington, D. C.: Association for Childhood Education, International, 1969.

Witmer, H. L. (Ed.) <u>Psychiatric interviews with children</u>. Cambridge, Massachusetts: Harvard University Press, 1946.

Wolman, B. B. <u>Contemporary theories and systems in psychology</u>. New York: Harper & Brothers, 1960.

Wolman, B. B. <u>Manual of child psychopathology</u>. New York: McGraw Hill Company, 1972.

Woltmann, A. G. The use of puppetry as a projective method in therapy. In H. H. Anderson, & G. L. Anderson (Eds.) <u>An introduction to projective techniques: And other devices for understanding the dynamics of human behavior</u>. Englewood Cliffs, New Jersey: Prentice-Hall, 1951.

ENVIRONMENTAL INTERVENTIONS IN EMOTIONAL DISTURBANCE

Melinda Wagner

TABLE OF CONTENTS

397

I. INTRODUCTION

The differentiating labels "ecological" and "sociological" were eschewed in this paper. Feagans (1971) distinguishes
between sociological and ecological theory when she states, "the
emphasis within sociology is almost exclusively on the environment
while ecology emphasizes the role of individual differences in any
outcome." This distinction, however, is not viable when discussing
intervention. It will be seen from the descriptions of interventions given in this paper that the majority of interventionists
from either school take the environment into account to some extent,
and turn their attention to the individual to a greater extent.

The common element in all the interventions reported here
is an emphasis on environment in the intervention plan, whether
in the statement of the problem, or in the course of action. Interventions will be ordered according to the degree to which they
stress environment.

Clarity might be aided here by a discussion of Rhodes
and Gibbins (1972) trichotomy of intervention types. These are:

(1) Excitor-centered interventions, which "aim their change-

effects almost exclusively at the excitor, the disturbed child;"

(2) Respondent-centered interventions, which "concentrate on

the other side of the transaction--the responding environment

or responding setting of the disturbance;" and

(3) Exchange-centered interventions, which "center intervention

upon the excitor-respondent exchange patterns themselves."

It has been suggested that sociological interventions fall into

the respondent-centered category, and ecological into the exchange-

centered category . In fact, however, many interventionists, al-

though seeing the problem (the disturbance) as emanating from the

environment, direct their attention (their "change-effects")

toward the child. This, in the author's mind, placed them in the

realm of excitor-centered interventions.

It was decided, therefore, not to deal separately with

sociological and ecological interventions, but to categorize them

according to their conception of the problem, and the direction

and form of their action. A continuum, based on this analysis is

presented in chart form on page 3. To determine the placement of

each intervention on the continuum, each was coded on the follow-

ing variables.

(1) Where does the interventionist view the problem as resid-

ing; where does he observe the problem? The coding possibil-

ities were:

(a) the problem is centered in some behavior or stage

of development in the child, or

(b) the problem is the interface between child and

environment.

(2) From where does   the interventionist perceive that the

problem emanates; what is the source of the problem? The

coding possibilities were:

    (a) the disturbing problem within the child emanates

from a problem in the environment, or

    (b) the source of the problem within the child is the

interface between child and environment.

(3) What is the object of the change action; what is the tar-

get of the action? The coding possibilities were:

    (a) action is directed toward a change in the child,

    (b) action is directed toward a change in the environment,

    (c) action is directed toward a change in the child and

the environment, or

    (d) action is directed toward a change in the interface.

It will be noted that action directed toward child, environ-

ment, and interface, respectively, corresponds to excitor-centered,

respondent-centered and exchange-centered interventions as described

above. The fourth type of target possibility, child and environ-

ment, was added because it was felt that there is a difference

between actually working toward a change in interface, i.e., "round-

ing a square child and squaring a round environment" simultaneously

and working on "both ends" of the excitor-respondent environment.

(4) In the case of action directed toward the child, does

the action utilize the environment to effect the change? The

coding possibilities were:

    (a) yes, the intervention does utilize the environment,

CONTINUUM OF INTERVENTIONS

Key:

Chd = Child
Env = A problem in the environment
If = Interface
Chd& = Child and
Env   Environment

Intervention	Problem viewed as centered in:	Problem viewed as emanating from: (The source of the problem)	Action is directed toward a change in:	In the case of action directed toward child, action utilizes environment to effect change:
Ecological Management; Students As Behavior Change Agents	If	If		
Conceptualized, No examples	Chd	If	If	
ReEd; Self-Enhancing Education	Chd	If	Chd&Env	Yes
Preventive Approach to Developmental Problems	Chd	If	Chd&Env	No
Street-Club Work	Chd	Env	Chd&Env	Yes
Conceptualized, No examples	Chd	Env	Chd&Env	No
Enhancing the Classroom Teacher's Mental Health Function; Mental Health Consultation	Chd	If	Env	
Family Interaction; Maternal Preventive Psychiatry; Maternal Care	Chd	Env	Env	
Conceptualized, No examples	Chd	If	Chd	Yes
Therapeutic Built Environment; Provo, Silverlake; Highfields; Industrial Neurosis Unit; Hawthorne Cedar Knolls; Maxim Gorky Labor Colony; Pittsburgh School Mental Health Program; Gheel	Chd	Env	Chd	Yes
Treatment of Non-Reading	Chd	If	Chd	No
Teaching Learning Skills; Social Adaptation	Chd	Env	Chd	No

or,

(b) no, the intervention does not utilize the environment.

The continuum should be viewed only as a tool for organizing diverse concepts and as an aid to understanding a field characterized by diversity.

A rationale for placement on the continuum will be given at the outset of the description of each intervention. This will be in the form of a paraphrase of the author's description of where the problem is centered, of the source of the problem, of the target of the change-action, and of whether action directed toward a change in the child involves use of the environment to effect the change.

Interventions can be categorized on the basis of where the action is directed. These groups of interventions are described by the major headings in this paper:

(1) Remediation Intervention

(2) Natural Community Intervention

(3) School Community Intervention

(4) Artificial Community Intervention (artificial in the sense that the community would not exist if it were not for the existence of persons classified as deviants)

(5) Artificial Group Intervention

(6) Architectural Intervention

(7) Family Environment Intervention

(8) School Environment Intervention

(9) Excitor-Respondent Intervention: Natural Group and Slum Environment

(10) Excitor-Respondent Intervention: Child and School Environment

(11) Interface Intervention

Many similarities will be noted in the techniques and processes utilized in the various interventions. For instance, it will be seen throughout the discussion of the interventions that those which utilize the environment in their actions toward the child include many of the same techniques. Comparisons of technique will not be made in the body of the text, but are provided in list form in the appendix, "Techniques Common to Several Interventions."

II. REMEDIATION INTERVENTIONS

The Remediation Interventions embody the idea that something is wrong with the child because of a problem in his environment or a problem in the interface between himself and his environment. Remediation Interventions direct their change action toward the child.

Social Adaptation

Meuron and Auerswald (1969), who espouse an "ecological systems" orientation, locate the problem in the child and define it as a lag in cognitive development. The source of the problem is a particular kind of family environment, in which there are deficits in language, characterized by limited vocabulary and language usage in patterned communication. There are also deficits in capacity to organize data, to plan, to make decisions as a group, and to resolve conflict. The action proposed by the Social Adapatation Intervention of Meuron and Auerswald is directed toward a change in the child.

The objective of the change action is to provide the child with the ability to maintain the self in a complex society. Meuron and Auerswald take the view that capacity to function in the complex systems of modern society depends on the ability to differentiate these systems, and on the development of cognitive

tools with which to identify, classify and integrate the messages
one receives from them.

The first step of the change action is a diagnosis of
the child's cognitive capacities, to discover whether the child
is developmentally behind the stage necessary for him to cope with
his social environment (generally school). If he is found to be
behind, a remedial curriculum geared to his needs for cognitive
growth is provided. If, after this experience, the child is still
unable to learn in the normal manner, an investigation is undertaken to discover if the child's difficulties are to be found "in
his soma, his emotional psyche, his family or some external system
such as his classroom   (Meuron & Auerwald, 1969)."

Teaching Learning Skills

Minuchin, Dollarhide and Graubard (1969) locate the
problem in the child. They identify the problem as a failure to
learn the rules requisite to school success. The source of this
failure is the type of family interactions and communication patterns which the child experiences. Specifically, family interactions and communication patterns are not of the type which aid
the child in perceiving which part of his behavior is disturbing
(i.e., parents' responses are global, erratic). The child learns
to pay more attention to the person with whom he is communicating,
and to this person's mood, than to what is actually being said.

The intervention action has as its target the child.

The objective of the intervention is to teach the child learning skills. Minuchin et al. contend that certain skills aid classroom learning, and that these skills can be taught. Although Minuchin et al. are concerned only with intellectual development, their emphasis on teaching learning skills, along with a standard curriculum, borders on the "whole child" concept which will be emphasized in other interventions. The "whole child" concept is the view that the educational process should include responsibility for the social, personal and emotional, as well as intellectual development of the child.

The intervention action directed toward the child consists of remedial class sessions which teach children listening skills, the significance of noise, taking turns, logic in stories and in conversation, judging and being judged, and role playing.

Treatment of Non-Reading

Staats and Butterfield (1969) locate the problem as "non-reading in a culturally deprived juvenile delinquent." The population on which they concentrate their efforts is the child who is unable to learn through traditional methods. The source of this inability is an inappropriate fit between the individual's behavior and the expectations of his environment; a problem in

407

the interface. Staats and Butterfield propose that problem behavior can arise because:

(1) Behavior that is necessary for adjustment in society is absent from the individual's repertoire,

(2) Behaviors considered undesirable by the society are present in the individual, or

(3) The individual's motivational system is inappropriate.

An inappropriate motivational system can be a function of defective conditions of learning, or of conditions of learning which were inappropriate for a particular individual. The action taken in the treatment of non-reading is directed toward the child.

The objective is to teach and maintain attentional and work behaviors necessary for learning to read. Reinforcement principles of behavior modification techniques are applied to the learning situation.

The training sessions are in the form of one-to-one tutoring, involving tokens with cash value. These tokens are used as reinforcement for correct responses and for attention. Staats and Butterfield emphasize the economy of this intervention. The only requisite for the trainer (tutor) is average reading skill. The suggestion is made that selected delinquents or prisoners could be utilized to train others. Physical paraphernalia required in the particular example given by Staats and Butterfield are: word lists on 3 x 5 cards, paragraphs from stories incorporating these words on 5 x 8 cards, and the story _in toto_ on 8-1/2 x 13 sheets of paper with comprehension questions included. In addition, tokens with cash value, (and money to back them up), visible containers in which to store the tokens, and charts to plot acquisition of tokens are necessary. The authors state that the cash outlay is not great. In the particular case cited, the student progressed readily and in four months had earned $20.31. Staats and Butterfield give statistical evidence of reading progress. So that the student would not come to depend on tokens, as he progressed, less reinforcement was given for more work (the stories became more difficult). Achievement did not decrease, however.

Training in reading aided the student's adjustment in school. (It is posited that his school work helped the reading training.) Disrupting behavior in school ceased. But it would appear that this student needed intervention into more than his learning-school environment. The training was ended after 4-1/2 months, due to the fact that the boy was sent to an industrial school for juvenile delinquent boys. This action was taken because of his disrupting behavior at the juvenile detention home where he had been living.

Natural Community Interventions identify a problem existing in the person. The source of this problem may be found in the
environment. The change action of the intervention is directed toward the problem within the person. A Natural Community Intervention
utilizes elements of a naturally occurring environment to effect the
change.

Gheel

The intervention performed by the inhabitants of the city
of Gheel in Belgium is built on a long tradition of interaction
with "lunatics," which began with a religious custom in the seventh
century. Originally, Gheel was a place of pilgrimage for the insane
to receive the miracle of St. Dymphna. Eventually, the inhabitants
of Gheel began to accept the seekers as boarders on whom they lav-
ished much hospitality, as was their custom. In the 1800's a doctor
provided centralization to the Gheelois custom and provided reforms
for some injustices which had crept in over the years. It is this
doctor's system, built on a people's custom, as it was reported by
Julia Byrne in 1869, which will be discussed here.

Dr. Bulckens intimated in conversations to Byrne (1869)
that the problem was to be located within the patient. It was felt
that traditional asylum treatment, if not the source of the problem,

410

would definitely worsen it. The target of the action is a change in the patient. This change is achieved through the use of a benevolent environment which does not differentiate a "normal" population from an "abnormal" population.

The type of client population served at Gheel is, in the main, an adult one. These persons suffer from "every form and degree of mental alienation." The boarders at Gheel are often persons who have been rejected by their families and communities. The objective of Gheel is to provide a resort for those persons who are "too mad to live anywhere else."

Because institutionalization, and the practices of labelling and grouping persons viewed as "insane" are considered to be irritants to the patient's condition, these things are eschewed at Gheel.

When a patient arrives at Gheel he is greeted by Dr. Bulcken's system, Le Patronage Familial, and by his establishment, L'Asile Patronal. L'Asile Patronal is a handsome and imposing building, kept meticulously clean. L'Asile Patronal serves as the base from which the Gheel system is directed. Each patient serves an initial probationary quarantine in L'Asile, during which time his placement in the Gheel community is decided. The patients are placed in categories based on the type of behavior which they manifest and the type of treatment deemed most beneficial to them and to the rest of the Gheelois population. Patient placement depends

411

on two aspects: the patient's "category" and the qualities of the
boarding families (the heads of which are called nourriciers). For
purposes of placement, Gheel and its surrounding environs have been
divided into six sections. The patient categories correspond to
these sections. The most docile patients are placed within Gheel.
The most violent are placed in the most distant localities, in the
area of small scattered farms. Each of these sections has a garde
de section who makes daily rounds, checking each household boarding
a patient and reporting to the head physician. The head physician
places patients with regard to the particular specialties of management of the nourriciers, and with an eye to matching interests and
occupations of patient and nourricier. He is also careful to place
together nourriciers and boarders who speak the same language
(boarders come from all over Europe), and who have the same social
class and similar tastes. The nourriciers are paid for their services by the friends or relatives of the patients, but the pay usually no more than covers the maintenance costs. As soon as he is
placed, the client ceases to be a "patient" and becomes a "boarder."

The healthy influence of family life is the prevailing
element in the Gheel system, Le Patronage Familial. A boarder remains with one family, unless adverse conditions develop, throughout
his stay at Gheel. A close watch is kept over the boarders through
the medium of the gardes de section. If it is decided at any time
that he requires treatment, he can be placed in L'Asile Patronal

for the necessary treatment and then replaced in the home of his foster family. The average length of stay for a boarder at Gheel is 1-8 years.

The process which most patients go through from their time of inauguration into their host family to the time of their "release" may be described as follows: generally, the patient has been scorned by those he knew; he has no one. At Gheel, and particularly within his family, he becomes the object of everyone's regard and attention. His position within the family is equal to that of all other members. He is well cared for. This attention causes him to rise in his own estimation. The boarder becomes interested in the joys and sorrows of his family. He can no longer think only of himself. As he comes to take an ever-increasing part in the life of the family, and dwells less on himself, he acts increasingly "normal." "Gradually he gains the level of those by whom he is surrounded, and often this simple and spontaneous resuscitation of moral vigor alone suffices to effect his cure   (Byrne, p. 62)."

Another influence on the boarder is that of occupation. All trades available at Gheel are available to inmates. Boarders of the working class are paid wages if they prefer money. Or, if they wish, they may be rewarded with tobacco, snuff, sugar, beer, gingerbread, or cakes. Their occupations and their status as functioning members of a family make the boarders feel useful and give purpose to their lives.

A third technique in the intervention consists of religious training. This is, of course, voluntary and usually is another part of a boarder's partaking in his family's activities. All church services are completely open to the patients.

A further technique of intervention used at Gheel is diversification of activities. "Change of scene and of ideas forms a part of their regime." These changes are as varied as circumstances permit. They may include walks in the country. The boarder accompanies his family on outings, and all community activities are open to the "inmates." Those whose condition is considered amenable to it are allowed to attend the public houses. The proprietor must abide by the law of Gheel to "allow no approach to excess in the matter of drink." The presence of the garde de section adds to the influence of this law.

Implicit in all of these techniques is the overriding freedom awarded to the boarders: freedom to be functioning members of a community; freedom to live useful and satisfying lives without being differentiated from their neighbors.

The medical staff of L'Asile Patronal attributes the cures which take place at Gheel to the healthy influence of simple and regular habits, the tranquil atmosphere by which the patients are surrounded, and the absence of restraint. The treatment afforded the patients is moral as well as physical. This treatment is possible due to the manner adopted toward the boarders by the population of Gheel. In most ecological and sociological interventions, the character of the staff is very important. At Gheel, the entire population is "staff." Byrne describes the character of the Gheelois as honest and simple rusticity. Byrne feels that the meeting of sane vis-à-vis insane is aided by the simplicity of the population and the lack of cultivation of their ideas. They treat their proteges with gentleness, forebearance and tact. The manner adopted toward the boarders by the population of Gheel is the "result of their long intercourse with the insane (Byrne, p. 148)."

"You are just like us. Forget about yourself. Be a member of our family and care about us, and we will care about you" is the message the people of Gheel give to their insane boarders.

The philosophy of Gheel, "if treated as normal, a person will be normal," is one which is common to sociological and ecological interventions. Here it is implemented by freedom; the patients "are contradicted as little as is consistent with the (individual) malady (Byrne, p. 13)." The patients are given a place in the life of a family. They share the joys and sorrows of this family. They participate in all the activities of their family, and yet they are free to partake of community life outside the realm of their family (an occupation, religious activities, etc.).

415

IV. SCHOOL COMMUNITY INTERVENTION

A School Community Intervention, like a Natural Community Intervention, perceives the problem which exists in the child as resulting from environmental problems. This type of intervention directs its change action toward the child. School Community Interventions utilize the school environment to accomplish this change.

Pittsburgh School Mental Health Program

This intervention views the problem as centered in the child. The children who are viewed as problematic by Stickney in his work with the Pittsburgh School Mental Health Program (Stickney, 1968), are the children who disturb teachers. The source of the problem is in the environment, specifically, a "pathogenic home situation." Stickney maintains that a "disturbed child is the delegate of a disturbed family." Stickney's intervention directs itself toward the child. The action directed toward the child utilizes manipulation of the school environment such that it becomes a therapeutic community to effect change in the child.

The objective of the intervention is that public schools become community mental health centers. Schools should be concerned with the mental health of all children, and of every learning aspect of each child. The school should become a therapeutic community fostering emotional, scholastic, and social learning. There is an emphasis, then, on training the "whole child." Schools are the ideal casefinding agencies. The school should be utilized as the coordinator of community services. All relevant agencies could come together there. This intervention stresses the value of the teacher, what he does, and what he could do.

Part of the Pittsburgh School Mental Health Program Intervention is the screening of all children prior to entrance into first grade. For a child found to be "disturbed" at this time, Stickney recommends small therapeutic milieus freely interacting with the large school environment. These special classes would have a dynamic population, rather than a certain number of "special class" pupils. For example, there might be a class size of 8 pupils, but several dozen different children utilizing the class in one week. Pupils are moved through these classes at a rate that will insure their early reintegration into the regular class.

Stickney maintains that a therapeutic program for disturbed children should begin with help in school subjects. The attributes of the special class teachers are of great importance in the construction of a therapeutic milieu. They must be good teachers who have demonstrated talent in their dealings with different children. The teachers should like children, be affectionate and humorous, be firm and consistent, and be relatively shockproof and nonpunitive. Special class teachers should be given special training and regular consultative support.

One of the advantages of this approach is that it maintains the child in his natural environment. Stickney cautions, however, that for children who have an untenable home situation, "squeeze-out" children, this program must not be utilized to keep them in school (and at home). In these cases an ecological diagnosis, measuring the school and home environments and the extent to which they accept the child must be utilized to determine the proper plan of action.

It is felt that more seriously disturbed children, "marginal (uncontainable)" children, and some "squeeze-out" children may require residential schools of moderate size. From the residential school they would move to cottage-style homes of 8-10 students with house parents. While residing in the cottages the children would attend nearby public schools. Re-integration of the child into his normal environment is again the emphasis.

A school could be built into a therapeutic community for all children by utilizing the procedures of the Pittsburgh School Mental Health Program. The program involved a staff of a coordinator, one person who served as psychiatric consultant and director, another psychiatric consultant, 3 social workers, a secretary, research associate and a clerk, 12 teachers and aides.

The intervention program consisted of two phases. In Phase I, crisis referrals were collected. Through these referrals

the staff was initiated into the school's complex subculture. A
definite method of consultation was employed by the program staff.
The staff would only answer joint referrals which were made by the
principal and the school social worker. In this way, roles which
already existed within the school culture remained legitimate and
were utilized, rather than resisted by the program's staff. The
crisis referral session operated as follows:

(1) The staff made it a point to hear everyone out. They
listened to the teacher's account of her problem with the
child, the social worker's account of her home visit, and the
psychological or testing data.

(2) The psychiatric consultant then made his best clinical
guess, diagnosing the problem.

(3) He then stated a plan of action. The diagnosis and the
procedures to be followed were explicitly stated.

(4) Finally, the consultant stated his intention to return
in one week, and did return to revise anything found to be
erroneous in the plan of action.

Phase II consisted of weekly case seminars concerning
pupils. These were viewed as educative for the teacher, a form of
in-service training. It was hoped that through these sessions the
teachers could become more informed, purposeful, and effective therapeutic agents. Their roles as therapeutic agents were considered
inseparable from their didactic tasks. These were large steps toward constructing a therapeutic community in the school.

V. ARTIFICIAL COMMUNITY INTERVENTIONS

The Artificial Community Interventions perceive a problem in the child, emanating from a problem in the environment.
Their actions, directed toward a change in the child, utilize special environments to effect this change. These interventions remove the person, who is defined by society as deviant, from his
natural environment and place him in an artificial community. The
communities are "artificial" in that their reason for being is the
re-socialization of "social deviants." The main goal of the Artificial Community Interventions is to provide the resident with a
role, a place in a community. The Maxim Gorky Labor Colony and
Hawthorne Cedar Knolls include academic education as a part of this
goal. The Industrial Neurosis Unit and Highfields do not.

Educative Approaches: Maxim Gorky Labor Colony

The Gorky Colony existed in the U.S.S.R. in the 1920's
under the directorship of Anton Semyonovich Makarenko (1951).

The problem population which made up the Gorky Colony was
a delinquent one: street waifs, highwaymen, burglars and pickpockets--
of 13 years old and older. Makarenko's book, The Road to Life gives
the impression that these boys and girls were a product of circumstances. The targets of the intervention action were the boys and
girls. The environment of the colony was utilized to effect change.

It is Makarenko's philosophy that the extent to which a waif falls short of the norm can always be probed and made good. "In a healthy collective he is sure--given the slightest spark of intelligence--to turn out a real human being." Makarenko has a definite idea of the type of human being he is striving to mold. To Makarenko, a real human being is a person with a communist personality, characterized by high intellectual standards combined with education and culture. He is a person who <u>uses</u> the high ideals he has internalized. He is devoted to principle, but regards principle as a gauge, not as a blindfold. He is possessed of a sense of humor, terseness of speech, dislike of ready-made formulas, the inability to lounge on sofas or sprawl over a table, and a gay but unlimited capacity for work, with none of the blessed martyr pose. Makarenko's ideal person has a sense of duty, honor, industry, and a high degree of social adhesiveness. Social adhesiveness is a complex trait which consists of common principles within a group, a constant awareness of one another, and perpetual consciousness of one high common goal. This consciousness constantly manifests itself in work toward this goal.

The personalities illustrated in <u>The Road to Life</u> demonstrate that this "ideal character" has many configurations. Makarenko developed a talent for "sizing up" raw material (the waif as he came from the street) and picturing the final product (the youth after experience in the collective). Makarenko wished to give the

youths the skills, pride, and self-confidence they need to take on
any role they might desire in society.

The colonists were aware that their potential station
in life was enhanced by their progress in the Gorky Colony. This
is illustrated by an exchange between a villager and a colonist
at a celebration commemorating the wedding of a girl colonist:

'Lads! Is it really true that you're the bosses here?'

'Of course we are!'

'What d'you need to farm the land for?'

'Don't you know what for? We'd have to be farmhands otherwise, and now we don't have to.'

'And what are you going to be?'

'Oho!...I'm going to be an engineer--Anton Semyonovich
(Makarenko) says I am, too--and Shelaputin is going to
be a pilot'
(Makarenko, Part <u>2</u>, p. 200)

Children were sent to the Gorky Colony by the various
bureaus of the government (Child Welfare, Social Education). The
colony was the only place of residence for the boys and girls.
Most were orphans or alienated from their families. A resident had
freedom of choice regarding whether he would remain in the colony
or leave it. The colony was self-supporting. It included dormi-
tories, a school, a theater, workshops (cobblers, carpentry, smith-
ing, a flour mill) and agricultural facilities for raising cattle,
hogs and farming the land.

In the Gorky Colony everyone acted upon everyone else. Makarenko chose the teachers and staff on the basis of their being real human beings. Makarenko made wure that these teachers were well-paid. The Road to Life demonstrates how very fully Makarenko's personality and the personalities of his staff were involved in the intervention into the boys' lives. This use of personality, involvement, and dedication is something which can be captured only in the dialogues, situations, and day-to-day dramas presented in Makarenko's "diary," The Road to Life. Specific techniques employed in the colony's "collective education" are described below.

Group Processes: the Detachment. The colony members were divided into detachments (groups), each with a specific work requirement. Each detachment had a "commander" chosen by the members of the detachment. The detachment was Makarenko's "basic technological feature" in the collective education of the colonists. The composition of each detachment varied little over time. Even if there was a turnover of persons, "the detachment is a collective, with its own traditions, history, merits, and reputation (Makarenko, Part 3, p. 280-281)." Each detachment had a numérical name, and a "speciality." The detachments were: First Detachment, cobblers; Second Detachment, grooms; Third Detachment, cowherds; Fourth Detachment, carpenters; Fifth Detachment, girls; Sixth Detachment, smiths; Seventh Detachment, Rabfak Candidates (Rabfak is the institution of higher learning); Eighth Detachment, field workers; Ninth

Detachment, millers; Tenth Detachment, hog tenders; Eleventh

Detachment, small fry. A rule, made by the colonists, was that all

work, pleasant or unpleasant, was performed by the detachments in

shifts, according to numerical order. A shift lasted one month.

A teacher was assigned to every two or three detachments.

"The function of these teachers was to stimulate within detachments

the concept of collective honor, and the desire to occupy the best

and most looked-up-to position in the colony (Makarenko, Part 3,

p. 282)."

Decision-making and power were emphasized at Gorky. The

detachment commanders had much decision-making power within the

colony. If there was a crisis involving whether or not a member of

the colony should be allowed to remain at the colony, the "Com-

manders' Council" would make the decision. Any decisions involving

the future of the colony as a whole were made by the Commanders'

Council, in meetings with the entire population of the colony in

attendance.

Collective Identification and Pride in the Collective. The

boys and girls who lived in the Gorky Colony were "Gorkyites." The

colony was not a place, not an institution, but a living, breathing

entity of people and material things which they built, renovate,

or worked hard to obtain; it was a collective. Makarenko's

charges didn't feel the stigma of being delinquents, but rather

pride in their collective. The feeling was "We are Gorkyites. We can do anything."

The colonists enjoyed a march through the town, complete with red banner and bugles playing a march. "People notice us in the streets, gather round us when we halt, ask us questions, make friends. The gay, smart colonists joke, rest, feel the beauty of their collective (Makarenko, Part 3, p. 399)."

Gorkyites came and went, but a Gorkyite was always a Gorkyite. Older members of the colony, who had gone away to the Rabfak (institution of higher learning) returned for special celebrations and at crucial moments when help or support was needed. They were not "outsiders" when they returned, but functioning members of the colony.

Provision of a Cause: The Interests of the Collective. Their pride in the collective was justly deserved. The need for a cause, for an identity was strongly felt by Makarenko. The colony had to be constantly on the move. It could not stagnate. It had to embody one goal while it worked toward another. This could be outwardly observed in the manner in which the colony transformed a tumble-down estate into a sort of "model farm" complete with high quality home-grown animals. As soon as the colony became entrenched at the Tripke Estate, it took up a new challenge: to transform a badly demoralized children's home at Kuryazh into a "new Gorky Colony." The challenge was, of course, met handsonely.

As they took on this new challenge, the colonists realiz-

ed that it was necessary to subordinate everything to the requirements of the collective. At this time Makarenko said, "It was a
joy, perhaps the deepest joy the world has to give--this feeling
of interdependence, of the strength and flexibility of human relations of the calm, vast power of the collective, vibrating in an
atmosphere permeated with its own force (Makarenko, Part 2,
p. 340)."

Each of the Gorky residents had his path in life, and
the Gorky Colony, too, had its path. The Colony's path was not
an isolated one. It crossed the paths of other groups. The collective "had formed complex social ties with other organizations--
Komsomol, Pioneer, sport, military and club. Innumerable roads
and paths had been trodden between the colony and the town, along
which thoughts, ideas, and influences travelled, as well as human
beings (Makarenko, Part 3, p. 881)." The path of the Gorky Colony
also crossed the path of the Soviet nation. Marching through the
town of Podvorky, on the way to Kuryazh, Makarenko "suddenly realized the vast historical significance of our march,...our colony
was performing a task which, slight as it might be, was nonetheless
acutely political, a veritably socialist task (Makarenko, Part 3,
pp. 19-28)."

The Komsomol organization, a communist youth club, was
part of the life at Gorky. This common political philosophy and
the fact that the Gorkyites were taking part in the "constructional

work" of their nation did much to unite the colonists.

The Gorky Colony's path was explained by Makarenko in this manner: "We must get rich, we must study, we must clear a path for ourselves and for future Gorkyites, must learn to live like true proletarians, and leave the colony true Komsomols, in order, outside the colony, too, to build up and strengthen the proletarian state (Makarenko, Part 3, p. 202)."

This path could not be followed, nor its goal reached, without discipline.

Conscious Discipline: The Pressure of the Collective.
Makarenko utilized his own interpretation of "conscious discipline." He stated that "the necessity, usefulness, obligatory character, and class significance of a given disciplinary measure must be made absolutely clear (Makarenko, Part 3, pp. 265-266)." Makarenko felt that this discipline whould develop from collective experience, as a result of the "friendly pressure of a collective."

He was in disagreement with the Soviety pedagogical theorists of his day who interpreted "conscious discipline" as meaning that discipline would emerge from "pure consciousness, from purely intellectual conviction,...from ideas." These theorists felt that conscious discipline could not result from adult influence. Self-discipline was required. "in the same way they reasoned that any form of organization for children is unnecessary and harmful, excepting 'self-organization,' which is essential (Makarenko, Part 3, p. 266)."

Discipline and the order of everyday life became the traditions of the collective. The collective was concerned with discipline and order not merely when infringement arose, but all the time, guided by the "collective instinct."

The Opening of Perspectives: Joy. Another technique used by Makarenko is his collective education of the Gorky Colonists, was "opening out of new perspectives." There were two methods of opening perspectives and heightening endeavor. One method was to establish perspective for the individuals, "with a certain emphasis upon his material interests (Makarenko, Part 3. p. 282)." Wages played an important role in this method. Makarenko, himself, believed in the concept of wages. It enabled children to gain something practical from education, rather than ideals only. But money for payment or reward was strictly forbidden by Makarenko's superiors in the Soviet bureaucracy. Makarenko, then utilized the second method of opening perspectives which consisted of "raising the tone of the collective, and organizing an elaborate system of collective perspective (Makarenko, Part 3, p. 283)."

Makarenko believed that tomorrow's joy was the greatest motivator. "Man must have something joyful ahead of him to live for. The true stimulus in human life is the morrow's joy. In pedagogical technique this not too distant joy is one of the most important objects to be worked for. In the first place, the joy itself has to be organized, brought to life, and converted into a possibility. Next, primitive sources of satisfaction must be steadily converted into more complex and humanly significant joys." The satisfaction of eating a sweet biscuit develops into the satisfaction based on the sense of duty. "To educate a man is to furnish him with a perspective leading to the morrow's joy. It consists in the organization of new perspectives, in the full use of existing ones, in the gradual building of worthier ones (Makarenko, Part 3, pp. 283-284)."

The Kuryazhites (the new Gorkyites) were shown the value of human personality, "the most joyful perspective of all," during a "Gorky evening." Gorky the man, as illustrated in his writings and his letters to the colonists, was shown to them. "They had never imagined that such a life was possible." They next day the new Gorkyites began to work. For now they saw a goal, and a purpose. "They made the most conscientious and stupendous efforts to overcome the sloth which is man's oldest heritage (Makarenko, Part 3, p. 287)."

Style and Tone. Makarenko identified wtyle and tone as important elements in collective education. Style is a delicate thing,
requiring constant attention. It is not rapidly built up. It depends on
the slow accumulation of traditions, conceptions and habits which
are accepted "by conscious respect for the experience of older
generations (Makarenko, Part 3, p. 264)."

The "detachment-commander" organization and the fact that
colony members wore uniforms, marched in lines, had "colors" and
a bugle, imparted a military style to the Gorky Colony. Its style
was military, but its deep-down organization was not. The hierarchical command structure of the military was lacking, and the list
of rules and punishments was lacking. One the one hand, expectations were definite. Everyone knew what was expected of him and
how to carry it through. Yet rules were situation-specific, not
absolute.

For example, two situations involving drinking were handled differently. One boy, depressed because his friends were
leaving for the Rabfak, became drunk on the day of their departure.
He went into the Director's (Makarenko) office. The Director sent
him to bed. At a different time a boy became drunk because he
didn't get his way concerning a personal problem. The Commander's
Council decided on "turning him out." He was required to leave the
Colony.

It must not be supposed from the military style that Makarenko was not concerned with emotion. He was very sensitive to the expression of emotions and "dreams." He noted the most subtle expression of emotion in boys who had lived most of their lives on the street and who were usually at first incapable of expressing emotion.

Tradition: Ceremony Insignia. Another characteristic of the Gorky Colony's style is that they did things in a grand and dramatic manner. Several celebrations were held annually by the colony.

The Feast of the First Sheaf was held annually on the 5th of July. The townspeople were invited to this feast. After the Gorky Colony's move to Kuryazh, the Feast of the First Sheaf afforded a special opportunity to display the new colony, and its agricultural methods, to guests. This particular celebration included costumed buglers on horseback, colonists with flowers in their buttonholes and traditional festive speeches made up in Commander's Council.

On the 26th of March, annually, the Colony celebrated the anniversary of A. M. Gorky's birthday. Most Gorky celebrations included the townspeople, but this particular one was for Gorky Colonists only. "Everything was very simple and intimate, drawing the Gorkyites still closer, although there was nothing domestic

about the forms of the celebrations themselves. We began with a
parade, solemnly bringing out the banner, speeches were made, and
then there was a solemn march past the portrait of Gorky (Makarenko,
Part 2, pp. 98-100)."

On one occasion of the celebration of Marxim Gorky's
birthday, the identification as "colonist" was legitimized. "The
title of 'Colonist' was only given to those who truly valued the
Colony, and worked for its improvement (both youthful residents
and staff). But those who lagged behind, who complained, muttered,
or played truant, would remain mere "charges"...At the same time
it was resolved: if a staff member did not receive this title during the first year of work, he would have to leave the colony.
Each colonist received a nickel-plated badge, made to our special
order in a Kharkov factory. The badge was in the form of a life
belt, inscribed with the letters "M.G." (Maxim Gorky), and on top
was a red star (Makarenko, Part 2, pp. 102-103)."

The colonists kept up a running correspondence with Alexei
Maximovich Gorky. The fact that this great man (Makarenko had considerable difficulty convincing the colonists that Gorky really was
a man, who was once a boy, just like them) identified with and
corresponded with the colony, gave the colonists a sense of worth
and seemed to make them want to work harder in school and to make
something of their lives.

The letters from Gorky were very dearly cherished by the colonists. They were read over and over again, with the admonition from a Commander with an eye to preservation, "Don't pass your fingers under the words. You've got eyes, you can read without your fingers (Makarenko, p. 237)."

At the Gorky Colony, the collective entity, collective pride, collective identity, collective tradition, collective interests and goals served to make tomorrow's joy a reality for hundreds of former street waifs.

Educative Approaches: Hawthorne Cedar Knolls

The staff of Hawthorne Cedar Knolls, a residential educative institution in New York, perceives the problem as existing within the child. Ninety per cent of the Hawthorne population, which consists of boys, aged 8-1/2 to 18, and girls, aged 13 to 18, have serious school learning problems, even though IQ's are not significantly different from normal. The older population are serious school management problems. There is some feeling that the environment is the source of the child's problem. It is reported that children who manifested problem-causing attitudes and values had grown up in "chaotic homes." The change action of Hawthorne is directed toward the child. It utilizes the environment by organizing the physical classroom, teacher-student relationship, and teaching techniques around the needs of the student.

433

The purpose of the intervention is to transform these young "failures" into functioning members of society. The goal of the intervention is to re-orient the values of the child, to shift cultural attitudes, and, specifically, to change his concept of school. At Hawthorne the child acquires skills and is stimulated by higher aspirations and achievements.

This task is accomplished at Hawthorne Cedar Knolls by the hour-by-hour management of the child in all phases of his life. Hawthorne is treatment (psychiatric) as well as education-oriented. The controlled environment produces an atmosphere of treatment and self-help. The school is oriented toward healing and understanding. The educative aspect of the treatment, as reported by Goldsmith, Krohn, Ochroch and Kagan (1965), will be described here.

One of the techniques utilized by the school is division of the population into separate classes based on age and needs. The "junior boys" class demonstrates a need for security. This class is given one teacher. Through this teacher the boys are exposed to consistent behavior and kindness from an adult. An effort is made to remove the element of competition from the classroom. All of the children at Hawthorne Cedar Knolls are also provided with the security of cottage life.

A second class is made up of older boys and girls who are not delinquents and who are considered more "fragile" than the remainder of the population. These students are motivated toward continuing a formal academic program. A modified core program on the 9th and 10th grade levels is prepared for them.

A third segment of the population is made up of older, aggressive, "extremely delinquent" boys. Contained therein are severe management problems. Their attitude toward school is a hostile one. These boys have no desire to continue their high school education. The work they do in the Hawthorne school is related to large projects. The boys acquire various skills and knowledge while working on a specific project. Control and physical work are the keynotes of this particular class.

The fourth class is made up of persons who fall between the last two class-categories. These are persons who are ambivalent toward school and who have experienced much failure. Here again activity classes are used, but with modifications. A defined class organization is present but it embodies a great deal of flexibility. There is flexibility with regard to curricular materials, the length of time spent on a particular activity and demands made by teachers for productivity. The goal is to provide a successful learning experience, and, by so doing, to encourage the student in his educational endeavor.

The most difficult teaching problem is provided by a fifth class of youngsters. They are intelligent, aggressive and delinquent. The set of experiences contrived for the handling of these boys is described in their teacher's daily anecdotal records.

Although his is a kind of "post hoc methodology," the activities are utilized in other interventions.

The problems of the boys, as they relate to the goal of education, were viewed by the teacher, Kagan, as follows: The boys' attitudes, values and beliefs were not those which would lead to success in school or in life. The boys believed that adults were negative, mean and selfish. The boys were apathetic, moody, and, underneath the delinquent bravado, felt worthless. They demonstrated a facility to utilize therapeutic phraseology to keep from doing things ("I'm disturbed today."). Along with this went a tendency to blame others for things they could not do. They displayed no serious goals or plans. This particular segment of the population felt a need for status as a socially acceptable group.

Kagan felt that the purpose of his intervention was to teach each youngster "that which was in line with his level of functioning, was of interest to him, and which he needed in order to stimulate some realisitic aspirations." In order to do this he had to address himself to each of the problems listed above.

So that the boys would learn that adults and adult values were not all negative, Kagan had to use himself to project the image of a "model" adult--friendly, helpful, and concerned. He maintains that his projection of the "model adult" image, his use of his personality with the students, was largely intuitive. Kagan respected the boys in his class and used the normal social amenities toward them. He was concerned that the size of his class did not allow him to devote sufficient individual attention to each boy. He showed each student his concern by, at least, a nod or a slap on the back.

So that each boy could overcome his belief in his own worthlessness, he needed to achieve tangible, measurable productivity. To aid the boys in developing a feeling of worth, Kagan emphasized the positive aspects of their behavior and achievements, and largely ignored the negative aspects. When a student performed well, the teacher communicated this fact to everyone at the residency who interacted with the boy.

Kagan also organized the physical classroom and his teaching techniques around the need to provide the boys with achievement. The physical plant was set up to provide comfort and control. The setting was divided into two areas, craft and academic. The latter consisted of four tables and chairs closely lining the walls. This was "in recognition of the preference of many of the boys to sit with their backs to the wall or off in a corner." As the boys manifested interests which could be translated into productive classroom experiences, activities and equipment were introduced to meet these interests. Kagan used ungraded texts so that there would be no stigma attached to the level at which a student was working.

To counteract the use of therapeutic phraseology and blaming others as explanations for failure, Kagan treated the unimpaired learners in his class with a certain amount of challenge. When they resisted performing, and utilized therapeutic jargon as excuses, he questioned them concerning whether they expected to solve their emotional problems in the next few years. When they answered in the positive, he replied, "Fine, you'll be healthy but unemployed." Kagan never utilized this technique with impaired learners. Instead he constantly encouraged them and reminded them of their progress. The teacher and the school supervisor made it difficult for the students to "pass the buck," to blame others for their own underproduction. As an example, if a boy complained that he didn't have something done due to lack of a reference book, the teacher would send him to the supervisor, who would make sure the student had the book in hand as soon as possible.

The intervention technique requires that the teacher be very explicit with the boys as to specific goals. The possibility of removal from class by the supervisor, due to lack of production, was omnipresent.

So that the boys would come to manifest serious goals and plans, they were "encouraged and helped to explore their interests and occupational goals even when these goals were rather fantastic." The teacher "slowly helped them modify these goals to make them more realistically attainable (Goldsmith et al., p. 284)."

438

To aid in providing status as a socially acceptable group, it was emphasized to the boys, time after time, that knowledge is equivalent to power.

What has been related here is an effort to "change the delinquent's concept of school" largely through accentuation of the positive--a positive and helpful adult, positive achievement, and positive life goals.

Noneducative Approaches: Industrial Neurosis Unit

Maxwell Jones, a pioneer in the area of the therapeutic milieu, sets down the record of his first efforts in The Therapeutic Community (1953). It describes the Industrial Neurosis Unit of the Belmont Hospital in England, which was under Jones' directorship beginning in April, 1947.

The staff of the Industrial Neurosis Unit view the problem as centered in the individual. They identify this problem as desocialization of the patients with severe character disorders. These are men and women who have experienced chronic failure. They are unable to hold a job and prone to cause disturbances; they are 'trouble-makers." The source of the patient's problem is to be found in the environment: "They are the symptoms of a sick society." "Inevitably they have developed anti-social attitudes in an attempt to defend themselves from what appears to them as a hostile environment." The action taken in the Industrial Neurosis Unit is

directed toward a change in the patients. The action utilizes environment to effect this change, since 'a healthy group life makes
healthy individuals."

The objective of the intervention is resocialization of
the patient. The ultimate goal is their resettlement   into their
own communities and jobs.

The average stay at the Unit is from 2-4 months. A patient's discharge date is decided by his psychiatrist. The patient's
psychiatric state and the availability of a suitable job are major
factors in this decision.

The therapeutic community of the Industrial Neurosis
Unit consists of carefully managed relationships within a closed
institution. There is a well-defined social structure and a well-
trained staff. The aim is to construct a unit culture, and to
give the patient vocational and social roles in this culture.

"Therapy "as conceived in the Industrial Neurosis Unit
includes the entire waking day of the patient and includes all his
contacts with other persons. Treatment is located in the interactions of healthy community life as experienced within the Unit.
In this view of therapy, the doctors, nurses, job supervisors and
other patients all play vital roles in the treatment.

The staff of the Industrial Neurosis Unit includes 4
psychiatrists, 1 psychologist, 2 psychiatric social workers, 2
disablement resettlment officers of the Ministry of Labor, 5 occu-

pational instructors. 1 research technician, and a nursing staff of 20.

The physical plant consists of 5 vocational occupational workshops--hairdressing, tailoring, plastering, capentry, and bricklaying--each with its own instructor.

Roles. Since roles are "an essential factor in the development of a therapeutic community (Jones, p. 49)," some space will be taken here to discuss the roles of the staff and patients. The agreement of the staff with the treatment program, and a certain set of staff attitudes are of utmost importance in a therapeutic community type of intervention.

An important member of the research staff is the D.R.O., the disablement resettlement officer of the Department of Labor. It is the D.R.O.'s role to give point and purpose to the psychiatric treatment and a work goal to the patient. The D.R.O. is a liaison between the patient's desires and the "limitations of the labor market for neurotics." Another responsibility of the D.R.O. is to attempt to make the interview with an employer (the culmination of the D.R.O.'s efforts) a successful one.

The patient has a relatively free choice of roles and associations. He is obligated to participate in the social situations created by the workshops and the discussion groups. The social and vocational roles which he is encouraged to take on while in the hospital "approximate as far as possible to what is found in the relatively healthy outside community." The patient group as a whole needs to feel that there is a positive group structure and discipline to guide them.

The nurse is seen as having three roles: authoritarian, social and therapeutic. In her authoritarian role, it is her responsibility to give the patient community a positive discipline. She must not, however, make decisions which should be made by the patients. In her social role she must give her patients a feeling of security and of being understood. She must not behave to fulfill her own sexual and social needs. The norm against patient-nurse sexual contact is a strong one. It is felt that the patients need non-sexual parent figures. In her treatment role, it is the nurse's duty to interpret or transmit the Unit culture to the patient. "The more she has accepted this culture, the more readily and competently can she fulfill her (treatment) role." One of the nurses commented that maintaining a balance between the authoritarian role, the social role, and the treatment role, is rather like walking a tightrope. She felt that the nurse's uniform and title helped her maintain the balance. Physical accoutrements and 'uniform' are important to the atmosphere conveyed by a particular milieu.

The nurses and doctors of the Industrial Neurosis Unit are acting to fulfill a particular treatment goal to a much greater degree than they are acting out the traditional professional nurse

442

and professional doctor roles. The relationship between doctors and nurses is one of "unusually good understanding." The fact of being members of a research team, acting in line with a particular treatment goal, and the stress on free communication, draws them together in a manner that the normal hospital hierarchy does not. The relationship found in the Industrial Neurosis Unit is sometimes difficult to maintain alongside other wards which use a more traditional approach.

The doctors do not dress the part of a professional doctor. There is no white coat and no stethoscope. There is an attempt to bring the doctor's role into a realistic perspective and to avoid the pretense that the doctor is a miracle worker. This is difficult to accomplish, however, as many patients view the doctor in this light. The doctor's role, vis-a-vis the patient in the Industrial Neurosis Unit, is social, supportive, exemplary, activating, and interpretive.

The doctors, nurses, and the D.R.O. attempt to utilize social therapy techniques to convert potential roles into actual social and vocational roles. The patients experience a definite pattern, a routine, in which these social techniques of therapy are spaced. This is possible due to the residential nature of the Unit.

At 8 A.M. breakfast is over.

9 A.M. fatigues are over.

9 A.M. - 10 A.M. a community meeting is held.

These meetings take varying forms throughout the week.

Monday is devoted to grievances.

Tuesday--films depicting job training, rehabilitation, social

problems are shown.

Wednesday--a discussion group is held.

Thursday--a discussion group is held.

Friday--a psychodrama is presented

10 A.M. - 12 Noon	Patients work.
2 P.M. - 4 P.M.	Patients work.
4 P.M. - 7 P.M.	Patients who are 'well enough' may leave the grounds.
7 P.M. - 9 P.M.	An organized social program prepared by a committee chosen from the patients is presented.
9 P.M.	Bed.

Therapeutic Techniques. Several different therapeutic
techniques are utilized in the Industrial Neurosis Unit. The
concept of the therapeutic milieu includes a bias away from psychoanalytic treatment. Relatively few of the patients in the
Industrial Neurosis Unit receive uncovering types of treatment.
Individual treatment is mainly along supportive lines.
There are however, facilities for "all known physical methods of

444

known physical methods of psychiatric treatment." Insulin and electrical convulsive treatments are used frequently.

The work therapy is considered an important part of the treatment. Despite the definitive nature of the workshops, there is no attempt to train for a trade. Rather, the aim is to return the patient to the habit of work. The conditions of work approximate as closely as possible semi-skilled or unskilled factory work. Maxwell Jones emphasized time and again that it is a patient's attitude toward work, rather than his aptitude which has the greater probability of predicting success in a job. Placement into a particular workshop in the hospital is not arbitrary. The decision is made by the patient, the psychologist, the D.R.O., and the patient's own doctor (one of the 4 psychiatrists). An attempt is made to fit his placement with employment prospects in the patient's home area. The D.R.O. and his contacts are indispensable in this attempt.

Unit discussion groups, documentary films and psycho-dramas are all considered educative in that they attempt to build a group attitude which will be incorporated into the Unit culture and internalized in the individual. The main principle behind these techniques is that "social problems and real life situations are either raised in discussion or acted out in psychodrama. The whole group attempts to arrive at a constructive attitude in relation to the problem raised." Their purpose is to change social attitudes in the desocialized patient.

445

Psychodramas are theatrical presentations of episodes from the patient's past life. The patient chooses the cast, writes and produces the drama. This involves one week of preparation. Occupations of the cast are suspended, rehearsals taking the place of work in their general routine. One of the values of the psychodrama is that it requires the patient to view all the roles of the participants in this particular episode of his life. Another value is the group experience. The presentation of the psychodrama is followed by a discussion led by a psychiatrist. During this discussion the 'director' of the drama has an opportunity to compare his attitude with that of others.

Other activities, such as beginners' dance classes, socials, and concerts are attended voluntarily by the patients and by the staff. Facilities for sports are available. These are conceived as a part of the treatment since they provide opportunities for creating social roles. Importance is attached to activities (e.g., dancing) which have 'social currency,' and can be utilized in the patient's relationship with the outside community.

Two types of therapy groups are set up to utilize group processes as treatment. Group A consists of 16 to 28 persons who meet for about an hour. The topic of discussion is chosen by the group. There is a tendency to relate to the group what might be related to the patient's doctor. The role of the leader (a staff member) is not an active one. The staff feels that the actual con-

446

tent of the group session is not of prime importance. Rather the
identification and interest generated are the positive factors.
The pervasive attitude of the group toward any one individual seems
to be "We are like you; it helps to talk."

Group B is made up of six people from Group A. This is a
more intimate and cohesive group. The feeling of belonging engendered in this small group session is an aid in reaching the major
goal of the Unit, i.e., to provide the patient with a social role,
a place in the community. The group remains cohesive outside of
the context of their regular meetings. It is felt by the staff
that social pressure, as experienced in a group, does appear to
bring about modifications in personality.

Culture. In addition to the social therapies described
above, there is a wider cultural aspect of treatment. The concept
of culture as it is applied in the Industrial Neurosis Unit is that
it is a cluster of socially determined attitudes and behavior patterns grouped and elaborated around structurally defined roles and
relationships. Jones believes that it is the internal assimilation
and integration of culture that is disturbed during the process of the
desocialization of the chronically unemployed patient population.
The efforts of the staff are toward the development of a suitable
hospital culture in which to resocialize the patients. The Unit
culture is to be realistic, to approximate real-life situations

447

and to aid the patient in his adjustment to these. The patients
who are admitted to the Industrial Neurosis Unit are generally
those who have no place in society. They come from broken homes
and are unemployed. The intervention is an attempt to absorb the
patient into the Unit community, which has developed a definite
culture of its own. In the Industrial Neurosis Unit, the culture
is a 'conscious' one. There is awareness of the motives behind a
pattern of behavior. The doctor does not make all the decisions.
Instead, the "aim is to achieve a communal responsibility in relation to all Unit problems whether they relate to patients or
staff."

In the Industrial Neurosis Unit, "attitudes tend to perpetuate through the most stable, united and permanent group, i.e.,
the staff." It is recognized, however, that the patients do a good
deal of acting on each other, and that the patients in residence
make a difference in the treatment experience. "It might be said
that the more the patient culture approximates to the Unit culture
as represented by the staff, the greater will be the effectiveness
in treating new patients." Some patients absorb the group culture
well, others to a lesser degree, and it seems probable that it is
the degree to which this initial identification can take place,
irrespective of the severity of the patient's illness, which determines the success of the intervention.

448

It would seem that the major contribution of the therapeutic community is social adjustment, social awareness; and it is
those who have problems in this area who will show the most improvement.

Noneducative Approaches: Highfields

The staff of the Highfields experimental treatment project for youthful offenders at Hopewell, New Jersey (McCorkle, Elias
and Bixby, 1958) views the problem as existing within the child.
The population at Highfields is described as "normal delinquent
boys." Their delinquency and their anti-social attitudes are identified as the problem. The source of the problem is to be found
in the environment. Case histories of the boys indicate that family problems and gang life contribute to their delinquency. The
goal of the intervention is to effect a change in the boy. Highfields utilizes its own environment to aid in this change.

The boys at Highfields are all adjudicated offenders.
When the court is confronted with a youth deemed suitable for
short-term treatment, it informs the boy that his sentence will
be suspended if he agrees to come to Highfields for from 1 to 6
months. When the boy is released from Highfields he is placed on
regular probation in his community. Since Highfields is an institutional setting, it is able to exercise some choice as to the
offenders it will treat. Highfields requires that a boy be at

449

least 16 years of age, with no previous institutionalization. Highfields will not accept homosexual boys.

Highfields is a small residential institution for 18
boys. The boys are removed from their community and live at the
house at Highfields.

The objective of the Highfields project is resocialization. Many of the boys' problems stem from their "conception of
self and others as hostile, aggressive, inadequate persons." The
Highfields program is organized to change these distorted images.

Highfields aims to make the life at the house a microcosm
of the way life should be in the 'real world'. The staff is concerned with helping the boys gradually work up to the standard of
the outside world, not with creating special 'institutional'
standards for them.

The Highfields staff strives to build security, informality and flexibility into their treatment program. There is an
absence of punitive or counter-aggressive attitudes on the part
of the staff. The progenitors of Highfields feel that, in order
to understand themselves and others, the boys need an informal,
easy experience in a social world.

The physical environment adds to the atmosphere. Highfields' setting is a reconditioned farmhouse on 400 acres, much of
which is heavily wooded. "In a sense, the entire facility represents a single, almost natural unit." There is an absence of

physical restraints such as walls, locks, bars or custodians. The physical accoutrements at Highfields also suggest informality in more subtle ways. There are no bulletin boards, signs, posters notices or labels. There is no period of quarantine, no uniforms, no school, no vocational training, no organized recreation. There is no rule book and no schedule of activities that account for every moment of the day.

There are only 2 inflexible rules at Highfields: 1) The boys are not permitted to leave the grounds unless accompanied by an adult. 2) The boys are not permitted to converse with the female patients at the Neuropsychiatric Institute where they work.

No effort is made to prevent escape. The only sanction against the boys walking away from Highfields is that it is a violation of probation.

Highfields is not a stigma-producing institution, whereas the reformatory, which is the alternative form of treatment for the boys, does produce a stigma. The threat of the reformatory acts as an unspoken sanction. "The reality of the reformatory often-times is sufficient to define the limits of conduct for the major-ity (McCorkle et al., p. 66)."

Informality and flexibility are manifest in the fact that the traditions and customs manufactured and maintained by the boys themselves provide the only structure in the social system represented by the house at Highfields. Informality and flexibility are also manifest in the fact that each action and reaction is considered as it arises. The staff must think about each act of the boys in terms of the objectives of the program, rather than in terms of a predetermined set of rules and regulations. It is extremely important, therefore, that the staff members accept and agree with the program adopted at Highfields.

The staff consists of a director, an intern and cottage supervisors who live at Highfields. A secretary and a work supervisor are daytime employees. The main function of all the staff is to "help the boys." The director plays a dual role as therapist and administrator. He is the guided group interaction leader. He keeps in close contact with county court officials. The intern is a trainee, a graduate student in sociology, who spends one year at Highfields. The cottage supervisors are a married couple with no previous experience working with delinquent boys. They relate to the boys in a spontaneous, non-institutional way. The boys relate to them as adults, not as carriers of a particular role. McCorkle et al. believe that it is the non-professional personnel which help most, understand most, and create the greatest impact on the boys. Requirements for the job of work supervisor are a bachelor's degree and experience with delinquent boys. The main tasks are to supervise the boys at work (in this, the work supervisor takes on the role of a boss, or foreman), and to take the boys to town on Saturday evenings.

452

There is an attempt to minimize differentiation of the boys at Highfields. There is no formal categorization, no trustees, no merit system. The roles, which the boys have established themselves, are simply "new boy" and "old boy." A boy is an "old boy" when he acts like he has learned something and is ready to go home.

There is free communication between staff and client. The boys are told that they "are welcome to ask questions of any employee at the house at any time (McCorkle et al., p.2)." The question to which the staff will not have an answer is, "When can I get out of here?" No set time for a boy's stay at Highfields is made. He must "work his way out."

A boy works his way out by

(1) living in the house at Highfields and participating in its social structure,

(2) participating in guided group interaction sessions,

(3) working at a nearby state hospital, and

(4) maintaining contact with his community.

Life in the house. The atmosphere is informal. The boys talk, as you would expect boys of sixteen and seventeen to talk, about girls and cars. There is no rigid rule against profanity. The talk is natural and expressive.

That problematic situations arise through the natural interactions of boys with boys, and boys with staff, is desirable.

These situations are thought and discussion provoking. The boys have a chance to judge and make decisions.

As part of the life at the house, the boys are awakened individually at 6 a.m. each working day by Mr. M_, the cottage supervisor. The boys have rotating KP duty, helping "Mom" (Mrs. M_) prepare means and clean the house. There are two "bed checks" every evening. Mr. M_ checks the room at 10 p.m. and talks with the boys as he does so. Mr. M_ makes another check at 11 p.m.

Work. The boys do agricultural work at the nearby Neuropsychiatric Institute from 8 a.m. to 5 p.m., Monday through Friday. They are supervised by the staff work supervisor, and paid fifty cents a day. The function of their work is the establishment of work habits, rather than vocational training. A boy may be suspended or fired from his job at the Institute. If this happens, he is required to work at Highfields, but he receives no pay.

Guided group interaction. The boys are divided into two groups of nine members for purposes of the guided group interaction sessions. The groups remain stable except when an "old boy" leaves Highfields and is replaced by a "new boy." The guided group interaction sessions are held in the evenings. The therapist (director) is active in these sessions. He plays a critical, supportive, guiding role.

The boys discuss whatever they wish. The therapist attempts to guide the discussion so that matters are discussed which relate to adjustment. The guided group interaction session is designed to break down the defenses of the boys, to get them operating toward their own adjustment.

Due to the lack of structure at Highfields, the boys complain that "everything a boy does can be a problem." This is exactly what is desired. It is these problems, disturbing to the boys, which are brought up and discussed at the guided group inter-action sessions. Each meeting is summarized by the leader (dir-ector). The boys are asked if they know why the content and tone of the meeting was as it was.

Requests to leave Highfields and return home are made within the guided group interaction sessions. Similarly, the decisions of the peer group and the director, as to whether a boy is ready to leave, are announced within the sessions. There is a turnover rate of about 5 boys per month. "These group shifts point to the fact that Highfields must be viewed in two quite different lights: on the one hand, as an abstraction, it is a firm, contin-uing program with a specific philosophy and definite goals. On the other hand, on the concrete level, it is a series of constantly changing groups each with its own structure and problems--a highly unstable culture, held together by fixed principles and aims."

The Highfields' staff emphasizes that a boy's success at Highfields depends to a great extent on who is there when he arrives, and if this population is one which will orient him and carry on the traditions. These conditions are termed "auspicious circumstances."

Contact with community. The boys at Highfields make a "recreational" trip to Hopewell, the nearest community to High-feilds, every Saturday. They are accompanied by the work supervisor. On Sunday, the boys may entertain visitors at Highfields. They may leave the premises only if an adult is included in the party.

In addition, the boys may be granted two or more three-day furloughs to go home. One of the boys explained the rationale behind the furlough as follows:

> There are reasons why boys get furloughs. They aren't gifts. A boy gets his first furlough to see what his problems are and he gets home on his second to see if he has solved any.
> (McCorkle, et al., p.29)

Another method of maintaining contact with the boy's home community is a monthly report which is prepared partially by the boy himself and partially by his group. This report is sent to the judge who placed the boy on probation, and to the probation officers. These reports do much to reassure the community of the boy's progress and to change their attitudes toward him.

How well the informal structure coupled with guided group interaction perform can be seen in these comments from a chapter entitled "The Boy's Own Story" which consists of several diaries written by boys after leaving Highfields.

> I figured I'd say the right things so Mr. M__ would think I was making progress and figuring out my problems. But after a while I found out it wasn't that easy and Mr. M__ wasn't so crazy after all...
>
> (McCorkle, et al., p. 128)

Another boy, Pete, relates that in the beginning he thought he would smooth talk his way through Highfields, but then discovered that he really had to work through his problems, and that this was satisfying. In a discussion a boy stated, "For me Highfields is a place where the boys are supposed to get some help (McCorkle et al., p. 15)."

The boys have, essentially, come to these conclusions 'on their own,' i.e. the functions of Highfields are not made explicit. Just 'figuring Highfields out' must give a boy quite a sense of accomplishment. Since involvement of the boy in the treatment process is a goal at Highfields, 'structurelessness' is a much more efficient technique than laying down a set of rules. Setting down in a didactic manner how the boy is expected to act, and how he is supposed to feel would remove the element of participation. 'Figuring Highfields out', learning its traditions and customs and adding some of his own, gives the boy a sense of involvement, and of belonging.

The Artificial Group Interventions, like previous types of intervention, identify a problem within the child which has resulted from a problem in the child's environment.   Artificial Group Interventions direct their change actions toward the child. These interventions maintain the child in his home community and utilize the human environment represented by an artificially formed group to effect change in behavior and attitudes.

The Provo and Silverlake Experiments

The Provo Experiment of Provo, Utah (Empey and Rabow, 1961), and the Silverlake Experiment of Los Angeles County, California (Empey and Lubeck, 1971) will be discussed together as examples of 'artifical group' interventions which leave the boy in his community and build up a group of adjudicated juvenile offenders for purposes of intervention.

The Provo and Silverlake interventions identify the problem as the delinquent behavior enacted by the youths.   Circumstances in the environment are the source of this delinquency.   It is a group phenomenon, a product of differential group experience in a particular subculture.   The interventionists believe that most   delinquents are concentrated in slums or in the lower class where learning situations limit their access to success goals

(which are the same as middle-class success goals). The strain
resulting from lack of access to internalized goals leads to identification with delinquent peers. This identification leads to
delinquent behavior. Delinquent behavior is viewed as a learned
way of coping with environmental demands. The Provo and Silverlake change action is directed toward the youth. A particular
kind of human environment is utilized to effect this change. This
consists of a peer group made up of adjudicated habitual offenders,
15-18 years of age, which meets at the Provo and Silverlake institutions.

The courts send these boys to Provo and Silverlake as an
alternative to incarceration. Provo and Silverlake do not accept
serious sex offenders, narcotics addicts, seriously retarded or
psychotic boys.

The objective at Provo and Silverlake is not to change
the individual's entire way of life, but rather to change the
normative orientations toward lawbreaking which the boys manifest.
The boys are expected to come to grips with their life alternatives
at Provo and Silverlake. It is felt that alternatives open to the
boys are limited since "in most cases, delinquents are lower class
individuals who not only lack many of the social skills, but who
have been school failures as well." The interventionists consider
that an emphasis on goals which could be reached through education

is impractical. Rather, the alternatives open to the boys are described as follows: they can continue their delinquent behavior and
go to prison, or "they can learn to live a rather marginal life in
which they will be able to operate sufficiently within the law to
avoid being locked up."

The intervention consists of two phases: Phase I
Intensive Treatment, consists of 3 hours a day 5 days a week and all
day Saturday spent at the institutional setting at Provo, or 1-1/2
hours, 5 days a week, at Silverlake. Phase II, Community Adjustment,
consists of employment in the community and maintenance of reference
group support.

There is very little structure or systematization
present at the institutions. There are no set standards to which a
boy must conform as criteria for release. There are no explicit
rules which would formulate a system which could be "beat." The
lack of formal structure also allows the boys freedom to define
situations for themselves; i.e. it promotes decision-making and
binds neither the peer group nor the interventionists to a particular action in a particular situation.

There is very little staff-client interaction. Anxiety is perpetuated in this way so that the boys will be kept off
balance and so that they will be left with no alternative but to
turn to their peer group for information.

The staff, consisting of a director, a group leader, a part-time tutor, a part-time work supervisor and a part-time cook, are selected on the basis of their capacity to implement the intervention strategy.

Group processes and work are utilized in the Intensive Treatment Phase. The key tool in the intervention is the peer group, made up of 10 boys. The peer group is the instrument by which norms are perpetuated, and through which important decisions are made. The peer group participates in guided group interaction sessions under the leadership of the director or the group leader. The guided group interaction session provides a place for questioning the utility of persistent delinquency. It is a place for learning alternative behaviors. It is a place for receiving recognition of one's personal reformation and for demonstrating a willingness to help others. There are certain sanctions inherent in the peer group which aid in the accomplishment of these things. For example, no one in the group is released until everyone is honest and until every boy helps solve problems; since the members of the peer group live in the community, they know of other members' outside activities and judge them; all members of the group realize that failure at Provo or Silverlake places them in the reformatory.

The work aspect of the intervention consists of physical work in and around the institutional building. This is considered an immediate attack on delinquent values and work habits.

In Phase II, Community Adjustment, the boy puts into practice what he has learned in Phase I. It is expected that the boy will want to find employment in the community. The decisions to find employment, and what sort of employment, are decisions which must be made by the boy. Some aid in finding a job is available, but the initiative must definitely be his. There is an attempt to maintain reference group contact to support the boy in his efforts.

Provo and Silverlake, then, utilze a peer group in an unstructured and non-residential institutional setting, under the leadership of a staff dedicated to program goals. These goals involve substituting lawful life goals for the delinquent ones held by the youthful clients.

VII.   ARCHITECTURAL INTERVENTION

Several social scientists concerned with the urban environment (e.g. Hall, Sommer, Parr, Wohlwill) have made strong statements about the deleterious effects of the physical environment.
They posit a man-made environment which does not fit human environmental needs as a cause for mental and social disorder. They support research to identify environmental needs and to discover
the optimum architectural and urban planning designs to meet
these needs. (One requirement may be that a person be allowed
some freedom to design his own environment.) In other words, these
theorists see a problem in persons which is caused by a certain
type of man-made environment, and wish to change the environment
in order to alleviate the problem. They have been, in the main,
concerned with urban planning and housing. Since research into
the optimum human environment, although fascinating, is in its infancy, it would be difficult to construct an intervention based
on it at this point.

Those architects who have written specifically about emotionally disturbed children make tamer statements concerning environmental influence. These authors (Bayes, Bednar and Haviland,
Abeson and Berenson) have as their goal change in the child brought
about by the usual special education techniques. They wish to build
a physical environment which will aid the use of these techniques.

It is the latter authors mentioned above, particularly the writings of Bayes (1967) and Bednar and Haviland (1969) which will be reported here.

This group of authors identifies the problem as existing within the child. Bednar and Haviland are concerned with children with learning disabilities. They divide learning disabilities into perceptual, motor, and psycho-social, but recognize that any one child may manifest learning disabilities of more than one type, and that one learning disability may exacerbate others. The source of the problem is seen as neurological or environmental (home situation) or an interplay of both. The target for change is the child. The authors wish to utilize the physical environment to effect this change in the child. The objectives of the architects is to build 'special environments' for 'special children' which, along with special education, will eventually enable them to return to their 'normal' milieu. The main concern of Abeson and Berenson, Bednar and Haviland, and Bayes is to design an environment which will promote the special education technique utilized, whatever that may be. Their philosophy is that "the educational decisions should shape the architecture and not the other way around (Bednar and Haviland, p.8-18)."

Bednar and Haviland state that built environments can be provided at three different levels:

(1) a 'comfort' level, which assures comfort for its users;

(2) a 'therapeutic'level, which provides not only comfort,
but enhances therapy, by viewing the physical environment as
an expression of psychological needs;

(3) a 'contributory' level, in which special features are
added so that the built environment is planned and designed
to facilitate specific approaches to special education.

The therapeutic built environment will be reported here. The contributory level could be exemplified by Hewitt's engineered classroom design, which provides for each side of the learning triangle
he utilizes: task, reward, and structure (Hewett, 1968). The
model for the engineered classroom is taken from examples of classical and operant conditioning.

Creating an environment requires three steps, which proceed
from abstract to concrete. The designer begins with a series of
environmental variables. Environmental variables identified by
Bednar and Haviland are space, light, color, sound, texture, cli-
mate, and shape. These variables are then forged into a series of
conceptualizations concerning the physical environment being designed. The final step is the selection of actual hardware to implement the design. Bednar and Haviland consider the notion of
'conceptualization' to be the most important because it synthesizes
the basic environmental variables in order to solve specific design problems. The conceptualizations which will be presented here
outline some broad roles which the built-environment can play in

465

educating children with learning disabilities. These conceptualizations and a few implications for actual hardware are reported here. It should be noted that the architectural examples are only a sample of those provided by Bayes and Bednar and Haviland. Bednar and Haviland caution that the examples are for purposes of illustration; the state-of-the-art of environmental and educational research has neither confirmed nor denied their relevance.

Conceptualizations

It will be noted that several of the conceptualizations seem contradictory. The way in which the contradictions might be compromised architecturally is mentioned wherever this was clarified by the authors.

1. Space-time identity. It is posited that a common characteristic of children with learning disabilities is an underdeveloped understanding of the space-time continuum. The child cannot grasp the meaning of time in relation to space and movement. Poor design features can reinforce a distorted sense of space-time. For example, moving through identical spaces or among identical buildings gives the impression of standing still. The environment can ameliorate the problem and help establish space-time identity. The child should be given a sense of where-he-has-been, where-he-is, and where-he-is-going. Bednar and Haviland list several architectural possibilities for accomplishing this. A few are: (a) Using a ray of sunlight across a modulated wall to demonstrate the passage

466

of time. (b) Laying out a child's daily path so that he remains 'oriented' both inside and outside the building. (c) Ordering architectural space on the basis of space-time interdependence rather than functional grouping, i.e., making activities which are adjacent in time also adjacent in space.

2. Ambiguity. Ambiguity should be avoided. Ambiguity leads to frustration, and frustration may augment already prevalent psycho-social problems.

Some ways of avoiding ambiguity in learning spaces for children with learning disabilities may include:

(a) Expressing environmental cues directly. For example, disclosing all light sources, natural and artificial.

(b) Using materials and assemblies in an 'honest' way. For example, avoiding materials which visually simulate other materials (imitation wood-grained plastic, brick-patterned linoleum, false fireplaces and false doors).

(c) Maintaining the structural integrity of the building, such as:

(i) Showing a simple transfer of load in the building's structural system, avoiding supports, cantilevers, and overhangs which seem to defy the forces of gravity.

(ii) Presenting the building as a relatively substantial piece of work. For security's sake, the building should be 'clothed' enough so that it doesn't look as if it can be dismantled in one afternoon by a handyman with a tool kit.

3.   <u>Articulation</u>. An articulated environment is one which displays the fact that it has different parts. All boundaries between spaces of different mood or function must be clear and positive. An articulated environment can be meaningful for special
education because:

(a) It can help the child recognize and prepare for changes
in activity and behavior.

(b) It can help with problems of sensory hyperactivity by
carefully controlling the kinds of physical stimuli associated with various learning tasks. An area for concentration
may be low in stimuli, and an area for reaction much richer
in stimuli.

(c) It can help with problems of dissociation by allowing the
student to perceive meaningful wholes rather than parts. The
amounts of clutter and visual noise, for instance, should be
considered.

4.   <u>Transition</u>. Transition can be thought of as the 'joint' or
'link' between things which have been articulated. The transition
space is the in-between realm; the place between two places. In
order not to contradict the principle of articulation, each transition area must be clearly expressed and articulated.

(a) The entrance to a building is a major architectural event.
Entrances should be positive and significant. They should
enhance the action of coming in and going out. An example
of a transition between outside world and inside living units

468

is provided at Aldo van Eyck's children's home in Amsterdam in the form of an interior street. The children's activities are protected here, but not limited. "Architecturally this is expressed by the use of external type materials and lighting. The walls are finished with the paviors often used for Dutch streets," rough, brown, and powerful. On the inside living units the walls are white, smooth, and softer (Bayes, p.14).

(b) Three general 'zones' of territoriality have been identified: private, intimate, and public. Spaces catering to these differentiated zones must be distinct, with easily crossed barriers.

(c) Transition spaces should be provided from corridor to classroom which allow the child to prepare himself for learning activity and from classroom to lunchroom which allow the child to prepare himself for the large group activity of the lunch room.

5. Decisions and alternatives. There are many decisions which the user of a physical environment must make in order to exist within it. The two extreme situations of environmentally based alternatives should be avoided. No alternatives may result in frustration. For example, a child may want to leave the room. He sees an exit which he cannot use (a large window, a firedoor, etc.) or cannot reach. Too many alternatives (or undemarcated alternatives) may also result in frustration. For example, a child sees many identical

rooms with identical doors and cannot decide where he should be. Or, a child sees many different activities proceeding simultaneously in a space and cannot decide which to join.

6. Consistency. Conceptualizations 1-5 have emphasized variety and punctuation. The built environment must also provide a degree of consistency for the child. "A thoroughly articulated environment can be (through careful design) a consistent one as well (Bednar and Haviland, pp. 7-10)." The child is learning to manipulate his environment. It should provide him with successful experiences in doing this. Consistency can help provide success. Consistency occurs on almost a subconscious or subliminal level. For example, it can be provided by:

(a) Door which generally swings the same way.

(b) Hardware on doors, windows, cabinets and toilet partitions which is not only simple to operate, but which is consistent throughout.

(c) Avoidance of seemingly meaningless differences in colors, textures, lighting patterns, and surfacing materials.

(d) Patterns and decorative motifs repeated through a building, as long as they have some inner significance for the child, may help in re-establishing rhythm and harmony with the child.

(e) Careful consideration of changes in the room such as furniture rearrangement, paint color changes, space use alteration, and shifts in lighting level and quality. These changes should not be made suddenly.

7. <u>Scale</u>. Relating a building to a child's scale is an important way
of giving him a sense of security and belonging.

   (a) The exterior of the building can be designed to appear smaller,
   to keep the building from 'looming' over the child as he approaches
   it. Careful attention to site development, earthwork, planting,
   steps and other features of the building's facade can all help to
   accomplish this.

   (b) Heights of blackborads, shelves windowsills, and stair railings
   are reference points for children and they can cause frustration if
   poorly located. Caution must be taken not to overdo scale accommodation, however. A 'miniature building' could make the adults
   in the school appear that much larger, and perhaps more threatening,
   to the children.

8. <u>Sociopetal-sociofugal</u>. This conceptualization is concerned with
the physical environment as a socializing mechanism. The sociolcgical
disposition of space in architecture can be discussed in terms of a
dichotomy. A "sociopetal" plan or arrangement of furniture encourages
the formation of human relationships. It draws people together and encourages them to interact. It is centripetal in tendency, bringing
people to the center. The plan arrangements of most home living rooms
are sociopetal in nature. A "sociofugal" plan discourages the
formation of human relationships by keeping people spatially distant
from one another.   It is centrifugal in tendency, propelling
people to the perimeter of the plan.   Airports and hotel

lobbies generally represent sociofugal plans. This aspect of environment can be utilized to 'program' a child's social interactions. An environmental design with this conceptualization in mind should:

(a) Control the number of people within sight at any one time, since visual contact facilitates interaction.

(b) Consider the size of the space in relation to the number of persons it houses; overcrowding and overconcentration are to be avoided.

(c) Allow different degrees of association between the child and others. "The growth of interpersonal relationships depends, in a community, on being able to slip easily and unobtrusively from one to another of three separate zones of sociability--complete privacy, the intimate group, the larger group." Bayes provides an architectural program for this in a circular form. On the periphery are twenty single rooms, allowing for privacy. These are subdivided so that in the next zone toward the center there are five spaces belonging to intimate groups of four people in each. In the center there is a communal area to facilitate the larger group activities (Bayes, p. 113)."

(d) Allow transition between zones of equal sociability without disruption. A child moving from one area of privacy to another (from a cubicle to a locker, for example),should not have to pass through a large group area (a corridor, for example).

9. <u>Privacy</u>. "Where private areas are to be provided, they must <u>be</u> private. Doors must be solid and properly hung with substantial securing hardware. The walls must be solid and insulated against acoustical intrusion   (Bednar and Haviland, p. 7-14)."

10. <u>Territoriality</u>. Territoriality may be conceived as a place of one's own and the accompanying establishment, identification, and defense of that place. Seats habitually chosen in a classroom, a regularly occupied place in a restaurant, as well as the space in one's own home or 'room' exemplify territoriality. A place of one's own preserves the personality of the individual and provides emotional security.

(a) Each child will assume (and should therefore be given) some territory of his own. In the case of a day-time school, a desk, a cubicle, or a locker. In the case of a live-in institution, a room, or if there are two or more to a bedroom, a 'bed place.' A sense of spatial ownership can be imparted through screens, or recessing of the bed. The protection of a child's privacy and right to his own possessions develops a feeling of responsibility and self-respect. It also helps others in the room to recognize the basic rules of individual rights and personal property.

(b) Children should be allowed to exercise the defense of their territory by personalizing it with drawings, color, writing, etc.

11.   Room significance. Rooms should provide a sense of enclosure
for the sake of emotional security.   There are two aspects to this
problem of 'containment':

(a) Architectural design should give a sense of enclosure,
security, and visual warmth.   It should not embody too open a
plan, and should provide adequate but not excessive windows.

(b) The plan should not be so rational that it avoids any
corners or cubby holes which satisfy a child's need for isolation.

Changes of mood, from elation to despair "should be respected
and an environment provided to meet them   (Bayes, p. 20)."

(a) To accommodate a despairing mood, an environment of curves
and warmth--quiet, rather dark, with enfolding chairs--should
be provided.

(b) To accommodate elation, the possibility of climbing to
high places should be provided.   Bayes states "If the form of
a room should be determined by the needs of the activities
which take place within it, the case for irregular shapes is
a strong one   (Bayes, p. 20)." Flexibility in use and in
feeling is easier to accomplish in a framework which is less
rigid than the rectangle.

12.   Usability. Human tolerance and adaptability to problems in
using environments is very high.   Exceptional children, however,
may not exhibit these high tolerance levels or adaptability.

Architectural barriers to usability must be eliminated so that the special children housed in the physical environment can use it to their fullest potential.

(a) Attention must be given to anything that the child must operate: doors, windows, rails, cabinets, blackboards, serving lines, lockers, desks, etc. The criteria in their choice are simplicity, honesty, unambiguity, and consistency.

(b) Nonsignificant barriers must be eliminated. Large panes of glass across circulation areas, many changes in levels, and poor location of fire and security doors can all present problems.

13. Movement. Movement through a building is an important aspect of using it. "A successful movement system will not only result in ease of circulation for the child, it will also increase his own confidence in his ability to cope with his environment. This is important in fostering a more positive self-concept   (Bednar and Haviland, p. 7-17)."

The avoidance of corridors in buildings for the mentally or emotionally disturbed is a recurrent theme. Corridors of limited length may be required, however, to avoid other planning defects (ambiguity in room use, for example). In ordering the movement system, the following points should be kept in mind:

(a) Environmental cues to movement can facilitate student circulation. Colors, shapes, textures, materials and graphics

475

can all be employed to accomplish this.

(b) A basically 'simple' circulation pattern can help the
exceptional child to remain oriented in time and space. Circulation paths should be well enough ordered to avoid ambiguity and to assist the user in making movement decisions.

The route that a child takes in going from one place to
another "should be carefully visualized in the design so that there
are changing vistas and a succession of experiences of visual significance   (Bayes, p. 19)."

14.   Character. Character, like scale, enhances the 'fit' of the
building to the occupants. Controversy has been prevalent concerning whether the educational environment for exceptional children
should be structured to resemble a home or a school. Bednar and
Haviland posit that if the above concepualizations can be translated into structural facilities, this environment will evolve its
own unique character. Bayes feels that there is a need for cultural familiarity and an environment not too dissimilar from the
occupant's background. In addition, buildings for children should
possess childlike attributes. There should be something to induce
fantasy, perhaps a playful sculpture or many whimsical shapes.
There should somewhere be tension and mystery; not dark corners,
but perhaps organic forms which are not part of the structure.
There should be something for the sake of laughter.

476

15.   Staff needs. A view expressed in Bayes is that "the provision of adequate and comfortable accommodation for the staff is the most important aspect of the whole problem, that if the staff are content the children will be better looked after   (Bayes, p. 27)." Adequate staff accommodations include a room to which they can withdraw at almost any moment and facilities for ease of communication between staff members.

Bednar and Haviland state that the above conceptualizations emanate from the learning disabilites themselves, and from the roles which the physical environment might play in actually ameliorating them. They may be thought of as "innate qualities of all environments for all children with perceptual, motor, and psycho-social disabilities   (Bednar and Haviland, p.8-11)."

16.   Program factors. There are additional factors, however, which must be superimposed on the basic conceptualizations if a specific planning and design problem is to be solved. These 'program factors' do not emanate from direct needs of the learner, "but rather they arise from the educational program in which the learner is placed. This program represents the viewpoints of the teacher, the administrator, the parents and the community   (Bednar and Haviland, p.8-11)." The program factors identified by Bednar and Haviland will be listed and explained very briefly here. It should be noted, however, that they must be considered if the environmental design is to be a practical and satisfactory one.

477

(a) "Changeability." Tailoring the physical environment closely
to the child's needs leads to the need to accommodate the change
which occurs within a child, and to the need to accommodate
the fact that the child population utilizing a built environment
changes. Within each conceptualization, the architect should
strive to provide a range of environmental interpretations.

(b) "Educational tools, equipment and media." The tools to be
used in the educational process should be considered integral
parts of the environment from the earliest stages of planning.
The particular types of environment which the tools attempt to
create (e.g., the 'perceptually directed' environment of a
sound movie) should also be recognized. The architecture should
be structured to facilitate the creation of these special
environments. Technical requirements must not be overlooked.
The educational tools may have implications for acoustics,
materials, cabinet work (for storage), and power outlets.

(c) "Flexibility." Bayes warns that excessive flexibility
within a built environment violates the conceptualization of
avoidance of ambiguity, and fails to provide for two all-
important needs--security and familiarity. The feeling of
permanence and solidarity must be reconciled with the flexibility
of light-weight moveable partitions and prefabricated panels.

Bednar and Haviland, however, feel that flexibility may
be desirable from the educational, as well as the economic, point

of view. If research substantiates the idea that children in
school could develop their relationship to the physical environment by changing it, and that a novel environment stimulates
an exceptional child to greater achievement, a changeable
environment, one which retains novelty, may be an advantageous one.
(d) "The site." Many of the conceptualizations concerning environment for special education can be realized out-of-doors,
as well as within the confines of the building. It is becoming
accepted that tactile experience is helpful in learning. The
outdoor site of a school can provide opportunities for this
factor. Direct educational experience with land which has been
adapted for teaching (botany, biology, physics, etc.) and for
experiences of beauty, recreation, and physical education can
be effective in special education.
(e) "Integration and segregation." This factor is concerned
with the degree to which children with learning disabilities
should be separated from children without learning disabilities,
and to what extent children with a particular type of learning
disability should be segregated. This educational issue has
an effect on architecture. This is the decision which will
determine which of a range of possibilities the architect will
provide: a few special features inserted into regular schools,
wings added to existing schools, small-scale special education
pavilions, or large campuses for exceptional children.

Because special education has no agreement on approach to be used with respect to children with learning disabilities, and because environmentalists are just beginning to isolate environmental variables and to evaluate their influence on behavior and emotions, educator-architect dialogue is difficult. The environmental conceptualizations and program factors presented here are a first step in the research and architect-educator-social scientist communication necessary to the construction of a therapeutic built environment.

Family Environment Interventions preceive a problem in
the environment as the source of the problem within the child.
They differ from preceding interventions in that they have as their
target of change the problem-causing environment represented by
the family.

Maternal Preventive Psychiatry

Spitz, in "The role of ecological factors in emotional
development in infancy" (1949) defines the problem as arrested
and regressing emotional development in infants. Since "emotional
development acts as the trailbreaker for all other perceptive development during infancy," arrested emotional development results
in arrested perceptual development (Spitz, p. 145). The reason
for this arrested development is to be found in the environment.
The particular factor which Spitz considers as crucial in the arrest of the emotional and perceptual development of infants is
the quality of emotional interchange with the mother or her substitute, from whom all early experience derives. Spitz emphasizes
that the problem of lack of healthy emotional interchange between
mother and child is determined by more than the qualities of the
mother.

> The particular ecological significance of this
> finding lies in the fact that this emotional inter-
> change is largely governed by culturally determined
> mores and institutions on the one hand, by social
> and economic conditions on the other (Spitz, p. 153).

It is Spitz's contention that industrial society tends to deprive

the child of its mother in early infancy. Spitz proposes to di-

rect the intervention at the two levels of the environment which

are viewed as problematic--the mother and the society.

On the level of the mother, Spitz would prepare the per-

sonalities of future mothers for motherhood. This would involve

social psychiatry, preferably begun before the birth of the child,

to remedy psychiatric conditions apt to damage the child. Some

potentially damaging psychiatric conditions are identified by

Spitz as neurosis, an infantile personality, periodic mood-swings,

and constant rapid shifts in attitude.

On the level of society Spitz advocates a re-arrange-

ment of legislation whereby social institutions would encourage,

rather discourage, mothers to spend more time with their children,

and education to prepare women for motherhood.

In this intervention, then, developmental arrest, which

has been posited as the problem in other interventions (Meuron

and Auerswald, 1969), is dealt with through intervention into the

environmental circumstances identified as the source of the

problem.

Spitz' position was further developed and elaborated by
M. Ribble (1943). Her view is that all infantile experiences are
of great importance to the direction of the infant's development.
In support of this position, she contends that the child is very
sensitive to the environment, that he lacks adequate organization
of his primary body functions to meet the demands of his post-natal
work, and that he shows great instability in these body functions.
She maintains that there must be a long period of very attentive
"mothering" if the infant is to develop normally physiologically,
anatomically, and psychologically. In each step in the development of her position, she has cited as evidence the "developmental
status" of the infant.

S. R. Pinneau (1950) has evaluated Ribble's contentions,
evidences, and conclusions in the light of most representative
and controlled physiological, anatomical, and psychological experiments, observations, and studies. Almost every one of her points
has been refuted by the results of these investigations. Those
not refuted are discounted in consequence of considerations more
in keeping with the known facts. "The most lenient conclusion
possible would deny the presence of scientific evidence substan-
tiating her general thesis, whereas a conclusion in keeping with
the material here presented and with its implications, points to
a direct refutation of the thesis itself   (p. 222)."

Vogel and Bell (1960) identify the problem within the child. A child who is labelled 'emotionally disturbed' in the context of the school environment, may have taken on the emotionally disturbed role due to his function as scapegoat in his family environment. It is the family which is the source of the child's problem. Vogel and Bell feel that the family is in the large part responsible for the emotional health of the child. Vogel and Bell emphasize not only the personalities of family members, (stressed in Spitz, 1949) but their interactions as well, particularly unresolved conflicts and interactions between parents.

Vogel and Bell intervene in the environment represented by these interactions. The therapy which they utilize consists of treatment of the family by a team of psychologists, psychiatrists, social workers and social scientists. The families are seen weekly in a psychiatric clinic and in their homes, over periods ranging from one to four years. There is some intimation that the child receives remedial treatment apart from his family, also. Vogel and Bell state that by the time a family is seen by the clinic, the scapegoated child has internalized the expectations thrust upon him to the extent that "it was difficult to effect change only by removing external pressures (p. 392)."

484

Bowlby, in <u>Maternal Care and Mental Health</u> (1952) defines
the problem as developmental retardation which manifests itself
physically, intellectually, socially, and emotionally. The cause
for this retardation, which may become apparent before the age
of one year and may last throughout life, is maternal deprivation
experienced in the child's early life. The environmental aspect
which Bowlby pinpoints as essential for good mental health is
"that the infant and young child should experience a warm, intimate and continuous relationship with his mother (or permanent
mother-substitute) in which both find satisfaction and enjoyment
(p. 11)." Vital factors entering into the particular effect maternal deprivation has on a particular child are: (a) the child's
age, (b) the length of deprivation, and (c) the degree of deprivation. Bowlby's study is primarily concerned with the complete
deprivation associated with separation from the mother figure.

Children under seven years of age are vulnerable to
developmental damage attendant upon separation from the mother.
From birth to three years of age is the most vulnerable time.
Children from three to five, although not as vulnerable as the
younger child, may be seriously damaged. From five to seven the
vulnerability diminishes. Adjustment to maternal deprivation
remains difficult at this age. Bowlby cites evidence which demonstrates the adverse effects of maternal deprivation.

485

Deprivation can have adverse effects on the development of children in three separate time periods: (a) during separation, (b) during the period immediately after restoration of maternal care, and (c) permanently. Once a child has experienced deprivation compensatory mothering is "almost useless if delayed until after the age of two and a half years." One particularly acute effect of maternal deprivation is the child's inability to form satisfying relationships. Bowlby and others have found this trait in "affectionless" delinquent adolescents who experienced maternal deprivation as infants or young children. Bowlby (1952, p. 35) states:

> ...it appears that there is a very strong case indeed for believing that prolonged separation of a child from his mother (or mother substitute) during the first five years of life stands foremost among the causes of delinquent character development... There is a specific connection between prolonged deprivation in the early years and the development of an affectionless psychopathic character given to persistent delinquent conduct and extremely difficult to treat.

It is interesting to note that in a review of the total population of Hawthorne Cedar Knolls (a school reported on earlier in this paper) cited by Bowlby, 14% had been in institutions before the age of four, 24% had been in foster-homes before the age of four. Only 25% of the Hawthorne Cedar Knolls population, extant in April, 1950, had been raised by both parents.

Bowlby is particularly concerned with maternal deprivation which takes place in Western societies, since he feels that alternative effective child-care structures are missing. The

486

extended family and close-knit community serve this function in primitive and peasant societies. Industrialized societies are characterized by "social fragmentation." The mother and father have a far heavier responsibility for the rearing of their child. In Western communities "it is emotional instability and the inability of the parent to make effective family relationships which are the outstanding cause of children becoming deprived of a normal home life (p. 82)." Note the vicious circle aspect of this argument. Since incapacity to make meaningful relationships is a characteristic of a damaged child, children deprived grow up to be parents depriving.

Bowlby's preventative action is directed toward the child's environment. His main concern is to ensure that the infant and young child experience a "warm, continuous relationship" in a "natural home group" (mother, father, child, siblings, if any) or in a setting as close to that ideal as possible. Bowlby advocates that societal institutions strive to insure the success of the family, rather than providing substitute homes, which do not provide the all-important one-to-one relationship. Bowlby's philosophy is that a bad home is better than a good institution.

Bowlby's report concentrates primarily on the relationship with infant and young child and mother. The father's role as economic and emotional supporter of the mother is assumed. The father's relationship to the infant is considered secondary.

487

In order to prevent the failure of families, Bowlby proposes direct aide to families and long term community programs.

1. Direct aid to families

    A. Socio-economic aid (Material, etc.)

        Material aid should be granted to keep the child in the care of a parent or relative, rather than institutionalizing him.

        1) Day care

            Day care as a means of helping the husbandless mother should be restricted to children over three who are able to adapt to nursery school. Until the child has reached this age, direct economic assistance should be given to the mother.

        2) Housekeeper service

            For fathers with motherless children a housekeeper service should be provided.

    B. Socio-medical aid

        1) Rest homes to which mothers may go with younger children should be provided

        2) Marriage guidance

        3) Child guidance

        4) Boarding school

            In the case of older children, 8 years of age and up, boarding school may be of some value. Such an arrangement may reduce tensions for both parent and child.

        5) Special education arrangements for maladjusted children. These would preferably be day schools where there is

"close contact between teachers and psychiatrists and special efforts are made to work with the children's parents and to arrange vocational guidance and after-care (p. 89)."

II. Long term community programs

A. Socioeconomic developments

1) Provision of family allowances

It must be recognized that greater economic vulnerability accrues to the family with x children. Provision of family allowances is therefore a "vital step in the right direction. . . .Since the mother of young children (under 5) is not free, or least should not be free, to earn, there is a strong argument for increased family allowances for children in these early years (p. 90)." (You can see that, in 1952, the author was not concerned with the population explosion.)

B. Socio-medical developments

Bowlby's long-term program of mental hygiene for prevention of family failure would be "psychiatric care of individual families writ large (p. 92)." This would include treating children, giving psychiatric help to parents, and early and effective aid to troubled families. For this undertaking vast numbers of workers trained in psychological medicine and preventive mental health are necessary.

Although Bowlby contends that "The right place for a child is in his own home, or, . . .perhaps in an adoptive home" he recognizes that there will undoubtedly be some children who will need care outside of their homes for some period of time.

Emergency foster-home care. Bowlby feels that the best providers of emergency, short-term child-care would be neighbors and relatives. The familiar surroundings would lessen the trauma experienced by the child.

Failing this sort of placement, the next best thing is boarding homes (foster-homes), i.e. private homes which care for children in return for subsistance allownaces.

Bowlby gives 3 principles of child-care placement.

(1) A clean cut cannot be made between a child and his home.

(2) Foster homes and institutions cannot provide children with security and affection they need.

(3) Realistic long-term plans are essential for the security of the child and the satisfaction of the foster mother.

The placement procedure should include case work with parents, case work with foster parents, and case work with children.

IX. SCHOOL ENVIRONMENT INTERVENTIONS

The School Environment Interventions perceive a problem
within the child. The source of the problem is in the interface
occurring between child and environment. These interventions are
similar to the Family Environment Interventions in that they have
the environment as the target of their change action. The environmental   context into which they intervene is the school environment.

Mental Health Consultation

Iscoe, Pierce-Jones, Friedman and McGehearty (1967) report "some strategies in mental health consultation" which were
tried in the San Antonio and Austin, Texas public schools.

Iscoe et al. list the factors which were viewed as problematic by their consultees (employees in the public schools) as
follows: 45%--child's emotional state, school motivation, ability
to learn; 14%--teacher's personal concern and anxiety; 14%--child's
home situation; 15%--teacher's professional uncertainty; 7%--role
conflicts and inter-personal relationships. It can be seen from
this that the problem is variously viewed as emanating from the
child, from his environment, or from the interface between the
child and his environment. The intervention is directed toward
a change in the child's school environment. "The emphasis is upon

491

developing and expanding the resources of the teacher rather than specific servicing of the disturbing child (Rhodes and Gibbins, p.35)."

The Child Behavior Consultant as developed by this intervention consults with teachers, nurses, principals, anyone in a school system who feels the need for consulting services. Thus, acting upon the child is the teacher, principal, or some other school employee with whom the child is normally in contact. Acting on this person is the Child Behavior Consultant. The Child Behavior Consultant does not meet with the child. The Child Behavior Consultant spends one-half day each week at the particular school to which he is assigned. The purpose of the consultation is to change the teacher or other consultee in such a way so that he can better cope with his own problems or the problems of the children under his care.

Personnel for the particular research project reported by Iscoe et al. were graduate students in a program of school psychology, who received additional training to prepare them for the role of Child Behavior Consultant. The suggestion is made that it isn't necessary that these trainees have doctoral degrees. Retired businessmen and mature housewives could be trained to be Child Behavior Consultants.

Paraphernalia required by the Child Behavior Consultant are paper and pencil tests, which are utilized for evaluation purposes, and to clarify situations in which the consultees require help. The consultee fills out testing instruments which measure his orientation to child behavior, present his autobiographical data and identify situations which are management problems for him. The consultant fills out forms which report the dimensions of each client (child) and consultee, and his manner of handling the case.

Since the purpose of the intervention is only defined in a very broad manner, i.e., to aid the consultee in coping with problems, the school personnel and the consultant do not always agree on the consultant's purpose. The strategy utilized is that the consultant allows himself to be 'manipulated' to the school's purpose. He will then be indispensable, and will be in a position to 'manipulate back' in order to bring about some changes he believes necessary.

This intervention considers the role of the teacher an important one. His value and the influence he has upon the children under his charge are recognized and emphasized.

It is probable that the thought required in filling out tests, the attention paid to the teacher and his problems, having 'someone to talk to', and the discovery that these problems are not unique to one particular child, classroom,or teacher, are major aids in enhancing the teacher's ability to cope, aside from any concrete advice from the Child Behavior Consultant.

Enhancing the Classroom Teacher's Mental Health Function

This intervention, proposed by Morse (1967), is also concerned with consulting services rendered to schools.

The intervention locates the problem within the child. Teachers with whom the interventionists worked stated that their problems were that children are difficult to manage due to 'acting out' behavior, or that they are difficult to teach "because they seem not to learn by procedures adequate for most pupils." The source posited for the problem behavior is the interface between the child and his environment. This formulation is based on life space theory, which says that the contemporary self and the contemporary environment interact to produce behavior. The targets of the change-action are the child's teacher and parents.

There are four overall goals toward which the intervention program addresses itself.

(1) Increase the teacher's sensitivity to individual and group psychological problems.

(2) Present diagnostic procedures which will direct teachers' efforts along more sophisticated and complete dimensions.

(3) Study the management of learning processes according to principles of good mental health.

(4) Translate the theoretical knowledge of psychology into practical action.

The staff of the program consists of mental health consultants who work with parents and teachers. In training, the consultant is given "heavy emphasis on matters relating to discipline and control, and the group setting for academic learning."

There are no specific techniques connected with this intervention, but rather a set of general principles. These must be followed and built into an actual program of action as the individual school situations dictate. The consultant, using profile tests, aids in building specific elements for use in the classroom.

This program assumes that the educational process must take into account the 'whole child.' "The adjustment and learning facets of the child's life cannot and should not be separated." The child's relationships with his teacher and parents have much to do with the manner in which the child adjusts. In this intervention, the teacher is considered the ultimate 'relationship agent' and the teacher's personality is considered a significant factor in this relationship. The program stresses intervention on the level of the teacher and the parents rather than directly on the child.

The stance of the program is one of problem-solving. Processes which aid in this endeavor are the following:

(1) The mental health consultant defines his relationship vis-a-vis the teacher and parents as one of a co-equal.

(2) The teacher is requested to produce a rough rank-order-

ing of problems, as he sees them. It is felt that the process of learning to formulate a problem is an important skill.

(3) The consulting staff searches for relevant psychological principles to apply both to diagnostic planning and to a proposed program of action. The teacher himself should create the concrete plan of action.

(4) There should be an evaluation of the action.

The target for intervention is decided upon in terms of the question, "Where can changes be made to support the child's capacity to learn and adapt?" Some common answers to this question are that changes can be made in:

(1) the nature of the adult-child relationships,

(2) the demands of tasks, and

(3) the nature of the peer or group relationships produced in the classroom.

In the proposed plan of action, "the external forces of the here and now, being under the jurisdiction of the teacher, are emphasized."

Evaluation of a research project embodying this intervention program indicated that it "helped adults, both parents and teacher, to develop a more defined and secure role in their work with children."

X. EXCITOR-RESPONDENT INTERVENTION: NATURAL GROUP AND SLUM ENVIRONMENT

Natural Group and Slum Environment Interventions perceive a problem within the child. The source of the problem is to be found in the environment. This intervention differs from previous interventions because it is bilateral. It directs its change action toward both the disturbing persons, as they occur in a naturally formed group, and the problematic environment represented by the slum milieu.

Street-Club Work

Aryeh Leissner (1965) reports on street-club work in New York and Tel Aviv.

The problem behavior in which street-club work intervenes is located within the child and is defined as socially disapproved behavior, i.e.,"any behavior which a given community at a given time considers in conflict with its best interests," regardless of court action. The disturbing populations with whom Leissner worked were delinquent street corner groups. A delinquent street corner group is defined as a loosely organized, fluctuating group whose hangout is a specific outdoor location, and whose norms and activities are primarily delinquent.

The source of the problematic delinquent behavior is considered to be society and its institutions, which provide unequal opportunities for adjustment, due to the youth's presence in the slum milieu. The slum milieu consists of the physical environment of the slum and the socio-economic and cultural background of the slum dwellers. Factors which are recognized by the street-club worker as contributing to the street corner group adaptation to the slum-milieu are the problems of adolescence, lower class values, ethnic discrimination, inadequate immigrant absorption (an element of which is slum clearance and relocation, or 'dislocation'), and conflict between parents and youth.

The majority of the street-club workers change action is directed toward societal institutions and the environment, however. Social action, not just adjustment of the group members to society, but actual change of the society, receives enough emphasis to warrant placing this particular branch of street club work in the category of interventions which work on both ends of the disturbing problem. Street-club work utilizes the environment and the group which is already in existence to effect the change.

The ultimate objective of street-club work is to reach out to youngsters who, due to a special set of circumstances, have not yet taken advantage of the opportunities for growth; this segment of youth requires a healthy growth process so that individuals will be able to assume the privileges and obligations of

adult status in the society. The specific purpose of the intervention is to change the attitudes and behavior of delinquent street
corner groups. The goal is to help youngsters cope with their environment and with their own fears, confusions and hatreds.

Street-club work is unique on the continuum chart because it is without a brick and mortar institution. It does not
work within the school, or build a new environment. The street-club
worker works within the natural milieu.

The atmosphere which is to be encountered in this milieu
can be felt in the following excerpt from Leissner's experience as
director of the Action-Research Project on Delinquent Street Corner
Groups in Tel Aviv. He contends that the tone is very similar to
that which he found in the slums of New York, and would probably be
the same in a slum area of any large city.

> Having been introduced by the worker, and having met some of
> the distrustful stares and curious questions of the youngsters,
> I settled down in the familiar position of the street club
> worker, my back comfortably supported by a wall near a coffee-
> shop,...observing the teenagers milling about noisily, rest-
> lessly...Around me there was the familiar 'sounding' and
> teasing highlighted by the bursts of laughter when one of
> the boys 'scored' with a smart remark. There was the
> boasting about the boy's exploits, the casual use of ob-
> scenities interspersed with 'you mother. . .' profanities...
> There was a small group of pretty, dark-haired girls
> across the street, keeping their distance, but very much
> aware of the boys who ignored them pointedly...This was an
> atmosphere of noisy banter, interspersed with periods of
> uneasy quiet...the surface bustle of friendly activity
> and the constant awareness of the tension underneath, the
> tension that was discernible in the overheard remarks of
> three boys in a huddle nearby who were discussing a 'job'
> they had pulled the night before. Lowering their voices

with a quick, distrustful glance in my direction, they were
saying something about 'police' and 'getting rid of the
stuff.' 'Trouble' was in the air in the midst of the joking
and jostling, the 'trouble' that lay in the worried look of
the street-club worker sitting at a table inside the coffee-
shop, talking earnestly, intensely, to a nervous, fidgeting
boy --the 'trouble' the Project worker recognized when the
three boys who had been whispering in a corner suddenly
walked off with set, purposeful faces and disappeared in
the dark of a small, unpaved side-street.
                                        (Leissner, 1965, pp. 2-3)

An interesting by-product of the lack of an institu-

tionalized setting is that the worker must gain a mandate from the

group before he can help them. The client group itself must sanc-

tion the attempt to offer it a service.

Conventional, structured group work settings deal
primarily with formed, 'artificial' groups which have entered
into an, at least rudimentary, a priori agreement with the
group work agency to accept its service under the conditions
of the agency's mandate. The street-club worker works exclusively with 'natural' groups in the physical setting of their
own choice...He has no outside power over the group--he cannot form it, he cannot choose the 'right' members; he cannot
'throw out' anybody, or--in our refined language--consider
anybody as 'unsuited for therapy.' They are there, they
are in the street; they have not asked for help and they are
not apprehended.   (Leissner, pp. 69-70).

This is one of the primary ways in which street-club

work differs from Highfields, Provo and Silverlake. The interven-

tion does not involve a captive audience, who are threatened to

some extent by probation or the reformatory. Since the street-club

worker does not structure the environment, he cannot set up oppor-

tunities for problem-solving and confidence-building to occur. He

must be constantly on the lookout for situations he can utilize to

meet his objectives. This kind of intervention requires a particular sort of staff. In order for the street-club worker to be able to establish helpful relationships, he must possess a 'power of acceptance,' and imagination to aid him using every opportunity to gain his ends.

The street-club worker feels that it is necessary to intervene into the entire group, as it exists on the street corner, because the delinquent subculture provides roles, expectations, obligations, rationalizations and reassurances so that "it is difficult to change or control one member's behavior without first changing the character of the entire group (Leissner, p. 18)."

The street club worker utilizes the following methods in reaching his goal of helping the group to adopt new values and norms which are "realistically related to their socio-economic and cultural background, and which serve constructive ends in the shaping of their future (Leissner, p. 78)."

(1) Establish a relationship of mutual acceptance and trust.

(2) Accentuate the positive.

(3) Limit, modify and prevent unlawful behavior.

(4) Open and create opportunities in social, economic and cultural life.

(5) Provide help in coping with modern society and in working through personal problems.

(6) Guide the group to seek positive relations with their community and with societal institutions.

(7) Provide a cause.

   Establish a relationship of mutual acceptance and trust.

The establishment of a relationship with a 'healthy,' benevolent

adult helps to overcome the negative attitude toward adults and

conventional society which is prevalent among disturbing youngsters.

The establishment of this relationship consists of two aspects:

(a) the acquisition of mutual acceptance and trust, and (b) the

clear definitions of the worker's role and function.

   There are certain prerequisites which aid the acquisi-

tion of the trust of the group. One of these is honesty. The

worker must be honest about his professional goal, which consists

of changing the group's behavior through discovering from the group

what causes the behavior and how to stop it. He also must be honest

in the 'model' he holds out to them. The expectations which he

conveys must be "geared to the realities and potentials of the

youngsters' personalities and life situations (Leissner, p. 85)."

The worker should be honest concerning his own limitations, values,

and feelings.

   A second prerequisite to gaining mutual trust and accep-

tance is that the worker convey his own acceptance of the group's

values, norms, and behavior. It is the worker's first, and probably

most difficult, task to show that "he accepts the boys on their own

terms, that he is honestly, and without prejudgment, trying to under-

stand who they are and why they are that way (Leissner, p. 88)."

"Getting acquainted means sticking around in the gang's hangout and

502

trying to make friends no matter what happens (Leissner, p. 86)."
At this stage the worker cannot interfere or voice disapproval. It
is of paramount importance that the worker demonstrate shock-proof-
ness and patience. The worker may utilize 'scenes' which are inevitably staged to shock him, to gain his ends. The gang will eventually ask, "What did you think?," and at this point frank discussion may ensue. The worker may thereby learn something about the
values and norms of the group which serve to condone their behavior.

The most important factor in the clear definition of
the worker's role and function is the worker's acceptability as a
person. The personal factor supercedes all intellectual explanations
of role and function in the process of becoming accepted and establishing relationships. Examples from Leissner's own experience
with street corner groups show that concrete demonstrations of help
is what it takes to gain the confidence of the group. The youngsters want to know all about the worker, and believe him to be a
'cop' or anything which he is not. They deceive, exploit, and test
the worker. An aid to the worker's goals is that the group attempts
to use the worker as someone who solves their problems. In order
to 'use' the worker in this way, the group must talk about their
problems to the worker. If the group assigns a purely functional
role to the worker, making him, for example, 'the guy who gets jobs
for us.' it is the worker's responsibility to overcome this. After
some attempts at giving the street-club worker an incompatible role,

the group will accept him as 'their worker,' and a relationship of
mutual respect is well on its way.

There appears to be a need felt by the gang, to have a
relationship with a knowledgeable, resourceful, trustworthy and
accepting adult. "The intervention of a trusted adult who advises
caution, settles disputes, and provides face-saving alternatives
undoubtedly results in the diminution of conflict behavior
(Leissner, p. 68)."

Accentuate the positive. In the street-club worker's
attempt to channel energies into satisfying socially acceptable
channels, it is important to realize that street corner groups
take part in activities which are not delinquent.

The average age of delinquency is 13-19. A youth at
this stage is teetering between childhood and adult status. Some
of the street-club workers relate that one minute they feel that
they are working with vicious adults, and the next with helpless
children, who only want to play. There is a make-believe aspect
to delinquency which can be put to use. A successful street-club
worker will instigate vivid, adventurous games which involve
planning and manufacture. An imaginative, exciting program will
channel off aggressive energies "that are often given vent in van-
dalism and brawling" and will "dilute delinquentness."

This make-believe, looking for adventure, aspect of delinquency is interesting when viewed in the light of an article by

504

A. E. Parr, "Psychological aspects of urbanology." Parr feels that lack of differentiation, variety and stimulation in the physical environment of the slum leads to understimulation, and a quest for novelty, which may end in the activities characterized as juvenile delinquency. Parr feels that there is a human need for variety (unanticipated experience, adventure). If it is lacking: (a) People may become dull. (b) People may resort to imagination. (c) People may deliberately or unconsciously create surprise by irregular and often unpremeditated actions. Juvenile delinquents may be adventuresome spirits in unadventurous surroundings.

Programs of sport and recreation are not a cure-all, but the street-club worker feels that they do help to fulfill important needs and to provide alternatives. They serve to "dilute delinquentness." It is interesting to note that sports and organized recreation were definitely not a part of the interventions of Highfields, Silverlake and Provo. The reason for this may be that these interventions included institutions that could in some measure circumscribe the activities of the boys, so that 'dilution' was not viewed as a paramount problem. These interventions also included threat; the boys were known, adjudicated offenders, and the interveners could 'afford' to be intense. Since the entire street-club intervention depends on the acceptance of the worker by the group, he cannot directly stop delinquent activities, but must first 'dilute' them.

505

To accentuate the positive, the street-club worker must
(a) accept the limitations of the subcultural norms, and (b) support the more positive and acceptable satisfactions the group
offers to its members, until the group is ready for attitudinal
change. Walking this tightrope, allowing just enough of the subculture to exist so that an activity will be acceptable and enjoy-
able to the group and yet prohibiting serious misbehavior, has to
be an intuitive activity on the part of the worker.

Limit, modify, and prevent unlawful behavior. The street-
club worker limits unlawful behavior in large part through his personal influence. He helps the youngsters gain insight into the
motives for their unlawful behavior. He points out the consequences
of this behavior and offers satisfying alternatives.

Open and create opportunities in social, economic and cultural life. The street-club worker must give concrete assistance
in gaining access to opportunities. He must face the realities of
problem situations which arise in the slum milieu and find working
solutions to them. One aspect of opening and creating opportunities
is to find employment for street-corner group members. The street-
club worker must first help the group to re-evaluate the unrealistic alternatives it has chosen. This must be accomplished before
work becomes salient. Leissner feels that an aid to the development of work habits is allowing the youngsters to work in a con-
genial, familiar environment, and to perhaps allow them to work

506

on group projects. In finding work for the boys, the street-club worker must teach them how to fill out forms, how to handle an interview and even how to graciously wait their turn.

Leissner is implicitly in disagreement with one aspect of the instilling of work habits as it is implemented at Highfields and in the Industrial Neurosis Unit. Leissner does not feel that any form of work will serve to instill work habits. He does not agree with the forestry work camp program, for instance, because when the youths return to Harlem, there are no trees on which to vent their newly-found skills. He feels that the work must not be meaningless to the youth. He fails to see how this would improve the general attitude toward work. Rather, Leissner's bias is toward community improvement work, which is meaningful because it is one's own community which is receiving the benefit of one's labor, and because the sorts of skills required (carpentry, plumbing, etc.) are necessary and useful ones.

Provide help in coping with modern society and in working through personal problems. Providing help in coping with modern society includes educating, counseling, and direct intervention. The street-club worker establishes a personal relationship with the personnel of the local police precinct who are likely to come into contact with the members of his group. The street-club worker is an advocate for the boy, and for rehabilitation under his influence as alternative to incarceration.

Guide the group to seek positive relations with their community and with societal institutions. The stree-club worker should
mediate between the group and its social environment. To do this, he
must bring about opportunities for better relations. Leissner perceives the street-club worker's action in this area as proceeding on
two fronts. In terms of the group, he attempts to make the members
more receptive to new contacts and experiences. He must also play
the part of an "advocate" who will explain the youngster's traits
and customs, problems and needs to interested persons and agencies.

Implicit in the street-club worker's attempt to mediate
between the group and its social environment is the realization
that the street-club worker cannot work in a vacuum. If the
street-club worker expects to reach his final goal, to obtain
lasting and deep changes in the values and behaviors of the street-
club group, he must be ready to help them face concrete issues,
such as inadequate educational facilities, ethnic and social class
discrimination in the access to the legitimate opportunity system,
exposure to destructive corrosive influences in the slum milieu,
and sub-standard housing. He is not encouraged to initiate and
provoke changes on his own but to help the youngsters in this
attempt.

Provide a cause. Leissner also stresses the need for a cause,
for an identity. A "cause" provides an idea or a set of beliefs
with which one can identify, and it also provides a means of establish-

508

ing and asserting one's identity. Leissner feels that the delinquent adaptations of street corner youth are attempts to meet this
need for a cause. The delinquent adaptation is unsatisfactory for
both youth and society, however. Providing something that tells
them who they are and what they stand for is one of the most difficult challenges for the street-club worker in today's society.
Leissner feels that street-club work should incorporate some of
the characteristics of the Youth Movement tradition as it exists
in Israel. In the early days of the Israeli nation, youth and
youth movements were very important. The rebellious, questioning
spirit which they engendered was valued. Now Israel is becoming
more like America, in that adolescence is viewed as inherently
trouble-prone and is treated ambivalently by adults. Few of
Israel's youth belong to youth movements today. Unfortunately
the Youth Movement tradition in Israel is a deprecatory factor to
street-club work. It is a tradition which tends to "depreciate
any youth-work approach which does not pursue specific ideological
goals with missionary zeal (Leissner, p. 72)." Leissner feels
that the Youth Movement could become a positive factor in street-
club work if its 'missionaryness' were 'toned down,' The Youth
Movement style inevitably involves some arrogance and exclusiveness.
Leissner feels that these are not necessarily negative qualities,
and at any rate they are better placed in a youth group with ideological goals than in a delinquent street corner group. Incorpor-

509

ating the Youth Movement into street-club work would serve to guide the rebeliousness, frustration and diffuse hostility of lower-class adolescents into more constructive channels.

The 'channel' into which Leissner would guide street-club work would be legitimate social action. The 'ideology' which Leissner advocates incorporating into street club work is militance against social malpractice.

Although the main emphasis is that the street-club worker aid the youth to cope, to adjust, to grow up and take on an adult status in the society, there is a definite trend toward an added emphasis on changing that society, on social action. Provision of power as a solution to the problems of the underprivileged is now, of course, the accepted rhetoric of 'action sociology' and social work but in early 1965 when Leissner was writing, it was a controversy-laden subject, and it would seem that Leissner was among the first to advocate experiments with power-providing solutions.

Leissner's approach appears to be a sensible approach to the isolation and helplessness of the street-club youth. It is a direct intervention into helplessness which says "here are our 'hopeless' problems and here's what we will do about them." The emphasis in this kind of group work, which is becoming more and more popular, is on more than an adjustment to society as it is. Part of this adjustment, of this gaining of status, and participation in society, is gained by attempting to change that part of society which has provoked isolation and denied status.

Leissner emphasizes, however, that the street-club worker engages in an exercise in futility if he works under the assumption that he and his street club can "effect the basic causes and change the societal system that is delinquent," i.e. neglectful, toward its lower-class youth. Delinquent behavior is feared and punished in our society. The street-club worker must aim to "change the attitudes that lead to delinquent behavior and to bring about the cessation of such behavior (Leissner, pp. 130-131)."

Child and School Environment Interventions perceive a problem within the child which emanates from a problematic interface between child and environment. It is similar to the previous type of intervention in that it is bilateral. This intervention has as its targets for change the disturbing person, the child, and the disturbing situation, the school environment.

Preventive Approach to Developmental Problems

Newton and Brown (1967) center the problem within the child. They identify it as a developmental problem which leads to the inability to cope with stress situations as they arise in school. The source of the problem is conceptualized as the interface which exists in the "complex transactional field that represents the child's life space." The solution to the problem is also to be found in this transactional field of the child's life space. The target of most of Newton and Brown's intervention action involves the child, his parents, and his teacher. It is from these "key people" that the child's most relevant role definitions emerge, and it is from them that he is most likely to receive the help that is the best possible for him.

The objective of the intervention is the management of stress through the enrichment and strengthening of parent-child and teacher-student roles. This is accomplished by providing key behavior agents (parents and teachers) with modes for handling stress and by relieving their anxiety about, but not their responsibility for, the child. The preventive approach to developmental problems in school children consists of three parts:

(1) A pre-school check-up for all children, which is meant to predict the child's ability to cope with school entry and future school stress, and to identify techniques which teachers and parents might be able to use in aiding the child to cope.

(2) Initiation of appropriate interventions. An intervention is defined as an activity intended to develop an environment favoring the acquisition and reinforcement of skills required for coping with the stress of school entry, and of the early years.

(3) Evaluation of the effectiveness of the intervention.

Pre-school check-up. The emphasis in this intervention is on "emotional first-aid." The function of the pre-school check-up is to provide a clearer picture of when first aid might be needed and of what kind of intervention it should include. The pre-school check-up is performed by a psychiatric team. The child is tested and observed by a psychologist. The parents are interviewed by a psychiatric social worker. The goal of the psychiatric team is to enhance the parents' confidence. The team emphasizes readiness, normality, and strengths which are already in use or available to be utilized in building coping skills.

Intervention. Newton and Brown's interventions utilized the concept of relativity in a significant way.

> There appears to be no one set of techniques that a teacher or parent must use to resolve a child's crisis. Rather there is a relative set of operations given this child, this situation, the feelings now generated by this situation, that must be performed to be effective.
> (Newton and Brown, 1967, p. 523)

The situation is relative, so the intervention should be relative, rather than based upon a set pattern or program.

In the project directed by Newton and Brown, several kinds of interventions were instituted as a result of pre-school check-ups. Specific case interventions were undertaken for individual children. Group interventions involved a particular subset of the project sample, made up of children with similar problems. A part of these interventions consisted of activities which "involve the development of new community and school resources and experiential possibilities."

An example of a group intervention is one instituted for a number of children whose problem was identified as weakness in social skills and inexperience in group functioning. The research team taught the parents of the children to relate potential school success to the child's need for increased social or cultural experiences. The parents were guided to lead the child to explore the world around him through informal neighborhood play groups, church programs, regular family outings, positive family separation, or pooled efforts by groups of parents to provide enriching activities. In addition, a new pre-school program was initiated by the City Recreation Department to provide increased social experiences for children whose parents were unable to provide supervised pre-school activites.

Because of their bias toward the relativity of disturbing situations and interventions implemented to manage them, Newton and Brown do not delineate specific methods utilized in their interventions. Some overall techniques, however, can be identified. These are commonalities which appear in Newton and Brown's explication of specific interventions and in the general beliefs and principles which form the basis for their work.

The major principles and the concrete activities which flow from them, may be mapped as follows:

(1) Involve the entire system.

    (a) Involve the parents.

    (b) Utilize the influence of the teacher.

    (c) Consider the attitudes of the teacher and his tolerance of particular problems of children when deciding on teacher-student placement.

    (d) Recognize and work within the 'school culture.'

(2) Emphasize normalcy and manage, rather than treat, stress.

    (a) Enrich already existing roles.

(b)   Emphasize strengths.

(c)   Promote fact-finding.

(d)   Provide models for management.

One of Newton and Brown's assumptions is that the entire school system must be taken into account in any attempt at intervention. This includes realization of the fact that each school has a particular and unique culture.

> It is necessary to understand and work within this culture if effective therapeutic interventions are to be feasible. For example, it is vital that principal-teacher modes of dealing with stress or problems be accepted as a point for beginning action. Interventions should be designed to supplement and extend school efforts rather than to supplant or merely evaluate them.
>   (Newton and Brown, 1967, p. 522)

Another major element in this program is the emphasis on normalcy. The interventionists insist that the child not be defined as abnormal or sick. It is Newton and Brown's contention that stress-coping skills are building blocks to maturity. Stress-coping skills are learned. The stress contingent upon school entry and early school years provides an opportunity which allows the child to learn them. It is not desirable, then, or even necessary, to treat the child or the stress-causing happenings. Rather it is desirable to manage the crisis.

> A major management technique is to focus on the strengths of the situation and the skills of the key behavior agents in order to reduce their anxiety, to enhance their positive influence, and to reduce the tension of the setting as a total field.
>   (Newton and Brown, 1967, p. 523)

Self-Enhancing Education

Self-Enhancing Education, as reported by Randolph and Howe (1966) is "a program to motivate learners." The problem is conceived by these authors to be children who are 'underachieving' and who manifest unproductive, repetitive behavior patterns. The reason for this is seen to be low self-esteem--negative feelings about themselves and about learning. The source of the low self-esteem and negative attitudes is thought to be the processes which the child's significant others (parents and teachers) utilize to teach him. Randolph and Howe posit that traditional teaching methods do not allow for enough involvement of the individual doing the learning. Randolph and Howe also describe six 'syndromes' manifested in parents, which they feel lead to low self-esteem and underachievement on the part of the child. Examples of these are a "Space Industry Syndrome;" parents are preoccupied with technological employment, which leads to emotional deprivation and isolation for the child. This leads to low self-esteem which manifests itself in lack of motivation and underachievement. An "Economically Disadvantaged Syndrome" is the problem of children confronted with affluence which they cannot have. This leads to lack of motivation.

Intervention into the family relationships receives a minor emphasis in self-enhancing education (SEE).

A combined involvement of family and school has greater promise in facilitating achievement. Even when the family

cannot be involved, it is possible, by SEE, to increase
the performance of children.
(Randolph and Howe, 1966, p. 8)

The major focus of self-enhancing education is to intervene into the teacher-student learning process. The purpose of the
self-enhancing education intervention is to provide a type of education which will allow for two-way communication. Self-enhancing
education strives to provide for the involvement of the child in
the purposes and the actual operation of his education. The goal
of SEE is to develop in the child stronger motivation, higher
achievement and socially productive behavior by expanding his self-
esteem, making him aware of self, and self-motivation. It is felt
that by achieving self-respect the child's interest can then turn
outward. He will be more ready to learn, and to care about and
get along with others.

SEE manifests a variety of 'sub-purposes' under the main
purpose of building the self-esteem of the child and bettering the
relationship between teachers and children. One of these is to
modify the perceptions of teachers and pupils so that they are more
able to accept differences. Another purpose is to lessen the psychological size of persons presently seen as admonishers, due to
the types of learning processes to which we subscribe. SEE wishes
to convey an impression of the teacher as a helping person, not an
admonisher. Another major purpose of SEE is to help the child develop social skills necessary for self-direction and self-control.

518

Self-enhancing education is concerned with the 'whole child.' SEE translates the 'whole child' concept into an intervention which looks and sounds curricular. The self-enhancing education intervention would take place in the regular classroom and would involve all pupils. The authors of SEE feel that low self-esteem is pervasive, that every child suffers from some degree of low self-esteem and that SEE can aid in heightening his self-esteem.

The influence of the teacher as an acting agent is emphasized. In the SEE program the teacher is perceived as a master teacher with guidance skills who acts as an agent for student growth. Skills which teachers should acquire are mentioned again and again throughout the explication of the SEE method given by Randolph and Howe. The most important of these are:

(1) be concerned and show your concern;

(2) listen actively by reflecting back the message given to you;

(3) involve the child.

The progenitors of SEE are interested in teacher-change.

> At times it is difficult to determine who is profiting the most from the learning opportunity, the adults or the children as they cooperatively restructure the learning situation. (Randolph and Howe, 1967, p. 8)

The SEE initiators are very much concerned that the teaching process be direct and forthright. A concrete example is the fact that the students are shown their scholastic aptitude tests and scores. The purposes of the educative process are spelled out to the

519

pupils, and the pupils participate in this attempt to personalize them. The teachers are discouraged from attempting to ascertain the motivation for a child's behavior, and are advised to confront behavior directly.

SEE proposes 12 specific processes which are designed to to raise self-esteem and to increase motivation and achievement by involving the child in solving his own problems, exercising self-control and self-direction. The SEE processes are geared toward helping children feel stronger and more adequate about their academic competencies, helping them feel physically adequate, and helping them feel accepted by their peers as worthy individuals. To raise self-esteem, the 12 processes which SEE utilizes are:

(1) problem solving

(2) self-management

(3) changing negative reflections to positive images

(4) building bonds of trust

(5) setting limits and expectations

(6) freeing and channeling energy

(7) overcoming unproductive repetitive behavior

(8) changing tattling to reporting

(9) developing physical competencies

(10) making success inevitable

(11) self-evaluation

(12) breaking curriculum barriers

Problem-solving. The problem-solving process nurtures participation. Each person contributes as a unique resource, of equal status
with every other resource. The problem-solving process exercises the
child's ability to think in various ways.

Self-management. Self-management overcomes the effects of
imposition and control. Learning opportunities are structured in
such a way as to encourage the child to control and direct himself.
Rather than special classes, special provisions within the regular
class are made for those who have difficulty managing themselves.
In extreme 'crisis' cases, the child, the teacher and the principal may
decide to send the child home. The parents' role in enabling the
child to acquire self-management is to provide just and stable
expectations.

Changing negative reflections to positive images. This process
overcomes the conception children have that adults see them as unworthy, weak, and inadequate. Strengths, as well as weaknesses,
must be indicated to the child. Either emphasizing mistakes only,
or ignoring mistakes, leads to feelings of inadequacy and lack of
motivation. The academic material that the pupil works on should be
at his 'growing edge.'

Building bonds of trust. Trust lessens the psychological size
of persons in positions of authority. It lessens the 'admonisher'
role of the teacher. Building bonds of trust requires the directness
of "congruent and forthright messages (Randolph and Howe, p. 72)."

Setting limits and expectations. This process defines specific intellectual areas within which the children can feel safe and
free to explore and set stable expectations. The children and the
teachers discuss the purposes of education. Together they come to
conclusions concerning the way in which a particular subject helps
to obtain these purposes. The purposes become 'personalized' to
the children.

Freeing and directing energy. In order to free children's
energy and to direct it into socially accepted channels, fears of
disapproval and failure that 'lock in' energy or cause it to be dissi-
pated in unproductive ways must be reduced. Children are encouraged
to originate their own goals and feelings and their own expressions
of them. This is achieved through acting, creative writing and
'moving to music.'

Overcoming unproductive repetitive behavior. This process
interrupts destructive behaviors and patterns which interfere with
learning opportunities. Teachers are encouraged to confront the
unproductive behavior directly and to set a clear expectation. The
teacher should demonstrate by his actions that he is a person who
is concerned with the child as well as with the child's work.

Changing tattling to reporting. Learning the difference
between tattling and reporting helps children to assume social
responsibility and to confront directly.

Developing physical competencies. Physical development enables children to overcome the low self-esteem that results from their concern about their physical adequacy. SEE uses a type of Movement Exploration which allows the child to respond individually, creatively, and at his own speed.

Making success inevitable. To make success inevitable, opportunities are structured which will provide a successful academic experience for the child. This produces feelings of adequacy in the child. The authors of SEE estimate that those children who will not benefit from a traditional school curriculum are one in four. They posit that diagnostic teaching is necessary. Diagnostic teaching involves (a) diagnosis of the learning problems of the child through various instruments, (b) design of individualized, sequenced curricular activities.

Self-evaluation. Developing self-evaluation overcomes the children's impression that their evaluation is done primarily by adults, which forces the child to work for adult approval rather than for self-improvement. In SEE the teacher is not the one and only evaluator. The students have accesss to answer keys. Since a purpose of SEE is to help the child develop social skills requisite for self-direction and self-control, these skills are subject to self-evaluation, also. Teachers and students set up a Bureau of Standards against which each individual can judge his efforts.

523

<u>Breaking curriculum barriers</u>. This process frees children to progress through educational opportunities as they are ready. Randolph and Howe posit that an open-ended curriculum is necessary. The positive attributes of this are enhanced if the teacher involves the pupils' ideas in the organization and operation of the curriculum.

Randolph and Howe provide a series of seven questions which are meant to be of help in getting SEE started in any particular classroom. In their book, Randolph and Howe also provide suggested activities (particular games to play, pictures to draw, signs to display) to pursue in connection with each question. Presented here are the "facilitating questions" and their purposes.

(1) Who are we?

By pursuing this question with her students, the teacher has a chance to help them feel that "the learning-opportunity activities are uniquely personal (Randolph and Howe, p. 120)."

(2) Where are we in space and time?

Beginning with the 'here and now; helps the teacher and the children relate the textbook materials to the world of things and people.

(3) Why are we here?

This question provides the teacher with an opportunity to involve the pupils "as unique resources in selecting goals, as evaluators of goals to be acted upon, and as co-planners in means to the desired ends (Randolph and Howe, p. 128)."

(4) What are our operational problems?

'The identification of operational problems is a cooperative process in which the children and the teacher take an active part."

(5) How can we solve operational problems?

Children should be allowed to vent their creativity on solutions to operational problems which they have helped to identify.

(6) How can we help ourselves to grow?

It is important that the child be aware of what is expected of him and when and how he has accomplished this expectation. Growth at an individual rate is the emphasis. "Whenever we can provide the child with standards of expectation for the specific learning activities, he can assume increased responsibility for his own assessment (Randolph and Howe, p. 136)."

(7) How can we assess our growth?

"The locus of assessment is in the child. He is made aware of what he is expected to accomplish in the learning experience. He has available standards by which he can judge his accomplishments. Grades, if used, represent the cooperative assessment of the student and his teacher (Randolph and Howe, p. 136)."

SEE hopes to increase the learning opportunities for both students and teachers. Through the 12 processes and the facilitating questions for beginning them in a classroom, the SEE program hopes to embark on a cooperative venture in which both teachers and students will become closer to the purposes of education, and in which each child's self-esteem is raised.

ReEd

The ReEd schools as reported by Hobbs (1966, 1967), Lewis (1967) and Weinstein (1969) are perceived as a 'new social institution.' The population in need of this new social institution is children who have been disturbing in regular schools.

The disturbing behavior can be observed in the child. Behaviors which were defined as problems when children were referred to ReEd schools are acting out, withdrawal, truancy or school phobia, and academic problems. Underachievement is also a problem manifested by the children served by ReEd schools. The children, ranging in age from 6-12 years, are of average or superior intelligence. Most are retarded 2-3 years in academic development.

The disturbing behaviors enacted by the child are thought to flow from the fact that the child has learned 'bad habits,' that he has acquired non-adaptive ways of relating to adults and to other children. The source of this non-adaption and bad habits is the quality of the interface between the child and his environment. This is identified on a general level as the goodness of fit between social institutions and the people they serve. More specifically, ReEd is concerned with the relationship between the child and his community and the child and his family.

Lewis identifies the source of the problem specifically as "discordant child-rearing systems." Lewis feels that the child's difficulties in ability, understanding, or motivation are connected to a discordance between the role prescriptions held by primary socialization agents and the role performance of the child. Misunderstanding of role prescriptions by the child are due to a breakup in the socializing systems. Increased concordance between the child's behavior and the expectations for his behavior held by his parents is a basic goal for ReEd intervention.

ReEd is a bilateral intervention in that it directs its change action toward the child and the environment represented by his family, his school, and his community. Although ReEd recognizes the problem as emanating from the interface between the child and his environment, the interventionists feel that removal from the disturbing situation for a time is a positive element. Intervention can then take place at 'both ends' in 'calmer water' than if the child was retained in his natural environment.

The environmental setting in which the child is placed is a residential institution, educative in focus. The children stay at the ReEd schools during the week and return to their homes on weekends. ReEd utilizes the environment as it exists in the simple, camp-like setting of the ReEd schools in its actions which are directed toward a change in the child.

ReEd is based on a 'systems concept' which is concerned with the functional adequacy of the total ecological system of which the child is a part. Hobbs provides a chart of the "ecological system, the smallest unit in a system approach to working with a disturbed child." This chart includes the child, the family, the community and neighborhood, the social agency, the school, and ReEd. Parents are not conceived as sources of contagion but as "responsible collaborators in making the system work (Hobbs, 1966, p. 1108)."

The goal is to make the system work without ReEd. The efforts will be directed toward lifting each component of the system above threshold with respect to the requirements of the other components. A goal of the ReEd intervention is to discover the ways in which the child and his 'real life' surroundings need to change in order to remove the discord between them and to undertake the changes.

Ideally the ReEd intervention works with the total ecological system of the child. Most information to be gleaned concerning its operation, however, has to do with the institutional aspects which are directed toward effecting a change in the child.

There are 40 children in each of the two ReEd residences, Wright and Cumberland. They are placed into 5 groups of 8 children each. The child lives and studies in this group of 8 students throughout his stay at ReEd. The average length of stay is six months.

The principle agents for action directed toward the child are two teacher-counselors for each group. One teacher-counselor is primarily a day-time formal teacher; the other is an after-school informal counselor, who works with the group as a whole. All decisions as to action to be taken toward the child are in the hands of the teacher-counselors.

Although the environment is structured at ReEd, and although the persons with whom the child will interact are controlled, ReEd does not include a completely structured day, with every hour planned to present a learning opportunity for the child. The teacher-counselor must be constantly on the lookout to provide the child with what he needs to help him re-enter his 'natural environment' and grow from normal contacts.

The teacher-counselors are people who have already taught in public school and shown sensitivity and a willingness to work with problems. The additional training required prior to becoming a teacher-counselor in a ReEd school consists of 3 academic quarters of course work and a practicum. They earn a Master of Arts degree in special education, with emphasis in the area of emotional disturbance. The practicum emphasizes: (1) clinical education with individuals; (2) small group teaching; (3) liaison work with families, schools and community agencies.

There are three other staff members who are important in the ReEd intervention, who do not interact directly with the child. These are the mental health specialist consultant, the social worker consultant, and the liaison teacher.

The mental health specialist consultant consults with the teacher-counselors. The social worker consultant consults with the teacher-counselors, the referring agency (which maintains contact with the child's family) and the liaison teacher. The social worker consultant also evaluates the community from which the child comes and intervenes for the purpose of providing any special community resources for a particular child. The liaison-teacher maintains a communication link between the ReEd school and the child's regular school. Although ideally communication flows freely among all the intervention staff, it could be said that the intervention of the teacher-counselors and mental health specialist consultants is primarily directed toward the child; the social work consultant and the liaison teacher intervene primarily into the child's home environment.

At ReEd, attributes of the staff are considered important. Personality characteristics and commitment to the program are both instrumental in ReEd's approach. The teacher-counselor is chosen through self-selection and careful screening. One of the basic requirements for a teacher-counselor is that he be a decent adult. Other requirements are that the teacher-counslor be "educated, well-trained, able to give and receive affection, to live relaxed, and to be firm. The teacher-counslor must be a professional, a person of hope, quiet confidence, and joy (Hobb, 1966,p. 1107)."

Since it would appear that intervention into the circumstances of the home community must take place on an individual basis, no processes or techniques for intervening into the child's home community are provided in the sources on ReEd intervention. Processes utilized in the intervention which takes place in the ReEd schools are provided in these sources.

A concern with the 'whole child' can be seen in the 13 processes which are used by the ReEd staff. Included within this list are processes to aid the child to gain in his feelings of self-worth, to gain academically, and to adjust himself to his environment so that he will be able to benefit from normal contacts. The processes are:

Time can be used. "The systems concept may entail simply observing when the family has regained sufficient stability to sustain a previously ejected child." The ReEd staff feels that to provide nothing more than a benign sanctuary for a child at a time of crisis is a worthy endeavor.

The provision of opportunities for success. ReEd attempts to contrive each day so that the probability of successful achievement for the child outweighs the probability of failure.

531

The provision of competence. Gaining competence affords the child respect in an achievement-minded society. To improve achievement in school is a goal at ReEd. "School is the very stuff of a child's problems and consequently a primary source of instruction in living (Hobbs, 1967, p. 347)." The gaining of competence is not restricted to school skills, however. Social skills are emphasized as well. These include anything from learning to swim to risking friendship. The acquisition of some unique competence helps the child assert himself as a person.

The development of trust. It is important that a child have a relationship with a 'good' adult, so that he will learn that adults are not all bad, and so that he will be able to learn from adults. The ability to learn from adults is impaired in the disturbed child because of his conception of adults as harmful. The goal is to help the child make a new distinction. Some adults cannot be trusted. Other adults can be counted on as predictable sources of support, understanding and comfort. The core experience in making this distinction is that of being "genuinely close to an adult without getting hurt." 'Intimacy-worthy adult,' is difficult to operationalize into staff training. There is no professional training which can render an adult trustworthy. Trustworthiness is something which is 'natural' in the healthy adult, who is the product of healthy relationships.

Feelings should be nurtured. It is important that the children learn to accept all of themselves without guilt.

The control of symptoms. Symptoms must be controlled, to ensure a child's acceptance by his community. The ReEd intervention is concerned that the child be able to gain affection, support, instruction and discipline from his normal "home" sources. The assumption is that the child is rejected by his family, friends, schools or community, largely due to behaviors which are unacceptable to them. At this point the ReEd intervention does not concern itself with the adequacy of the family or community. but rather accepts some accommodation to them as a *de facto* requirement in the child's life. At ReEd symptoms are removed or altered through reconceptualization or reconditioning.

The teaching of middle class values. Middle class values are important to the child's acceptance by middle class teachers. The 'middle class values' which the child must learn include good manners, cleanliness, good language, bookishness, and the need to work and to achieve.

The development of cognitive control. Gaining cognitive control provides the child with the ability to shape his own behavior by self-administered verbal cues. The teacher-counselors work to help a child learn what the useful signals are. The teacher-counselors do this informally through events which occur naturally throughout the day and formally through the council ring or pow-wow which takes place each night. In the evening council ring,

533

the children, in a group, are helped to consider their day, the rights and wrongs, how to handle similar situations tomorrow. This is a time of talking things over. The goal of this activity is insight, not the insight which precedes the reorganization of the personality, but rather insight into one's relationships with the community.

The group. The youngsters at ReEd remain in the same group, living and studying together, sharing experiences, for the duration of their stay at ReEd. The group is considered to be an important source of motivation and control.

Ceremony and Ritual. Ceremony and ritual provide order, stability, and confidence. These are considered important in the ReEd intervention because many of the children have lived chaotic lives. The groups into which the children are divided take on names, the Whipporwills, or the Bobcats, etc. They also take on certain traditions, and become renowned for being good at one thing or another. The powwow or campfire ring is a form of ritual, besides being therapeutic.

The provision of physical experience. Physical experience is considered to be a basis for the greater awareness of self. "The notion is that the physical self is the armature around which the psychological self is constructed (Hobbs, 1967, p. 352)." Programmatically, this idea has been realized in such activities as swimming, climbing, dancing, tumbling, clay modeling, canoeing, building a tree house and walking a monkey bridge.

The development of community ties. The development of community ties is undertaken so that the child can see the worth and obligation of participation in the community surrounding him. This idea had been operationalized in field trips to fire, police, and health departments. Membership in the YMCA, a children's museum, a playground group or settlement house may also be useful in this respect.

The knowing of joy. This is considered by ReEd to be important and therapeutic for the child. The intervention at the ReEd schools includes opportunities whereby the child can experience joy. How do these joyful things happen? "They probably require most of all to have them come to pass a sensitivity on the part of the teacher-counselor to what it is that means a lot to a particular child, and some ingenuity in arranging for things to happen (Hobbs, 1967, p. 353)."

The ReEd schools, then, are an attempt to take into account the whole child and his surrounding ecological system. It is a bi-lateral intervention in that it intervenes into both ends of the child-environment relationship. What is reported here is primarily the 'child' end of that intervention.

In an evaluation of ReEd written by Laura Weinstein, it is stated that in actual practice ReEd appears to effect more change in the child than in other parts of the system. Increased concordance between the child's behavior and the expectations for

535

his behavior held by his parents is a basic goal for ReEd intervention. Data suggest that the increased concordance which did take
place was due primarily to improvement in the child's behavior.

XII. INTERFACE INTERVENTIONS

The Interface Interventions differ from other interventions on the continuum chart in that they are based on the assumption that the disturbing problem cannot be identified in the behavior of the child, but only in the mismatch between the child's behavior and a specific environment. The problem exists in the interface, in the lack of 'goodness of fit' between the child and his
surroundings. These interventions correspondingly direct their
actions toward a change in the interface situation. The goal of
these interventions is to reduce the conflict inherent in a mismatch of child behavior and environment.

Students as Behavior Change Agents

The intervention reported by Graubard, Rosenberg and
Miller (1971) and Cook (1971) views the problem as existing in
the interface between the child and his environment. Problematic
conflicts were identified in three interface situations occurring
in school: the conflict between special education children and
regular teachers, the conflict between a teacher's tolerance for
noise and "children's spontaneous noise level," and the conflict
between special education children and 'normal' children. The
action which took place was directed toward a change in the interface. "The behavior of neither the behaver nor the perceiver in
isolation from this interface is the target." The targets were the

537

regular teachers and the regular class children, with the special class children implementing the change-action. By acting on others, the special class children changed their own behavior, so that the actual effect was an overall change in the interface.

The objective of using students as behavior change agents is to improve the social adjustment of special education students. "Deviants" are taught to modify the behavior of "normals." Social skills are taught so that interfaces can be changed in a manner positive to the deviant. Providing students with a powerful technology for improving their social relationships leads to self-enhancement. Skills which allow one to change others are necessary for self-protection.

The intervention is exemplified in the four experiments which were conducted in a regular school which includes special education classes. "Special Ed" children are in special classes for part of the day, and regular classes for part of the day. The change in the interface between conflicting groups is the most significant factor in these experiments.

Experiment I: Children modify teacher behavior. This experiment took place in a regular class in which special education children were enrolled. The problematic situation was the interface between special education children and regular teachers which resulted in clash and conflict. The objective was

to establish a positive relationship between individual special education students and the teachers. The targets for the intervention
action were the regular teachers. The acting agents were seven special
education students, called "behavior engineers" who were 12-15
years of age.

Each 'engineer' (special ed student) was assigned two
'clients' (teachers). Each engineer had the responsibility of accelerating praise rates and decelerating negative comments and punishment directed toward him by the teachers.

The engineers were instructed in behavior modification
theory and techniques by special education teachers. Cook emphasizes
that good teaching techniques as well as a good base of knowledge
in operant theory and behavior modification techniques are required
by the staff in this 'training' stage of the intervention. Intervention techniques were taught to the special class children through
the use of simulation, role-playing, review of video tapes, and
discussion.

Management techniques which they learned were: maintaining eye contact, asking for extra help, making reinforcing comments,
smiling, sitting up straight, nodding in agreement, making the 'ah-
hah, I understand it now' reaction, breaking eye contact during
scolding, ignoring a teacher's provocation and asking for extra
assignments. Students were taught to use these techniques contin-
gently, i.e., as responses to the teachers' behavior toward them.

539

Positive (reinforcing) techniques were used in response to behaviors which it was desired to increase. Negative (extinguishing) techniques were used in response to behavior which it was desired to decrease.

The "behavior engineers" kept their own records of praise comments and critical comments. These were spot-checked by special education teachers. The entire activity took place without the awareness of the regular class teachers who were the "targets."

Statistics recording praise and criticism rates pre-experiment, during experiment, and post-experiment (during extinction) show that these management techniques utilized by the special ed student engineers did accelerate praise rates and decelerate negative comments and punishment by teachers. These statistics also showed that teachers need a high level of reinforcement to maintain this situation.

Experiment II: Changing tolerance for noise. The problem here was defined as the conflict between teachers' tolerance of noise and "children's spontaneous noise level." The objective was to raise the teacher's tolerance for noise. The target of this intervention were teachers with skill in modifying behavior and maintaining quiet, well-controlled, structured classrooms. In this case, the acting agents were supervisors and superintendents, who would be perceived by the teachers as observers of high prestige. The action was to bring in these observers, in groups, for the purpose of demonstrating the particular teacher's tolerance of noise and the freedom of self-expression which she allowed to her children. The teacher was told that these visits would occur and that their purpose was to show her classroom as a model of self-expression.

The high prestige observers utilized rewards such as praise, reinforcement, and modeling. "Positive (as defined by the goals of the experiment) aspects of the teacher's performance became an underlined focus." As the teacher was praised for her tolerance of noise and freedom of self-expression in her classroom, the noise level and freedom of self-expression increased.

Experiment III: Deviant children change normal children. The problem in this case was the interface between "normal" children and special class children. The normal children teased, ignored, ridiculed, and scapegoated the special education children. The objective of the experiment was to make the meeting of normal student and special ed student more palatable to the special class children. The targets were "normal" children. The acting agents were special class children. The special education teachers explained and illustrated operant theory to the children. The special ed children made a list of their peers who made school unpleasant for them and described their behavior. The special ed children recorded data on negative and positive contacts with other children throughout the experiment. The basic techniques used were verbal praise (positive contacts) and ignoring (negative contacts). Each child's "plan of action" was engineered with his special class teacher on an individual basis. When special class students were successful in increasing positive contacts and decreasing negative contacts they were rewarded with candy.

Experiment IV: Changing the perceptions of normals toward special education classes and children. The problem here was viewed as the loss of prestige suffered by special education children and the concommitant harrassment they are subjected to—the stigma of being in a "special class." Also problematic was the isolation of the special ed room from the mainstream of regular education taking place within the school. It was the goal of this experiment to make special education classrooms a "focal point of positive attention for the entire student body and school." The basic action taken here was the instituting of contingencies. The special ed teachers and students worked together on this. "Reinforcing" activities were instituted in the special ed room. These activities were available to regular students on the condition that they participate in them with special students. "These activities include wrestling, boxing, fishing derbys, craft classes, pottery, listening to music, ice skating and other exciting trips."

These rather simple applications of behavior modification techniques had a major effect on the normal power structure existing within the school Because behavior modification was applied, it had the effect of reversing, or at least equalizing somewhat, the balance of power.

> Currently, establishment groups such as teachers, normals, and high-status children retain control over the power structures within the schools. It has been demonstrated that this control may be neutralized by developing the capacity to change others' behavior in those groups usually regarded by society as being in need of change.
> (<u>Graubard</u>, et al, 1971)

It is interesting to note that students who took part in the experiments as 'behavior engineers' did not view themselves as manipulative or in positions of power. The typical students' perception of the experiment to change teacher behavior (Experiment I) was, "We're trying to be nice to the teachers, so they will be nice to us (Cook, p. 25)." A typical student reaction to the experiment to change peer behavior (Experiment III) was, "If you have these skills it helps to make more friends (Cook, p. 35)." The authors emphasize that the skills which the special education students were learning are skills which 'normal' children already know and use.

Ecological Management

The Ecological Management form of intervention is based on two articles by Rhodes: "Psychosocial learning" (1967) and "The disturbing child: A problem of ecological management" (1969).

This intervention views the problem as centered in inter-face. The problem focus emphasizes the agitated exchange between the child and the person to whom his behavior is disturbing. This agitated exchange is seen to flow from the fact that the content of behavioral prohibitions and sanctions in a culture are "fre-quently discrepant with the natural propensities in the individual." The intervention action is directed toward the agitated environ-mental product, i.e., the interface. Ecological management is a planned intervention, so the programmatics which will be described have not been implemented in a total program as such.

The objectives for the intervention action are planned on two levels. In the short term this action consists of entering into a disturbing situation and changing it. Here the concern is with the interaction between a particular child and his human environment. In the long term the action consists of modifying the socialization process. In that respect, the concern is with the interaction between individuals and culture.

The operationalization of the short-term objective consists of re-education of the child and his relevant human environment. Rhodes stresses the importance of the person who would perform the re-education task. This would be a 'new breed' of special teacher. The teacher must not only educate the 'dis-turber' but must also educate those who are disturbed by his ac-tions. The teacher would need to be free to enter into the child's total life situation so that he might alter the process of transmission of culture. He must constantly search out "the right relationship between the self and the culture" from a position of much less than total immersion in this culture.

In the school situation, this teacher would not be a 'special class' teacher. Rather he would be a 'team teacher' with a regular teacher in a regular classroom situation. His role in the school would be as a 'buffer' and as a model of the way to respond to the child.

In the home setting he would also be a buffer and a model of how to respond to the child so as to reduce disturbance. He would accomplish this task vis-a-vis the family and the "immediate community of responders" through demonstration, example and interpretation.

The long-term goal involves a change in the transmission of culture. Rhodes feels that the method of transmission of culture is problematic. At present it is haphazard . To "change the way in which we transmit culture and the way we teach the child to relate to the culture." Rhodes posits that entirely new types of educative institutions will have to be implemented.

This institution must be concerned with the 'whole child.' It must teach him both how to deal with knowledge and fact, and how to live in a complex society. This will necessitate a shift away from the concentration on subject matter and the single classroom teacher. Resources now available will have to occupy a more central position. These include counseling and guidance, school social work, school psychology, special education, pupil personnel services, and child development specialists. These resources should be utilized to give the child a better understanding of the relationship between himself and his culture.

Two examples given by Rhodes of the type of educational facility required to operationalize this task are the educational park and the children's institution. The educational park would be an educative complex, resembling a miniature campus of a university. It would include students from several socio-economic backgrounds and from several neighborhoods. It would consist of two divisions, equal in emphasis and power. One division would be instructional, resembling the form of instruction we now have. It would include education specialists. The second division would be concerned with social-personal (psychosocial) learning and with the relationship between individual and society. It would consist of behavioral science specialists. Some of the goals of this portion of the educational park would include socializing the individual for mastery of modern metropolitan life; prevention of social disaffection or extreme social deviance; renovation or remediation of children or youth whose behavior or living patterns are dissonant within the existing culture. The psychosocial learning division could be subdivided into functional units for the above three goals. The director of the educational park would have equal training in the social sciences and in education. "Each child would be scheduled into both areas according to his life needs."

Another model for reorganization of the existing educative pattern is the children's institution, a third force external to the home or to the school which would augment and supplement the functions of family and school. The model for this is found in a self-contained collective town in Denmark. It is a planned community built expressly with human needs in mind. The children's institutions, whch are a part of this community, "serve children from birth through the age of twenty-one. They are staffed by specially trained educators and provide a practicum training facility for college students preparing for the educative profession. The institutions include a creche for infants, a nursery school, a kindergarten, a 'spare time home' for children of school age, a special teen program, and a youth program for the 18-21 age group (Rhodes, 1967, pp. 216-217)."

In order to fulfill the functions of socializing the individual for life in a complex society, prevention of social deviance, and remediation of persons whose behavior is dissonant within the culture, we need to provide a social instrument through which all persons have equal opportunities to learn social mastery. Rhodes provides some explication of certain processes which should be utilized within this instrument, exemplified by the educational park or children's institution.

547

In general, Rhodes feels that self-understanding processes such as group-psychotherapy, sensitivity training and guided
group discussions should become a part of education. He describes
the characteristics of some of the elements of this plan.

Characteristics of contrived experiences. Experiences must
be programmed which allow the child to function in a group, so that he
will be able to develop group skills. Experiences must be programmed
which allow the child to take on a variety of roles. Materials must
be utilized which provide a sensory experience for the child. Opportunities for the learner to be active must be provided in contrived
experiences. Social-personal (psychosocial) learning in children
"demands activity that is directed toward a meaningful environmental
experience."

Characteristics of goals in social learning. The context of
learning must be consonant with the life of the children. It must
include incidents which they understand and a temperament which they
sense. If the context familiar to the children is unacceptable to
the society in which the children are required to live, the change to
an unfamiliar but socially acceptable context should involve step-by-
step procedures.

Characteristics of consequences. The educative task is to
"manipulate the environment during the learning phase so that it
provides satisfaction to the individual in return for modifications
of his behavior toward social ends." For this behavior to be maintained

548

society must live up to its end of the bargain by providing continuing personal satisfaction in exchange for socially contributive
behavior once the learning phase has ended.

Characteristics of the emotional content. The previous processes have emphasized the context and culture of individuals. This
process is concerned with the internal dynamics of the individual
himself. Social and emotional learning must be in concert with the
internal dynamics of the child. The teacher must utilize these dynamics as a bridge between child and society. The teacher must also
not reject any of the dynamics which he finds inside the child. To
do this, to deal with the child in terms of the child, rather than
in terms of one's self or one's cultural traditions, the teacher must
place some distance between himself and his culture, his biases and
prejudices. To effectively intervene into the conflict-causing interface, then, is to provide a means whereby the transmission of culture
from generation to generation is carried out utilizing the knowledge
that we have, so that each child has an equal opportunity to learn
what is required of him, but so that he can gain some freedom from
cultural prohibitions which conflict with his internal dynamics as
well. The educative institution would attempt to educate the whole
child, and to deal with the "right relationship between the internal
dynamics of persons and the external characteristics of social
systems (Rhodes, 1967, p.228)."

XIII. CONCLUSION

Historical Factors in Intervention Implementation

Cultural relativity has been posited as an important element of social deviance and ecological theory. The conviction is that deviance is relative; a culture chooses the behaviors it will glorify, and those it will damn. Cultural relativity is an important consideration in the implementation of intervention as well. The particular behaviors we consider deviant are relative not only to the time and place, but to the way in which we define these activities and to our conception of their cause. The institutions we set up to deal with these behaviors, and the interventions utilized within them, are relative.

Some of the factors in this relativity which serve to delimit intervention are discussed by Rhodes and Gibbins (1972). One of the factors involved in the programmatic aspects of an intervention is the theory extant in the locale of the proposed intervention.

A much more important role, however, is played by the people in the community, their perception of threat, and the way in which they define this threat. For example, is the problem juvenile delinquency or drug abuse? If it is juvenile delinquency, is the cause sickness, sin, deviance, or an unwholesome family life? The process of building an institution for intervention might be mapped this way: the threat as perceived by the populace leads to their anxiety; this anxiety as perceived by politicians leads to funding; the funding leads to the construction of institutions which are built in the image of the threat as defined by the people.

A third, very important factor is the fact that once the institutions are set up, the actual buildings built, they have a life of their own. They are self-perpetuating. Even if a community changed its ideas and wished to turn a prison into a rehabilitation center, the barred windows, thick doors and walls would continue to emit the aura of punishment and the atmosphere of isolation.

Rhodes and Gibbins feel that what we now have in the way of institutions is a result of a complex historical and ongoing process "which can be relatively independent of specific scientific knowledge or a particular program planner (Rhodes and Gibbins, p. 18)."

It must be recognized, therefore, that there are many factors, other than theory, which impinge on the form an intervention eventually takes. Ecological and sociological interventions were often breaks with tradition at the time of their inception. The break away from the medical model, the "sick role," and the cure was in itself an innovation in the mental health field. A few of the more interesting examples of these breaks with tradition and of impinging historical factors will be taken from interventions reported in this paper.

551

In 1869, the village of Gheel and the hamlets and farms immediately surrounding Gheel had a long-established tradition of taking in people of "all mental alienations" as boarders and treating them as especially well-cared-for members of the family. It must be remembered that at this time in European history the "insane" were subjected to isolation and physical restraints of the chain and straight-jacket variety, in insane asylums of the type that made Bedlam (the popular name for the Hospital of St. Mary of Bethlehem in London) a synonym for chaos. Just a few miles distant from the haven at Gheel, prejudice and cruelty toward "lunatics" was the recognized norm of the day.

Anton Semyonovich Makarenko resigned from his beloved Gorky Colony due to criticism from the Bureaucrats of the 1920's. He had turned street waifs into proud colonists who, on an individual level, became medical students, pilots, or good party workers. His principles were those of proletarian duty, cultivation of the sense of honor, and industry. These were not accepted by the pedagogical theoreticians of his day.

Maxwell Jones writes of the difficulty of maintaining a therapeutic community, utilizing free and open communication, in a hospital ward adjacent to the traditional hierarchical system, with its communication from doctor to head nurse to nurses to patient.

Jones also provides a discussion of the political and historical reasons for an emphasis on social methods of treatment in the 1940's in Britain. This emphasis was partly due to the strain on psychiatric services caused by the war. Another factor was the "changing cultural pattern in Britain." Jones views this as a growing willingness to accept social responsibility on the part of the community; the growth of a social conscience. Jones posits that this can be seen in the political realm, especially in the legislation known as the Disabled Persons (Employment) Act of 1944, which aids disabled persons to secure employment, and under which the Industrial Neurosis Unit was implemented. Jones points out that one of the "social conditions" prevailing in Britain at the time was full employment, and the "social responsibility" might not have been so readily assumed if competition for employment had been greater.

The implementation of guided group interaction in the rehabilitation of delinquents (utilized at Highfields, Provo, and Silverlake) is partially a function of an historical process. During World War II, psychiatric services were severely strained by the number of men requiring treatment. Group psychotherapy began in this context. Dr. Lloyd W. McCorkle had participated in this. As director of Highfields, McCorkle utilized the same concepts under the rubric of guided group interaction, changing the name basically to avoid the feeling in the minds of the boys that there was something wrong with them which required therapy or treatment.

Aryeh Leissner, a street-club worker with experience in New York and Tel Aviv, recognized the historical and political contingencies upon the type of intervention which was instituted to "handle" juvenile delinquency. Leissner's discussion of these demonstrates the way in which anxiety in the minds of the populace can have a determining effect on the target of the intervention.

> The specialized social group work service known as the 'street-club worker' or 'detached-worker' program developed during the 1950's in the United States in response to the growing realization that there existed in the urban poverty areas a large segment of the youth population which could not be reached by the conventional methods of group work in the Settlement House, Community, or Youth Club settings. These youngsters, mainly lower-class adolescents congregating in street corner groups or gangs, adhered to delinquent values and norms, which they expressed by unlawful, destructive and self-destructive behavior.
> (Leissner, 1965, p. 67)

Leissner also demonstrates an awareness of political and social influences on the way in which the street-club worker will be allowed to pursue his goals. Leissner writes of the difficulty of pursuing a course of gaining rapport with a street-club, which involved tolerating delinquent behavior and strict confidentiality. This process is hindered by public opinion and some law enforcement officials who feel that the street-club worker's function is to control and report delinquent behavior. In his work with the law enforcement agencies and the courts, the street-club worker attempts to establish a personnel of the local

554

police precinct who are likely to come into contact with the members
of his group.

> The degree of understanding and cooperation which the worker
> obtains depends upon a number of factors: the worker's ability
> to explain his professional functions and to convey his under-
> standing for the responsibilities and complexities of the
> policeman's job; the personal attitudes of the individual officers
> with whom he deals; the attitudes of the commanding officer
> of the precinct and, last but not least, the public pressure
> exerted upon the police at any given time due to dramatic
> incidents of youth crime, press campaigns against 'young hoodlums,'
> etc.   (Leissner, 1965, p. 121)

Another negative factor impinging on the Tel Aviv street-
club worker's goals is party politics. The corruptness and false-
hoods of the politicians "strengthen and perpetuate the cynicism
and antisocial attitudes of the youngsters, and greatly reinforce
their tendency to regard conventional society as basically corrupt
(Leissner, p. 74)."

The program factors which are of concern to physical
environmentalists--changeability, educational tools, flexibility,
the site, integration, and segregation--(Bednar and Haviland,
1969) are accommodations to parental and community concerns, as well
as to education theory.

Those who advocate a "whole child" approach to education posit
that "the limitation of education to content-oriented instruction
is much more by public design than by educational philosophy
(Rhodes, 1967, p. 213)."

These are just a few of the more obvious and interesting
examples of historical factors which impinge on intervention im-

plementation. Environmental interventions were at times break-
aways from tradition and popular demand, though they continued to
remain under the influence of the historical process.

The Elusive Community

A question which nags at the mind concerns the "Community" interventions (Gheel, Pittsburgh School Mental Health Program,
Gorky Colony, Hawthorne Cedar Knolls, Industrial Neurosis Unit,
Highfields, Provo and Silverlake and to some extent ReEd). These
interventions create a community within which they impress upon
its members the interdependence of human beings, and individual
responsibility for the community. The distressing question is,
"Is there a community to go home to?" When the client of the
community intervention returns to his natural milieu, is there a
community willing and waiting for him to vent his new skills?
This is a problem which may vitiate the viability of this type of
intervention.

Since, from the experience of the "Community" interventions, it would seem that healthy groups do make healthy individuals, the lack of healthy groups in the home communities is indeed
problematic.

Although it is the goal of the Industrial Neurosis Unit
to construct a culture in which real life problems connected with
work situations and with relationships with others will arise,

will be discussed and worked through, one must ask to what extent
the supportive atmosphere of group life, and of membership in a
community, which the patient has learned to accept and to which
he has come to contribute, will exist in the real community to
which he will return after his stay in the Industrial Neurosis
Unit.

Joy Tuxford, who participated in a follow-up study of
patients in the Industrial Neurosis Unit six months after discharge, saw an absence of community life in the "real world" to
which the patients had returned. This is a problem which Ms. Tuxford posits as causing emotional disturbance as well as hindering
the re-integration of the treated person into society. She viewed
the problem of absence of community as being a result of lessened
responsibility of one member in a group to another, plus the increased responsibility of the state in family relationships. She
wrote,

> It seems to me...from the...experience I gained of the
> community structure in all parts of London, that there
> was in most areas a real paucity of group life; mainly
> due, I felt, to the fact that in many cases there was no
> real geographical cohesion and no focal point on which
> the inhabitants could center their emotions. In addi-
> tion, there appeared to be no social cohesion from within
> the group. Problems which arise within a group of small
> communities are nowadays solved outside the group. There
> has been a decline in the individual awareness of the role
> required of each group member and their relationships to
> one another. This has led to disintegration of the group
> and thereby the support given by the group to the individual
> has in part disappeared.
>   (Jones, 1953, p. 96)

557

Some of the boarders whom Julia Byrne met on her tour of Gheel seemed to have been abandoned by their own communities and families. She saw persons who had lived as boarders at Gheel for 14, 18, and even 30 years.

McCorkle, Elias and Bixby state that Highfields provided black adolescent boys with sorely needed self-esteem. Statistics which are dichotomized between races show that on a percentage basis, the black residents of Highfields had a lower "unsuitable for residence" rate than whites. That is, percentage wise, fewer black residents were returned to court while living at Highfields than white residents. And yet in a chapter entitled "Community Adjustment" which concerns rates of success and failure (recidivism) after leaving Highfields, McCorkle et al, state that although blacks made a better adjustment while staying at Highfields, they failed in greater proportion than whites in community adjustment. Blacks had a proportionately higher recidivism rate. It would seem that these statistics are an indictment of society-at-large and its failure to continue to provide the opportunities for self-esteem found at Highfields.

Leissner, the street-club worker, discusses slum clearance and the devastating effect it has on community feeling. This clearance and resettlement which involves displacement and dispersion of the community residents destroys "whatever vestiges of social organization remain in the slum community." Thus the res-

558

idents of the newly built housing projects "find themselves in a community that is not only new and alien but lacking in patterns of social organization to which they may link themselves and through which they might develop a stake in community life (Leissner, 1965, p. 58)." Leissner feels that the low-income housing projects of large cities are de-personalized and decommunized.

> In Tel Aviv and in New York I have heard boys and girls from relocated families speak with resentment of their new homes, although in most cases, there is little doubt that the dwellings they had left were greatly inferior to those to which they had been moved.
>
> The key to this lies, perhaps, in the fact that these youngsters feel that they 'are being moved' without having much choice or say-so in the matter. In New York, as well as in Tel Aviv, the process of relocation is experienced as a process of dislocation, mainly because, in many cases, it is not accompanied by a process of socio-economic and cultural absorption into established society. Many of the youngsters and their families prefer to stay in the relative safety and familiarity of their slum, rather than to move to new, 'exposed', unfamiliar surroundings.
> (Leissner, 1965, p. 58)

Some light may be shed on this observation by an article by Fried and Gleicher, "Some sources of residential satisfaction in an urban slum." These authors studied the effects of renewal and relocation. They feel that we need to understand the meaning of the slum's physical and social environment. The data which they provide toward this end are based on a probability sample of residents from the West End of Boston who were facing relocation. The authors found marked residential stability both within the West End and within the dwelling unit. They also found that the

West End was the focus for positive sentiments. The geographical cohesion which Joy Tuxford found missing in London was present in these respondents, and was centered around the local area of the West End. Fried and Gleicher found a sense of local spatial identity, local social relationships, and of local places. The authors emphasize the negative aspects of urban renewal. There are personal and social consequences to living in a slum, and to being removed from that slum by exterior forces, which are largely unknown. Leissner says "In both cities I have found that slum inhabitants have actually rejected better housing, because their cultural traditions were not even discussed with them. The attitude of 'you should be grateful for what you are given. . .,' so often encountered by the 'objects' of slum clearance, is often met with resentment and defiance (Leissner, p. 59)." This is not to be interpreted as a 'pro-slum' position. It is, however, a position negative to urban slum clearance which treats people like warehouse objects to be moved at the city's convenience.

Rhodes, in the Ecological Management Intervention, states that society must live up to its side of the bargain when a child is giving up socially disapproved behavior. The society must continue to provide the child with the rewards and praise for socially approved behavior which he receives at the time of learning these behaviors. This reciprocation of society is the important variable in the problem being considered here. There must exist a community made up of individuals who are willing to depend on one another and to take responsibility for one another if the social skills and group feeling learned in the "community" interventions are to be a viable means of combatting disturbing behavior.

TECHNIQUES COMMON TO SEVERAL INTERVENTIONS

I.   Techniques Which Promote Self-Worth and Demonstrate the Worth of Others.

   A.   Clients are provided with a place in a community.

      1.   Gheel.
      2.   Gorky Colony.
      3.   Hawthorne Cedar Knolls.
      4.   Industrial Neurosis Unit.
      5.   Highfields.
      6.   ReEd.

   B.   The client population is formed into groups for the purpose of demonstrating the interdependence of human beings and to utilize group pressure for change.

      1.   Gorky Colony.
      2.   Industrial Neurosis Unit.
      3.   Highfields.
      4.   Provo, Silverlake.
      5.   ReEd.

   C.   Ritual, ceremony and tradition are utilized to promote a feeling of belongingness and to perpetuate order and stability.

      1.   Gorky Colony.
      2.   Industrial Neurosis Unit.
      3.   Highfields.
      4.   ReEd.

   D.   Clients may make decisions concerning other clients, in order to utilize peer pressure and to aid the feeling of helping one another.

      1.   Gorky Colony.
      2.   Highfields.
      3.   Provo, Silverlake.

   E.   A relationship of trust with an adult is developed so that youngsters may learn to learn from adults.

      1.   Gorky Colony.
      2.   Hawthorne Cedar Knolls.

3. Highfields.
4. Street-Club Work.
5. Self-Enhancing Education.
6. ReEd.
7. Maternal Care.

F. The life alternatives held by the youngsters are considered.

Youngsters are encouraged to explore their goals, even if they appear unrealistic. The philosophy has a "the world can be ours" feeling.

1. Gorky Colony.

Client goals are respected. Clients are helped to modify these goals in line with realistic employment opportunities.

2. Hawthorne Cedar Knolls.
3. Industrial Neurosis Unit.
4. Street-Club Work.

Only realistic goals are considered. An emphasis on education and on goals which could be reached through education is considered impractical.

5. Provo, Silverlake.

G. The need for power is considered and programmed.

Youth Club (political) organizations are utilized to provide a legitimate social cause, and an outlet for identification.

1. Gorky Colony.
2. Street-Club Work.

The philosophy that "knowledge is power" is instilled.

3. Hawthorne Cedar Knolls.

Decision-making and wielding power over one's own life is emphasized.

4. Highfields.
5. Provo, Silverlake.

Behavior modification techniques are taught.

      6.   Students as Behavior Change Agents.

H.   Experiences are contrived which aid social, personal and emotional development, in order to train the "whole child."

      1.   Pittsburgh School Mental Health Program.
      2.   Enhancing the Classroom Teacher's Mental Health Function.
      3.   Self-Enhancing Education.
      4.   Ecological Management.

I.   "No-fail" opportunities are provided to aid achievement, self-confidence, and self-esteem.

Success in scholastic opportunities is provided.

      1.   Hawthorne Cedar Knolls.
      2.   Self-Enhancing Education.
      3.   ReEd.

Success in manipulating environment is provided.

      4.   Therapeutic Built Environment.

Success in employment opportunities is provided.

      5.   Industrial Neurosis Unit.
      6.   Street-Club Work.

J.   Experiences of Joy are provided.

      1.   Gorky Colony.
      2.   ReEd.

K.   Physical competencies are developed to aid self-esteem.

      1.   Self-Enhancing Education.
      2.   ReEd.

II. Techniques Which Afford the Child Greater Acceptance in His Natural Environment.

A.   Problems which occur in the institutional setting are utilized to teach coping with "natural" life situations.

1. Gorky Colony.
2. Industrial Neurosis Unit.
3. Highfields.
4. Provo, Silverlake.
5. Preventive Approach to Developmental Problems.
6. Self-Enhancing Education.
7. ReEd.

B. Behaviors which are disturbing to the community-at-large are specifically identified and attempts are made to lessen them.

1. Hawthorne Cedar Knolls.
2. Self-Enhancing Education.
3. Street-Club Work.
4. ReEd.

C. Work habits are established.

1. Gheel.
2. Gorky Colony.
3. Industrial Neurosis Unit.
4. Highfields.
5. Provo, Silverlake.
6. Street-Club Work.

D. Social skills are taught.

1. Industrial Neurosis Unit.
2. Preventive Approach to Developmental Problems.
3. ReEd.
4. Students as Behavior Change Agents.

III. Techniques Which Help the Child Recognize and Repair Relationships With Environment.

A. Group processes are utilized for the purpose of gaining insight into one's self and one's relationship with family and community.

Guided Group Interaction.

1. Highfields.
2. Provo, Silverlake.

Group Therapy.

3. Industrial Neurosis Unit.

565

Council Ring (powwow).

    4.   ReEd.

B.   Responsibility to community is taught.

    1.   Street Club Work.
    2.   ReEd.

IV.   Techniques of Which the Main Purpose is to Aid the Administration of the Intervention Program.

A.   Personal properties of the teacher or interventionist are considered important. Staff is chosen with this in mind.

    1.   Gorky Colony.
    2.   Industrial Neurosis Unit.
    3.   Highfields.
    4.   Street-Club Work.
    5.   ReEd.
    6.   Ecological Management.
    7.   Maternal Care.

B.   The entire staff must be in concordance with the intervention program and its goals.

    1.   Gheel.
    2.   Gorky Colony.
    3.   Hawthorne Cedar Knolls.
    4.   Industrial Neurosis Unit.
    5.   Highfields.
    6.   Provo, Silverlake.
    7.   Self-Enhancing Education.
    8.   ReEd.
    9.   Ecological Management.
    10. Maternal Care.

C.   Interventionists recognize and work within the extant school culture.

    1.   Pittsburgh School Mental Health Program.
    2.   Preventive Approach to Developmental Problems.

D.   The worth of the teacher and the breadth of his influence is emphasized.

1. Pittsburgh School Mental Health Program.
2. Mental Health Consultation.
3. Enhancing the Classroom Teacher's Mental Health Function.
4. Preventive Approach to Developmental Problems.
5. ReEd.
6. Ecological Management.

E. Strengths present in the child or in his life situation are emphasized.

1. Hawthorne Cedar Knolls.
2. Street-Club Work.
3. Preventive Approach to Developmental Problems.
4. ReEd.
5. Maternal Care.

F. Lack of defined structure is utilized so that there is no system which can be "beat," so that problems will arise which have to be thought through and resolved, and so that decision-making can occur as opposed to merely following a set of explicit rules.

1. Highfields.
2. Provo, Silverlake.
3. Maternal Care.

G. A form of threat is utilized to bring desired results.

Removal from class is a threat.

1. Hawthorne Cedar Knolls.

Remandation to a stigma-producing institution (reformatory) is a threat.

2. Highfields.
3. Provo, Silverlake.

Abeson, A., & Berensen, B. Physical environment and special
education: An interdisciplinary approach. Arlington,
Virginia: The Council for Exceptional Children, 1970.

Abeson, A. The physical environment: A brave new world. Council
for Exceptional Children Selected Convention Papers.
Arlington, Virginia: The council for Exceptional Children,
1969.

Bayes, K. The therapeutic effect of environment on emotionally
disturbed and mentally subnormal children. Surrey, England:
Union Brothers, Ltd., 1967.

Bednar, M. J. & Haviland, D. S. The role of the physical environment in the education of children with learning disabilities. Troy, New York: Center for Architectural Research,
Renssalaer Polytechnic Institute, March, 1969.

Berensen, B. The planned environment: An educational tool.
International Journal of Educational Science, 2, 123-125.

Bowlby, J. Maternal Care and Mental Health. New York: Schocken
Books, 1966.

Byrne, J. C. Gheel: The city of the simple. London: Chapman &
Hall, 1869.

Cook, C. Students as behavior change agents, report of a site
visit. Visalia Unified School District, Visalia, California
Fall, 1971.

Empey, L. T. & Rabow, J. The Provo experiment in delinquency
rehabilitation. American Sociological Review, 1961, 26,
679-695.

Empey, L. T. & Lubeck, S. Silverlake experiment, testing delinquency theory and community intervention. Chicago: Aldine,
1961.

Fried, M. & Gleicher, P. Some sources of residential satisfaction
in an urban slum. American Institute of Planners Journal,
1961, 26-27, 305-315.

Goldsmith, J. M., Krohn, H., Ochroch, R. & Kagan, N. Changing the delinquent's concept of school. In Long, N. J., Morse, W. C. & Newman, R. G. (Eds.) Conflict in the classroom. Belmont, California: Wadsworth Publishing Company, 1965. 278-285.

Graubard, P. S., Rosenberg, H. & Miller, M. B. Student applications of behavior modification to teachers and environments or ecological approaches to social deviancy. Lawrence, Kansas: Second Annual Invitational Conference on Behavior Analysis in Education, Department of Human Development, University of Kansas, May, 1971.

Hall, E. T. The hidden dimension. New York: Doubleday and Co., Inc., 1969.

Hall, E. T. The silent language. Greenwich, Connecticut: Fawcett Publications, 1959.

Hewett, F. M. The emotionally disturbed child in the classroom. Boston: Allyn & Bacon, Inc., 1968.

Hobbs, N. Helping disturbed children: Psychological and ecological strategies. American Psychologist, 1966, 21, 1105-1115.

Hobbs, N. The re-education of emotionally disturbed children. In Bowen, E. M. & Hollister, W. G. (Eds.) Behavioral science frontiers. New York: John Wiley & Sons, 1967, 335-354.

Iscoe, I., Pierce-Jones, J., Friedman, S. & McGehearty, L. Some strategies in mental health consultation. In Cowen, E. L., Gardner, E. A. & Zax, M. (Eds.) Emergent approaches to mental health problems. New York: Appleton-Century-Crofts, 1967, 307-330.

Jones, M. The therapeutic community; a new treatment method in psychiatry. New York: Basic Books, 1953.

Leissner, A. Street-club work in New York and Tel-Aviv (Impressions and observations upon group work with lower class delinquent street-corner groups). Tel-Aviv: Action-Research Project on Delinquent Street Corner Groups in Tel-Aviv, February, 1965.

Lewis, W. W. Project Re-ed: Educational Intervention in discordant child-rearing systems. In Cowen, E. L., Gardner, E. A., & Zax, M. (Eds.) Emergent approaches to mental health problems. New York: Appleton-Century-Crofts, 1967, 352-368.

569

Makarenko, A. S. The road to life (an epic of education). Moscow: Foreign Language Publishing House, 1951, Vol. II & III.

Meuron, M. & Auerswald, E. H. Cognition and social adaptation. American Journal of Orthopsychiatry, 1969, 39, 57-67.

Minuchin, S., Dollarhide, P. & Graubard, P. S. A project to teach learning skills to disturbed delinquent children. In Graubard, P. S. (Ed.) Children aginst schools. Chicago: Follett Educational Corporation, 1969, 357-371.

Morse, W. C. Enhancing the classroom teacher's mental health function. In Cowen, E. L., Gardner, E. A. & Zax, M. (Eds.) Emergent approaches to mental health problems. New York: Appleton-Century-Crofts, 1967, 271-289.

McCorkle, L. W., Elias, A., & Bixby, F. L. The Highfield's story: A unique experiment in the treatment of juvenile delinquency. New York: Henry Holt and Co., 1958.

Newton, M. R. & Brown, R. D. A preventive approach to developmental problems in school children. In Bower, E. M. & Hollister, W. G. (Eds.), Behavioral science frontiers in education. New York: John Wiley and Sons, 1967, 499-527.

Parr, A. E. Psychological aspects of urbanology. Journal of Social Issues, 22, 1966, 39-45.

Pinneau, S. R. A critique on the articles by Margaret Ribble. Child Development, 1950, 21, 203-223.

Proshansky, H. M. Ittleson, W. H. & Rivlin, L. G. (Eds.) Environmental psychology: Man and his physical setting. New York: Holt, Rinehart & Winston, 1970.

Randolph, N. & Howe, W. A program to motivate learners: Self-enhancing education. Palo Alto: Educational Development Corporation, 1966.

Rhodes, W. C. The disturbing child: A problem of ecological management. In Graubard, P. S. (Ed.) Children against schools. Chicago: Follett Educational Corporation, 1969, 17-29.

Rhodes, W. C. & Gibbins, S. Community programming for the behaviorally deviant child. In Quay, H. C. (Ed.) Psychopathological disorders of childhood. New York, 1972, 348-387.

Rhodes, W. C. Psychosocial learning. In Bower, E. M. & Hollister, W. G. (Eds.) Behavioral science frontiers in education. New York: John Wiley & Sons, 1967, 207-229.

Ribble, M. Disorganizing factors of infant personality. In S. S. Tomkins (Ed.) Contemporary psychopathology. Cambridge: Harvard University Press, 1943.

Ribble, M. Infantile experience in relation to personality development. In J. Hunt (Ed.) Personality and the behavior disorders, II. New York: Ronald Press Company, 1944.

Ribble, M. The significance of infatile sucking for the psychic development of the individual. In S. S. Tomkins (Ed.) Contemporary psychopathology. Cambridge: Harvard University Press, 1943.

Sommer, R. Personal space: The behavioral basis of design. Englewood Cliffs, New Jersey: Prentice-Hall, Inc., 1969.

Spitz, R. A. The role of ecological factors in emotional development in infancy. Child Development, 1949, 20, 145-155.

Staats, A. W. & Butterfield, W. H. Treatment of non-reading in a culturally deprived juvenile delinquent: An application of reinforcement principles. Child Development, 1965, 36, 925-942.

Stickney, S. B. Schools are our community mental health centers. American Journal of Psychiatry, 1968, 124, 1407-1414.

Vogel, E. E. & Bell, N. W. The emotionally disturbed child as the family scapegoat. In Bell, N. W. & Vogel, E. E. (Eds.) A modern introduction to the family. Glencoe, Illinois: The Free Press, 1960, 382-397.

Weinstein, L. Project Re-Ed: Schools for emotionally disturbed children--effectiveness as viewed by referring agencies, parents and teachers. Exceptional Children, 1969, 35, 703-711.

Wohlwill, J. F. The physical environment: A problem for the psychology of stimulation. Journal of Social Issues, 22, 1966, 29-38.

COUNTERTHEORETICAL INTERVENTIONS IN EMOTIONAL DISTURBANCE

Douglas Burke

TABLE OF CONTENTS

I. WHAT IS COUNTER THEORY?

This paper discusses what countertheorists have to say about schools and emotional disturbance, and what they would do about them.

"Counter theory" is not clearly a separate body of theory. The writers discussed here disagree with each other, as well as with other, established writers. In fact, the most satisfactory definition of "a countertheorist" seems to be a definition by extrusion: a countertheorist is someone whose work, though derived from a recognized tradition, is not generally accepted as "part of the field" by the authorities in that area. For example, A. S. Neill bases his work on a psychoanalytic framework, but is not accepted by most psychoanalytic authorities.

Counter theory is what countertheorists say and do. Usually it begins with the school or the child and works back to the theory from there. It means a bent toward the humanistic ideas of writers like Abraham Maslow. It is a tendency toward freer education, more in the hands of the student and less determined from above than in most models. Often it means a spirit of rebelliousness and innovation. And it is not so much a body of theory as it is a praxis.

A. Where Countertheorists Agree

Actually, no single statement describes all countertheorists. There are, however, related sets of ideas and concerns, about which they mostly agree.

Most countertheorists have a humanistic perspective.
They reject the Freudian view of man as having innate tendencies
that are disastrous, unless fundamentally reshaped by socialization, and contained by continuing mechanisms of control. They
also reject the behaviorist view that man is innately shapeless,
and amenable to almost any kind of environmental control. Instead, they feel that man is healthy by nature. Maslow writes
that man "has needs, capacities, and tendencies that are genetically based, some of which are characteristic of the whole human
species...and some of which are unique to the individual...these
needs are on their face good or neutral rather than evil
(Maslow, 1962)."

Countertheorists agree that drastic changes are needed
in the schools. They don't think that schools succeed in promoting either intellectual or emotional growth in students. Usually,
they see this as a systemic problem, not as a series of small
problems to be solved one by one.

They criticize school curriculum severely. Some want the
curriculum to be more "relevant"; others want students to determine
it; others prefer that it be individualized. Some want to do away
with learning divorced from practice. There are differences in

focus, but not really disagreements.

Countertheorists don't like the way schools label students. Lively kids may be seens as "acting-out" trouble-makers, or creative ones as "stupid" for giving an unexpected answer. Labeling usually justifies unequal treatment or segregation and is frequently based on racism, sexism, or class prejudice. Many countertheorists agree that some labels are inevitable, but they want fewer and better ones than we have now.

Countertheorists worry about alienation. In schools, students are often alienated from their teachers, from each other, or from their own "educational" activity.

Countertheorists also want to change power relations in schools. Their plans differ in detail, but countertheorists generally agree that there would be more intellectual and personal growth if students had more control over their own education.

They have comparatively little to say about the problem of "emotionally disturbed" children, because they question the assumptions behind the label. They often see "normal" children as equally "disturbed"--disturbed when they reach school or disturbed by the process of school itself. Disturbance is a characteristic of the system, not just of the participants in it.

B. Where Countertheorists Disagree

Some of the differences between countertheorists
are disagreements; others are merely differences in focus.

Where Does the Problem Lie?

Countertheorists work at different levels of analysis.
No theorist sticks to one level consistently, but it is possible
to identify different levels where different writers focus most
of their attention.

Some writers look mainly at the individual. They discuss
the individual student, or the relationship of student and teacher.
The concept of "emotional disturbance" is likely to appear in their
writings.

Others look mainly at the classroom or the school. They
examine ways that students relate to each other, and see the classroom as a functioning social unit. Often they see a need for changes
in classroom structure.

Some writers see schools as just a part in the whole
social system. What's wrong with schools follows logically from
the functions assigned to schools by society. Consequently, extensive change in the society is inextricable from school reform.

What About Deviance?

At least three trends of thought can be distinguished.
The most extreme view holds that deviance is to be celebrated; it
is the surest manifestation of man's precious individual nature.

More commonly, writers ask, "Who cares about deviance?" For them, social norms are not very important. Behaviors can be good or bad, effective or ineffective; but whether they are conformist or deviant just doesn't matter. A third view holds that there is such a thing as healthy normality which is to be desired--but it is not the same thing as conventional normality. From this point of view, the whole society is deviant from the ideal.

What Kind of Learning Matters?

Countertheorists differ about the relative importance of emotional and intellectual learning. Some writers clearly are concerned with one or the other; some are in between. On the whole, counter-theorists are more concerned with emotional well-being than are most educational writers.

Should There Be Separate Institutions Called Schools?

A few writers, like Everett Reimer, hold that the existence of designated educational institutions does more harm than good. Others don't go as far, but agree that the divisions between "life" and "school" should be reduced as much as possible. Some do not address the question. There is agreement, at least, that compulsory attendance should be abolished.

The issues discussed above demonstrate some of the differences and agreements between countertheorists. They provide the background against which the ideas and techniques recommended by countertheorists will be compared in the sections that follow.

This paper discusses interventions and methods described by countertheorists. Part IV is organized around foci of interventions; for instance, there is a section on how to deal with reading, and another on how to structure the classroom. This organizational scheme makes it possible to draw comparisons of different ideas.

But there is a price to be paid for this manner of organizing the paper. The work of one person or one project tends to be reduced to unconnected fragments. One may read on one page what a given author says about reading, on another what he says about classroom structure, on still another his suggestion for surviving political pressure. Yet, one may not be able to identify the author, find out who he is or from what experience he is speaking. Therefore, in this section of the paper, I would like to introduce you to the writers. The reader is urged to follow up his interest in these people by reading what they have to say in its original form.

Sylvia Ashton-Warner taught in an isolated school in New Zealand. Her students, the youngest children in the school, were both white and Maoris (the original inhabitants). The impetus that first moved her toward innovation was the cultural gap between the races.

She found the whole curriculum and style of teaching inappropriate to her Maori students. For instance, standard reading material was completely without interest or meaning for them. Another problem was that they were livelier than European children. There was a tremendous gap between their lives at home and the comparatively inhibited school.

To combat these problems, Ashton-Warner developed methods and theories which can be applied more widely--in fact, they have implications for all children. Her method, called Organic Teaching, is discussed in her book Teacher (1963). Her new book, Spearpoint: Teacher in America (1972), discribes her experiences in an American free school. It gives a revealing picture of what happens to her methods when they are transplanted into a different culture and a different institutional setting. Organic Teaching needs adjustment in many of its details, she says--but the essentials survive, and they still work. She also expresses some disagreement with the extreme "freedom" of the free school where she worked; she perceives it as fostering domination by the children.

Ashton-Warner sees a child's mind as "a volcano with two vents: destructiveness and creativeness (1963, p. 29)." Her methods aim at opening the creative vent. Examples of them will be found in several places later in the paper.

Another countertheorist is A. S. Neil, whose school, Summerhill, has been for decades one of the world's outstanding examples of radical innovation in education. His books about the school may have done more to popularize radical views than any others.

Summerhill is a "free" school. This means that there are a lot of things its students don't have to do--including for example, going to classes, or wearing clothes. There are also a lot of rules that they do have to obey, because of the necessities of community life. These are decided by all the members of the school, each with one vote.

Neill's objective is to turn out happy people; academic achievement is a good thing too, but it is definitely secondary. As he sees it, repression causes most people to be unhappy. Therefore ,letting people do what they want is a major step toward making them happy. Obviously he assumes that, left alone, people are neither shapeless nor basically bad, but fundamentally good and creative.

Although achievement is a secondary goal, Neill says that there is no serious conflict between achievement and the leniency of Summerhill. He believes that forced learning is slowly done, used with difficulty, and quickly forgotten. However, in an atmosphere of freedom, children can make up years of work in weeks or months if they so desire.

Countertheorist Paul Goodman, has quite a bit of experience in education, including teaching at experimental Black Mountain College in North Carolina, as well as more conventional college teaching. But his discussion of education comes less from practice, and more from theoretical reflection.

Goodman's books, Growing Up Absurd (1956) and Compulsory Miseducation (1962), have been two of the most influential books about what's wrong in education. What is less well known is that he also has concrete suggestions to offer, especially in the second book. Some of them are quite drastic; a few are not. As far as Goodman himself is concerned, none of them is as dangerous as leaving things the way they are.

In a sense, these three writers are central to educational counter theory. They represent--though the choice is somewhat arbitrary--pioneers in the field. Their work, partly because they have been at it for a long time, helps to form the context and the background within which others work.

A number of countertheorists have come from the ranks of public school teachers. In this paper, four such men are included.

Jonathan Kozol got fired from teaching in Boston and wrote a book about it. <u>Death</u> <u>at</u> <u>an</u> <u>Early</u> <u>Age</u> (1967) is a description of his experience in a mostly-black school, and it's primarily a book about racism. There is little that is radical about it, except that Kozol insists on seeing clearly in spite of social pressures. In fact, Kozol was fired for doing no more than consistently applying conventional liberal wisdom in an illiberal setting.

Since being fired, Kozol has worked in a newly-established "free school" in ghetto Boston. His new book, <u>Free</u> <u>Schools</u> (1972), is about that school and others like it. It is a biting book, which gives some of its sharpest criticism to "radical educators" who are so anti-authority that they can never get anything done, or who put their schools so far away in the country that they have nothing to do with making social change. Kozol's main theme is the balancing

act between conventional practicality, which never attempts
enough change, and dogmatic idealism, which pays too little
attention to the obstacles to get very far.

Herbert Kohl taught in Harlem. The system he found was
terribly destructive, but it did not do its damage so much
through the individual racism of teachers. Neither did it weed
out good teachers to the same degree as did the Boston schools.
Kohl found it possible to make changes that turned a hateful
school experience into an exciting one for his sixth-graders.
Then the children went on in a system that had not changed, and
lost what gains they had made. At the end of his book, 36
Children, Kohl (1967) seems almost sorry to have reawakened these
children to face a second death.

But he has some things to say about how to teach. In
The Open Classroom (1969) he distills his own experience into a form
others can use.

James Herndon (1968;1971) writes about both black and white
schools. As he sees it, they're not very much different, except that
what's wrong is so much sharper and clearer in the black schools.
There, you can't miss it. The other difference is that when he
succeeded with an unconventional approach, the black school fired
him (The Way It Spozed To Be), while the white school--some years
later, it should be said--tolerated him as an oddball (How To
Survive in Your Native Land).

Herndon's books have a reputation for their engrossing
humanness. He is willing that children should be as they are. Most

of them he likes. Some children do nothing but make trouble for him, and dislike him as well. As far as Herndon is concerned, that's their right, just as it is his right to dislike them back.

John Holt's work has been in white middle-class schools, the envied "good" elementary schools of our society. While he agrees with others that lower-class black and white schools are the worst ones, he finds quite enough to worry about where he is. Much of Holt's thinking and insight came from an opportunity to spend a good part of a school year in a classroom, not teaching but just watching. He was able to learn things that he never learned while teaching. For one thing, the teacher is busy. His intellect and emotions are caught up in what he is trying to do at the moment. He cannot respond to anything "extraneous" to the moment. In addition, he can't see the classroom as it is, because the kids respond to his authority by showing him only certain things.

Holt is best-known for his book How Children Fail. He points out that children cannot respond to schools as places for learning because they are too involved in fear and authority relationships (1964, pp. 43-44).

> A teacher in class is like a man in the woods at
> night with a powerful flashlight in his hand. Wherever
> he turns his light, the creatures on whom it shines
> are aware of it, and do not behave as they do in the
> dark. Thus the mere fact of his watching their behav-
> ior changes it into something very different. Shine
> where he will, he can never know very much of the
> night life of the woods.

How Children Learn (Holt, 1967) is mainly a look at children before they get to school. It poses the question: What do schools do to turn so many bright, lively people into stupid, difficult ones? The Underachieving School (1972) and What Do I Do on Monday? (1970) consider how to change things.

Elliot Shapiro also has worked in the public schools, but he has made his name as a principal, not as a teacher. Nat Hentoff's Our Children Are Dying (1966) describes Shapiro's work as principal of P. S. 119, in Harlem, in the first half of the 1960's. Shapiro seems to have achieved his success in two ways: first, he worked very hard, cared a lot about the children, and attracted to the school teachers who would do the same. The second is more unorthodox: he worked to unite the community and the school. He tried to put the school to work meeting community needs, and to put the community to work generating pressure to obtain resources for the school.

George Dennison (1969) and Herbert Grossman (1972) worked in small experimental schools for disturbed or "problem" children in New York. Both of them were both teachers and "administrative" decision makers in their schools. George Dennison helped to run First Street School on the lower East Side. The object of the school, which was financed by a small foundation grant, was to give successive, humanistic education to children who weren't making it in regular schools--some who had been expelled, others who had quit, a few who finally quit when they found this alternative. The extraordi-

588

nary thing about the school is not that it succeeded in teaching about twenty difficult children, with four or five teachers --but that it did so on a per-child budget that was approximately equal to that of the New York City school system! Dennison proposed the Street School, not as an expensive pilot program for problem kids, but as a financially viable model for the whole school system.

The school Herbert Grossman describes in <u>Nine Rotten Lousy Kids</u> was quite different. Grossman and his colleagues set out to show that they could run a successful school for very disturbed children whom no other school would handle and who otherwise would certainly be in institutions. Costs are not discussed in the book, but obviously they were high--though presumably lower than the financial and social costs of institutionalization.

There is nothing that stands out as "radical theory" in Grossman's school. In fact, the school was not built around a theory ; "We tried to do whatever was best for the kids." But the result of mixing this partly instinctive approach was some very unorthodox practice.

Some countertheoretical writing does not describe particular experiences in particular schools, but discusses ideas generally. A few books of this kind deserve special introduction here.

Neil Postman and Charles Weingartner both taught in public schools. The title of their book, <u>Teaching as a Subversive</u>

Activity (1969), is very much to the point; they proceed from the assumption that most of what usually goes on in schools is positively harmful to the development of intelligence.

As well as making an attack on education as it stands, Postman and Weingartner build a theoretical base for a new model of education. They draw upon the work of Korzybski, Sapir, and Whorf in linguistics, and on McLuhan's writing about media, to demonstrate that science has developed new ideas about man's learning and understanding, ideas which show conventional schools to be mistaken and obsolete.

They have specific recommendations for what ought to replace traditional education. They want an education based on discussion, not lectures; on questions, not answers; on the people in the classroom, not on a curriculum. They give dozens of suggestions for change, at all different levels in the system, from asking a class "What's worth knowing?" to requiring all teachers of English to teach math instead. Some of these suggestions, which the authors conveniently list, will be found in an appendix at the end of this paper.

Everett Reimer and Ivan Illich at CIDOC (Centro Intercultural de Documentacion), their center in Cuernavaca, Mexico, are studying modern institutions, especially schools. Reimer (1971), in School is Dead, and Illich (1970), in De-Schooling Society, have similar criticisms to make of the way schools work in our society.

They see the school system and society as being deeply intertwined, with flaws that are very deep and common to both. Thus,
Reimer argues that schools are more successful at teaching rote behavior, respect for authority, and acceptance of meritocratic ideas than
they are at educating human beings. And this, he says, is the real
purpose of schools: they provide a classificatory scheme and a
rationale for the unequal distribution of wealth and power.

There is a chicken-and-egg quality to this vision: the
dehumanizing and authoritatian qualities of schools derive from the
needs of a similarly dehumanizing and authoritarian society; but they
also help the society take that regrettable shape.

If this is true, then it is useless to think of attacking
these properties of schools without attacking the same features in
the larger society. What's more, one ought to expect fierce resistance
to changes that threaten the society at large. Reimer argues that
work in schools makes sense precisely because they are a weak point
in a wider system of which he disapproves.

This Book Is About Schools (Repo, 1970) is a collection of
articles from This Magazine Is About Schools. This Magazine is
published in Toronto. It serves as a vehicle for outsiders, radical
thinkers and workers to communicate with each other, and it is more
concerned with the observable realities of schools and children than
with the abstractions of "education." Reading it is a startling and
refreshing experience.

This _Book_ contains articles ranging from "Childhood in an Indian Village" by Wilfred Pelletier to "The Psychiatrist: a Policeman in the Schools," by Thomas Szasz. Other material that has appeared in _This Magazine_ includes the original publication of the notorious "The Student as Nigger, by Jerry Farber.

Charles Silberman became famous with a book about civil rights crisis in Mississippi and the South, called _Crisis in Black and White_. After several years of full-time study and travel concerning education, he published _Crisis in the Classroom_, another significant book. In over 500 exhaustively-documented pages, Silberman discusses the proposition that most schools today are failing badly; but that some are succeeding, and are doing so in ways that other schools can imitate. He also discusses the education of teachers in this context.

Silberman's own ideas about schools are provocative and they deserve both reading and discussion. But the most valuable thing about his book is the thoroughness of its survey. A vast number of experiments involving new directions in teaching are brought together here under one cover; and the people who are doing these things are given a good opportunity to speak for themselves. Some of the experiments have not been much publicized and others, like the British Infant Schools, are widely known. Of particular interest is the discussion of North Dakota's New School for Behavioral Studies in Education, a wide-open experiment that grew out of a budget crisis in a low-population state.

Peter Knoblock teaches in the Special Education Department at Syracuse University. His work is characterized less by a stance of opposition to things as they are, and more by a positive thrust. Knoblock's work is largely concerned with applying to the problems of education the insights and practices of what is sometimes called the "Human Potential Movement."

Knoblock represents, in this paper, a whole group of countertheorists who are often overlooked. These people use theories related to those of Maslow and the "Third Force" in psychology; many of their methods come from t-groups and group relations laboratories. They concentrate directly on human experience, and on maximizing genuine interactions and understanding between people.

Knoblock and Goldstein, in The Lonely Teacher, give a good example of this approach. They report on the experience of a group of special education teachers brought together to discuss problems and experiences from their teaching. Characteristically, the group achieved many helpful insights--the biggest one being the great importance of the loneliness that teachers face. They also reported that the greatest value of their meetings did not come from the intellectual product, but from the interpersonal experience of the meetings themselves.

III. COUNTERTHEORETICAL INTERVENTIONS

Part I of this paper has attempted to map out the theoretical ground occupied by countertheorists, to identify the kinds of general positions they take. Part II has introduced some countertheorists, telling us who they are, where they work, and what kinds of experiences lie behind their ideas. The last two sections of the paper discuss ideas about specific problems and situations in schools.

The division between the two parts is somewhat arbitrary. Part IIIA might be called "things that countertheorists worry about;" it discusses school concerns which are not easily operationalized into suggestions for change. Countertheorists have done things about these issues: issues like racism, teacher personality, and emotions in the classroom. And they hope that other educators will, too. But for these issues, more than those in Part IIIB, it is impossible to write anything approaching a "recipe;" those who wish to follow countertheoretical ideas will have to work out many of the details for themselves.

Teacher Personality

Many writers on education have tried to devise techniques, rules, or systems of teaching which are "teacher-proof." The assumption behind these attempts (explicit or implicit) is that there are things that a teacher should do and ways that he should act, and that these can be codified so that every teacher will be able to do them efficiently, without letting his own personality get in the way. There may be a conflict between teacher role and teacher personality; therefore, a clear definition of what teachers are supposed to do will help them to keep their teaching behavior relatively "uncontaminated" by personal idiosyncrasies. Ideally, then, the influence of teacher personality is, and ought to be, slight.

Most countertheorists disagree, on both counts. For them, teacher personality always has an effect, though often a bad one. Further, teacher personality should have an effect, preferably a good one. Therefore, it is important to get hold of the right kind of teachers, who will have helpful personalities, rather than trying to "train out" the effect of personality.

Countertheorists, then, think that an appropriate personality is legitimately considered an important qualification for teaching. Weingartner and Postman suggest requiring "each

teacher to provide some sort of evidence that he or she has
had a loving relationship with at least one other human being.
If the teacher can get someone to say 'I love her (or him),'
she should be retained...spouses need not be excluded from
testifying   (Teaching as a Subversive Activity, Weingartner
and Postman, 1969)."

Countertheorists say that teachers should see their
job as more than teaching subject matter. The job includes
being a model, someone to look up to, someone to identify with.
It's part of the role whether teachers think it is or not;
they'll do better if they're conscious of it. Like Weingartner
and Postman, William Glasser (in Schools Without Failure) holds
that it matters whether teachers care about the children. He
says that it is necessary for a caring teacher to avoid con-
flict-ridden, failure-threatening situations. This is especially important in the primary grades, since kids spend so much
time with their teachers, and are so emotionally attached to
them.

For "disturbed" children, especially, teachers should
see emotional changes as more important than the imparting of
intellectual wisdom.

Countertheorists are appalled by the racist and otherwise bigoted teachers who appear in the books of countertheorists
who have been in the public schools. For instance, the teachers

596

in Kozol's book who talk about "this kind of children" (meaning black) for whom different treatment is appropriate, never admit that what makes a child "this kind" is simply skin color. And the teacher in Kohl's school who told his children "You are animals." And the administration of a school in Silberman's book, which discouraged a black student from trying anything ambitious, nearly laughing in his face--and then, when he succeeded in spite of them, used his case as an example of how well blacks could do in their system.

No one will recognize himself in these descriptions. But the problem is there, hugely important, and calling for as much emphasis as it can get. It has been suggested that members of minority groups should judge whether teachers are prejudiced.

The existence of racism is well-known. Less widely recognized or documented, is sexism. For example, elementary school readers depict little girls planning to be nurses or wives, boys planning to be doctors; mothers who do nothing, and fathers who work.

Finally, one very specific suggestion from Herbert Kohl's The Open Classroom: treat yourself as a person in the classroom. At the start of the year, don't just ask the children what they did all summer. Tell them what you did too, who you are, and what you like doing. And let that be a precedent for the rest of the year.

Grades

Countertheorists do not like grades. Nor do they like required courses, required attendance, or most of the other examples of control in schools. Some of them pay more attention to the subject than do others; but they do not often disagree substantially.

The criticism is a simple and familiar one, which can be found, for instance, in Summerhill or Teaching as a Subversive Activity. Countertheorists complain that these systems of control, which are intended to measure, enforce, or define what education is, end up measuring something other than education. They draw students away from the real process of education by rewarding them for doing something irrelevant to education.

If one conceives of education as taking place within the student, it is easy to see a discrepancy between grades and learning. As long as there is a discrepancy, grades will involve some injustice. But the problem is worse than that: grades are not just an informative statement, but a reward system. Consequently, they shape the behavior of students. Instead of seeking to learn and understand, students may cheat, or engage in blind "answer-grabbing" in order to get good grades.

The rationale for required courses is that there are some things everyone ought to know about, and that taking a course will fill this need. But, say the countertheorists, such courses don't work. A student in a required course usually does not try to learn, but to pass; and usually he finds a way to pass without learning much. What's more, requirements perpetuate the notion that passing courses is what education is all about.

Postman and Weingartner say that requirements are part of the vaccination theory of education: when you have been through a course, you have "had" it, and you are immune from having to "have" it again. This sounds absurd, but it also sounds like the way most schools work.

A familiar argument is that grades are needed to give a student information or to reward him for his performance. Countertheorists say that grades measure the wrong thing. Some go further. Postman and Weingartner, for instance, argue that if a student can't tell for himself how he is doing, then he shouldn't be in the class.

Grades are also defended as performing the necessary function of evaluation: employers, other schools, etc., need to know how well the student has learned. Many countertheorists do not discuss this argument. They would probably say that if evaluation is necessary, someone other than the teacher should do it. Evaluation should be based on task performance rather than classroom behavior. Reimer says that grades, credits, and degrees do not measure anything that matters, but that they serve a function in pretending to measure these things. Such credentials serve as a justification for the uneven distribution of wealth and power in our society. Hence, he opposes any educational evaluation system even if it does not intrude harmfully into the learning process in the classroom. (A direct test of ability to perform on a job is another matter.)

What would countertheorists do about grades? The literature on this subject is scanty. Some countertheorists do not discuss it at all. The ghetto teachers have more urgent problems. Ashton-Warner, Dennison, and Grossman, work in environments without grades. But beyond that is a political problem: some of the grading innovations that teachers have introduced have to be kept quiet because of disapproval from higher-ups. So it is not a well-researched subject.

Postman and Weingartner (1969) call for abolishing grades; less emphatically, John Holt agrees. This is hard to do in itself. What's more, like some other suggestions it leads straight into difficulties that call for wider systemic change. Without grades, students could distribute their energy among courses as they pleased, without fearing negative sanctions. They might do so little in some courses that it would be silly to say they were "taking" those courses at all. Soon it would be hard to say what a "course" is in the first place.

Some changes come more easily. Professor Arthur Pearl of the University of Oregon suggests that deadlines on work ought to be abolished. This would create a grading system of "pass" or "haven't passed yet." A student would be allowed to do his work over as long a period as he wished, without penalty.

A milder version of the same thing is the "pass-no pass" system, which rejects the idea that to attempt a course without succeeding is worse than not trying it--which is what failing grades imply. Under "pass-no pass," a course not passed is not recorded. This can be done without abolishing deadlines.

Many teachers, especially in public schools, do not have the freedom to make these changes. There are others, which can be implemented in one classroom. Nearly all call for some audacity.

Pearl describes an option which he gives his students: "In my classes, students can always ask for a sample of ten students to be drawn at random to determine the legitimacy of their grievances--either about tasks to be performed or evaluation of the worth of those tasks." To do this, a teacher has to have faith that he and his students have substantially the same goals in mind. For instance, Pearl would be disconcerted if a jury held that each student should judge what is worth doing for him, and therefore, no work can be required.

The following four methods of handling grades were tried in Psychology 101 in the University of Michigan, among other places. Results were hard to evaluate. Students spent most of their time in other classes, with usual pressures to produce. This may have served to distort the amount of time and effort allotted for the psychology course.

The contract system. teacher and student negotiate a contract at the beginning of the term, about how he is to be graded. He may choose one of a set of alternatives the teacher presents, or he is free to write his own. There is room for discussion of the grade at the end of the term. But it is clear from the beginning who has the final power to decide the grade.

Uniform grading. a teacher can remove the question of grades from classroom performance by announcing uniform grades at the outset: usually all A's, sometimes all B's. There is nothing subtle about this system. The teacher who uses it must be prepared to stick to it. He should expect some students to seize the opportunity to do no work at all.

Student grading. there are two variations. Students may grade themselves, in which case, again, some will take advantage of the system. Or they may grade each other. This lets the teacher avoid discomfort, but it may make students more tense about grades than before--especially since they usually must stay near some pre-assigned average, and hence are competing with each other.

A-incomplete. A teacher may expect every student to earn an A, and leave his grade at "incomplete" until he has done it. This avoids unequal grades without lowering standards. It also angers students who don't want to do so much work.

No system of reform-within-one-classroom is very satisfactory. One reason is that grades continue to be a genuine tool for the acquisition of goods and status outside the classroom. One teacher cannot remove the power that grades possess. But some of these systems can make the classroom less threatening by making grading less mysterious and more predictable to students.

Emotions

Children and teachers are all people with emotions. Everyone recognizes that but not everyone thinks that emotions deserve special attention in the classroom educational process. Countertheorists generally think they do. Whatever a teacher wants to do, emotions are involved; if she doesn't deal with them they may get in the way. But, even more, for philosophical reasons: emotions are seen, not just as a complicating factor encountered while pursuing education, but as a big part of what education is about.

It is particularly clear in schools for disturbed children that out-of-control emotions are obtrusive. Teachers have to decide how to handle them. The staff at Herbert Grossman's school decided that urgent emotional growth had priority over academic learning. Thus, when kids were too upset to function well in class, teachers looked for chances to talk about what was going on emotionally, instead of just trying to calm them down enough to go ahead with the lesson. The same thing happened in Dennison's First Street School. In both schools, the exceptionally low student-teacher ratio facilitated attention to emotions.

The Pennsylvania Advancement School introduced psychological learning techniques as a major part of its curriculum. Described by Farnum Gray, in an article in Radical School Reform (Gross and Gross, 1969), this school taught underachieving students, many of them black. It was assumed that these students did not function well in schools because schools were not the thing that mattered to them especially emotional concerns about authority, family, race, and violence. Therefore, teachers employed encounter group techniques, game-playing, and other devices to open up these difficult subjects for discussion

For example, after some play-acting around the subject of aggression, the teacher introduced a new "game."

George (the teacher) told the group:

> New task. Think of something that you're afraid of.
> Now become specific in your head. Specifically.
> You must come up here and show us fear. Now concen-
> trate specifically on what you could be afraid of.
>
> Now wait a minute; that's only half the job. Some-
> time, while one person's up here being afraid of
> something, I will go to somebody else and tap him
> on the shoulder. His job is to go up and help the
> person who is afraid--help him to not be afraid
> (Gross and Gross, 1969, p.315)."

Once these critical subjects were dealt with openly,

teachers at the school found that they could not only lead the

boys to change personally, but also that teaching in conven-

tional subjects came more easily.

The kind of teaching which uses techniques drawn

from activities like encounter groups, requires risk-taking

and personal involvement from the teacher   The negative and

violent feelings of students are seen as a block to their

functioning, as something to be alleviated by whatever tech-

niques will do the job. But often these feelings are a legi-

timate response to oppression. Perhaps they should not be dis-

solved, but steered into action. Students are hurt if they are

paralyzed by their feelings. They are also hurt if teachers

try to smooth away feelings without changing the situation that

gave rise to the feeling. And of course if the situation re-

mains unchanged, the feelings will come back, as Kohl found out in Harlem (<u>36 Children</u>).

Richard Jones, (1968), in his book, <u>Fantasy and Feeling</u>
<u>in Education</u>, discusses how to bring emotional concerns into more
conventional educational material. His methods are designed
to be used with course material about social sciences, and for
contrast, he compares with methods advocated by Jerome Bruner,
whom he considers one-sided.

One of Jones' most striking examples concerns a course
on Eskimos. This was an experimental course taught at a well-
to-do white school in Massachusetts, with materials specially
prepared by experts in the field, to help students think like
anthropologists. In showing how widely different customs are
derived from similar human needs, it described how the Netsilik
Eskimos slaughtered animals for food and skins. It also described
the occasional practice of geronticide and female infanticide under
hard conditions.

Jones felt that students were put in a bind by treating
these emotional things in a very intellectual way. He proposed
that students should talk about their feelings while watching
the bloody killing of an animal, or while hearing about how a
baby might be left to die of exposure. When a teacher did this,
she got a lively response--and not a frightening one. Both
she and Jones felt that the students, when they didn't have to
bottle up their strong emotional response to what they were learning,
were better able to respond to the intellectual content. Even

606

more important to Jones, they also took the course more seriously, being aware that they were really discussing other human beings. Only by contrasting their own feelings of revulsion with the feelings of an Eskimo at the bloody death of a walrus--his only source of food--did they really achieve the original objective of the course.

Herbert Kohl and James Herndon both ran into a surprise in teaching their ghetto kids. By accident, they began talking about fairy tales. In both cases, most of their students had not heard some of the most familiar stories. Although they were "too old" for such stories, they responded to them powerfully. Herndon found that filling in this gap was worth doing for its own sake, but also that play-readings of Cinderella generated some of the most exciting intellectual discussions of his teaching year.

Much of Sylvia Ashton-Warner's book Teacher is about emotions in the classroom. It is plain that her own emotions and those of her pupils play a fundamental part in her method of teaching. She says, "I see the mind of a five-year-old as a volcano with two vents: destructiveness and creativeness. And I see that to the extent that we widen the creative channel, we atrophy the destructive one. And it seems to me that since these words of the key vocabulary (her method of teaching reading, discussed later) are no less than the creations of the dynamic life itself, they course out through the creative channel, making their

607

contribution to the drying up of the destructive vent (Teacher, pp. 29-30)."

In his book The Lonely Teacher, Peter Knoblock focuses on another emotional issue: the emotional needs of teachers. The group of teachers with whom Knoblock met, found that they all experience a powerful, draining sense of loneliness. When they had too little interaction, too little support and approval from colleagues or administrators, they found that their teaching was disrupted by their needs for approval and support from the students, and in some cases their lives at home suffered from their emotional fatigue.

Knoblock's book talks about how teachers can help themselves in this situation. In part, they can set up patterns of interaction that reduce the amount of loneliness they carry into their classrooms. In part, they can make some kinds of expression of their own emotions and needs more legitimate and less disruptive in classes. His discussion is insightful and helpful, but does not lend itself easily to the making of recipes for other teachers.

Countertheorists discuss emotion in the classroom using different terms, but without much disagreement. All would agree that emotions belong in the classroom, that they should be considered legitimate. They concede that there is some risk involved, that some emotions will be unpleasant ones. But they see the denial of emotions as being destructive and unnecessary. They do expect that there will be more good times than bad times.

Relevance

Everyone agrees that education should be relevant. The difficulty is in making this cliche come alive, in giving it specific and concrete meaning.

For example, in Schools Without Failure, Glasser describes how he asked a classroom full of students to name something other than schoolbooks that they had read. None of them could. When Glasser pointed out a comic book and commented that what the owner probably did with it was to read it, the children were dumbfounded. They had not realized that the thing called "reading" that they did in school was connected with what they did with comic books, or signs, or cereal boxes. Obviously their schools did not seem very relevant to them.

The most electrifying moment in Kozol's Death at an Early Age occurred on the day that Kozol brought in a book by Langston Hughes, and read poetry from it. First, there was the physical existence of a book with a black man on the cover; this was new, and intensely meaningful to many students in the class who had never seen such a thing before. Second, there was the relevant subject matter of the poems. It is clear from Kozol's description that hearing the poetry made his students interested

(Teacher, 1963).

And the same lesson comes from a different setting, peasant communities in northeast Brazil, where Paolo Freire found that he could teach literacy to peasants in six weeks. He did it by teaching them about the society that oppressed them, and by helping them see literacy as a tool for changing their situation. The same peasants appeared unteachable by any other means.

All of these examples--especially that of Freire--suggest that the deadness and lack of relevance of much teaching is not because most teachers and educators just lack imagination. It may be that the subjects which are most meaningful to people are the same subjects that threaten our present social order. This is particularly true if people have an immediate need to make radical changes in their society. In the case of Freire, the peasants were existing at the lowest level of survival in our hemisphere. As a result of his efforts, Freire found himself kicked out of the country.

Postman and Weingartner (1969) recommend that we ought to ask ourselves simply "What's worth knowing?" To do this properly is difficult, because it means trying to escape the mind-set imposed by established education. Thus, it is cheating to ask yourself, "Well, why is history worth knowing? And what about math?" The question should be asked as if schools and curriculum did not already exist, as if you are faced with the task of defining what schools should do with children, in order to help them become effective adults.

The reader is invited to undertake to answer this question for himself. Anyone who wants to know how Postman and Weingartner answered the question will find some of their answers in an appendix at the end of this paper.

in the written word as never before. They saw that written words could speak to them about their concerns--and more, that they could be written by black people.

Kozol's description of his fellow teachers and of the administration show why this sort of violation of the prescribed curriculum got him fired. The Boston school system appears divided between 'liberals,' who wish black people weren't black (poor things) and would rather not talk about the whole subject, and, on the other hand, the 'racists,' who simply don't feel that black people were worth worrying about. Neither viewpoint gives rise to teaching techniques that are relevant to black people.

There are striking examples of what happens when teachers encourage students to write about things relevant to themselves. Herbert Kohl (36 Children, 1967) asked his kids to write about the blocks where they lived. They came alive:

> I live on 117 Street, between Madison and
> 5th Avenue. All the bums live around here.
> But the truth is they don't live here they
> just hang around the street. All the kids
> call it "Junky's Paradise." Because there
> is no cops to stop them. I wish that the cops
> would come around and put all the bums out
> of the block and put them in jail all their
> life. I would really like it very much if they
> would improve my neighborhood. I don't even
> go outside to play because of them. I just
> play at the center or someplace else. (p.48)

Just as intense is the writing of Sylvia Ashton-Warner's students, when they write about their own lives in a Maori village

B. Proposals for Change

The following section is the "how to do it" section of the paper. Here specific ways to teach or to change things are grouped by topic. The reader can compare different ways of doing things, each coming from a different countertheorist.

Actual interventions are presented, rather than general discussions of philosophy or education. For instance, you will not find discussions of John Holt's view of what "good learners" are like, or Postman and Weingartners' descriptions of how children work. You will find descriptions of various methods for teaching reading and writing.

The organization by topics gives a fragmented character to the discussion; for some writers, it is quite difficult to understand their total message without reading their ideas together, and of a piece. Some of the suggestions cannot be implemented bit-by-bit; or, they lose some of their character if they are. Hence, I repeat Rousseau's warning in the Preface to Emile, which Silberman also quotes (Crisis in the Classroom, 1970, p.4):

> People are always telling me to make PRACTICAL suggestions. You might as well tell me to suggest what people are doing already, or at least to suggest improvements which may be incorporated with the wrong methods at present in use.

Thus a reader who likes an idea ought to follow it to its source, and to learn what kind of program for change the idea originated.

Reading

If any academic subject is central to the schooling

process --especially for students who have trouble in school--
that subject is reading. When a book is written to attack schools
for ineffectiveness, it is called <u>Why</u> <u>Johnny</u> <u>Can't</u> <u>Read</u>. Contro-
versies rage about the relative merit of phonetic vs. look-see
methods of teaching. So many students seem stymied by reading,
that massive searches are launched for sources of organic
difficulties to explain the problem--in as many as thirty per
cent of all children! To all this William Hull answers that
teaching is to blame. "If we taught children to speak, they'd
never learn (Holt, 1964)."

Countertheorists have some very concrete plans for
how reading can be taught more effectively. One of the most
celebrated is that developed and described by Sylvia Ashton-
Warner, called <u>organic</u> <u>reading</u>. It is used in one form or another
by several countertheorists.

Ashton-Warner began her innovative work in teaching
reading when she found that the regular "Janet and John" reading books
were impossibly inappropriate for her Maori children, She used
organic reading in conjunction with the regular books, to help
link Maori and white culture; but there is no reason it must
be limited in this way.

Organic reading starts with the assumption that kids
should learn to read the words that matter to them. Ashton-
Warner, in her book <u>Teacher</u> (1963, p.43) describes the process

I call a child to me and ask her what she wants.
She may ask for 'socks' and I print it large on
a card with her name written quickly in the
corner for my own use. She watches me print
the word and says it as I print, then I give
it to her to take back to the mat and trace the
characters with her finger and finally replace
it in the cover nearby. I call them one by one
until each child has a new word.

The word is treated as a physical thing, which the child is

able to possess. Each word appears on its own card, "and if

you saw the condition of these tough little cards the next morning

you'd know why they need to be of tough cardboard or heavy drawing

paper rather than thin paper (Teacher, 1963)."

The words that the child chooses to learn--or, to "have"--

are called his Key Vocabulary, and they aren't much like the words

in the standard reading books. Instead of being bland, simple

words that appear a lot in English usage, or words that resemble

each other phonetically, these words are full of life, full of

excitement, love, and fear. As Ashton-Warner sees it, people act

in two modes, and most words in the Key Vocabulary belong to one

or the other, to love (creativity) or to fear (destructiveness). The

example she gives are vivid ones: ghost, Mommy, Daddy, spider,

police, kill, butcher, knife, kiss, love, dance, darling, beer...

She teaches these words as 'one-look words,' A child is presumed

to know a word forever, once he has it on his card. If sometime

later he doesn't know it, the card is thrown away; it wasn't time

for him to learn that word yet, no use pushing it.

Teaching in America, Ashton-Warner found that children did not begin with the same vivid words as in New Zealand; instead, they were interested in dogs, cats, friends' names, and objects. She found also that they often learned by phrases, or pairs of words, instead of single words. The methods did not change, but the experience of using them did. She felt herself working "from the outside in" with American children, working closer to their inner selves, while with Maori children it went "from inside out." The children made their personalities felt--and they learned.

That is Ashton-Warner's method: to teach the words that children want to know, and to do it by giving them the words on individual cards. But she has more to say about what happens in the classroom.

Children teach each other their words; they sit in pairs and show them to each other, and test each other. The teacher tests them, too, and keeps track of each child's pile of words. She discards ones that he forgets, and when his pile gets too big, she discards some of the ones he's had the longest. And when he's learned enough, he goes on to the next group. He should know "at least forty words...but promotion depends not on the amount of intake but the rate of intake."

The method becomes a little more complex, as reading and writing are combined. The description of children writing, then

616

reading each other's work, will be described in the Writing

section of this paper.

Other authors who have set out to apply Ashton-Warner's

ideas to their own teaching, report that the method works. This

is true, for example, in Dennison's book, and in a report on the

Boardman school in Boston (Radical School Reform). The methods

used in some British Infant Schools--a very diverse set of

schools--are similar.

One other countertheorist has developed independently a

method which is quite similar in its immediate mechanics, but

worlds away in the context in which it is practiced. Paolo Freire,

is the Brazilian who worked with the dirt-poor peasants of north-

east Brazil, before he was deported for his effectiveness.

Instead of Maori children, Freire worked with adult peasants.

But the method, which he calls "dialogic education," is similar.

The main point is to teach the words that are uppermost in the

students' minds and hearts--Freire calls them "generative

words." Further, Freire calls for education in which students

and teachers learn, discuss, and change together.

The words that Freire's Brazilians chose to learn were not

the same as Ashton-Warner's Key vocabularies. They were words

like these: land, landlord, rent, food, and police--political

words, words that led to action, and trouble for the status quo.

How much of this difference in content flows from Freire's dif-

ferent students, and how much from the different teachers, is hard

617

to say.

Freire reports that about fifteen per cent of the peasants in a place could learn to read in six weeks, using this method. Further, he says that learning to read is part of a circular process: for a peasant to read, he must change himself and his life; to do these things, it is necessary that he learn to read. That is why it is essential that the process be carried on in self-directing groups of people who know each other, live in similar ways, and can help each other make these momentous changes.

Writing

The general statements that countertheorists make about writing are similar to those they make about reading. But they have some specific ideas and experiences that are well worth reporting.

For instance, Kohl, in 36 Children, let children write things that were entirely private. He gave out notebooks that no one, including the teacher, could look into without permission. The sense of real ownership which this created apparently helped awake interest in writing. And Kohl found that kids did quite a lot of writing. They showed it to him, to each other, and even wanted to publish some of it. It was much better writing than anything they had done under other conditions.

Ashton-Warner's method is different. Her students' writing was not private; she walked around while they were writing, to correct and criticize. Then she had them read to each other. But she

618

confined corrections to technical questions, of spelling, legibility, and the like. The content was none of her concern. Her students, too, wrote lively stories, about their real lives. Perhaps this method worked so well for them because they were younger than Kozol's students, not yet turned off to the school's version of literacy; perhaps her personality helped. With young students, she has used it successfully in both New Zealand and America.

One final example is Herndon's experience with slambooks. In the ghetto school where Herndon taught (The Way It Spozed To Be, 1968), there was a season for slambooks, like the season for marbles in Tarkington's Penrod books. Every student made a slambook--a book with a page devoted to every kid in the class, on which other kids could write comments and instead of signing their comments, they were identified by a code known only by the book's owner. A lot of excitement surrounded reading comments and finding out who wrote them.

All this was spontaneous, and officially forbidden. Teachers made great efforts to stamp out slambooks. Herndon did not. He compared the elaborate, accurate sentences he found in a slambook with the stumbling, careless efforts kids made on written assignments. It appears that teachers in his school were trying to stamp out an effective vehicle for literary expression, and to introduce some very distasteful ones instead.

Math and Science

The general recommendations that countertheorists make about

619

education apply to math teaching as well. Teachers should make the subject concrete, alive, responsive to the particular needs and interests of the students and soon. The specific discussions of how to do it are somewhat sparse, and tend to be centered around the use of teaching materials,

The most-favored materials for math appear to be the Cuisenaire rods. These are wooden rods of differing lengths, and colors which correspond with their lengths. Their cross section is about 1 cm. by 1 cm. and lengths go from 1 cm. to 10 cm. With them, children can learn many arithmetical principles. John Holt's How Children Fail (1964, pp. 123-136), gives an unforgettable description of how Dr. C. Gattegno used these rods in teaching a class of retarded children.

> With no formalities or preliminaries, no icebreaking or jollying up, Gattegno went to work. It will help you see more vividly what was going on if, providing you have rods at hand, you actually do the operations I will describe. First he took two blue (9) rods, and between them put a dark green (6), so that between the two blue rods and above the dark green there was an empty space 3 cm. long. He said to the group, "Make one like this." They did. Then he said, "Now find the rod that will just fill up that space." I don't know how the other children worked on the problem; I was watching the dark-haired boy. His movements were spasmodic, feverish. When he had picked a rod out of the pile in the center of the table, he could hardly stuff it in between his blue rods. After several trials, he and the others found that a light green (3) rod would fill the space.
>
> Then Gattegno, holding his blue rods at the upper end, shook them, so that after a bit the dark green rod fell out. Then he turned the rods over, so that now there was a 6 cm. space where the dark green rod had formerly been. He asked the class to do the same. They did. Then he asked them to find the rod that

would fill that space. Did they pick out of the
pile the dark green rod that had just come out of
that space? Not one did. Instead, more trial and
error. Eventually, they all found that the dark
green rod was needed.

Then Gattegno shook his rods so that the light green
fell out, leaving the original empty 3 cm. space, and
turned them again so that the empty space was uppermost. Again he asked the children to fill the space,
and again, by trial and error, they found the needed
light green rod. As before, it took the dark-haired
boy several trials to find the right rod. These
trials seemed to be completely haphazard.

Hard as it may be to believe, Gattegno went through
this cycle at least four or five times before
anyone was able to pick the needed rod without
hesitation and without trial and error. As I
watched, I thought, "What must it be like to have
so little idea of the way the world works, so
little feeling for the regularity, the orderli-
ness, the sensibleness of things?" It takes a
great effort of the imagination to push oneself
back, back, back to the place where we knew
as little as these children. It is not just
a matter of not knowing this fact or that fact;
it is a matter of living in a universe like the
one lived in by very young children, a universe
which is utterly whimsical and unpredictable,
where nothing has anything to do with anything
else--with this difference, that these children had come to feel, as most very young children do not, that this universe is an enemy.

Then, as I watched, the dark-haired boy saw!
Something went "click" inside his head and for
the first time, his hand visibly shaking with
excitement, he reached without trial and error
for the right rod. He could hardly stuff it
into the empty space. It worked! The tongue
going round in the mouth, and the hands clawing
away at the leg under the table doubled their
pace. When the time came to turn the rods
over and fill the other empty space, he was
almost too excited to pick up the rod he wanted;
but he got it in. "It fits! It fits!" he
said, and held up the rods for all of us to see.

Many of us were moved to tears, by his excitement
and joy, and by our realization of the great leap
of the mind he had just taken.

After a while, Gattegno did the same problem this
time using a crimson (4) and yellow (5) rod between the blue rods. This time the black-haired
boy needed only one cycle to convince himself
that these were the rods he needed. This time he was
calmer, surer; he knew.

Again using the rods, Gattegno showed them what we
mean when we say that one thing is half of another.
He used the white (1) and red (2), and the red
and the crimson (4) to demonstrate the meaning
of "half." Then he asked them to find half of
some of the other rods, which the dark-haired
boy was able to do. Just before the end of the
demonstration Gattegno showed them a brown (8)
rod and asked them to find half of half of it,
and this too the dark-haired boy was able to do.

I could not but feel then, as I do now, that
whatever his I.Q. may be considered to have
been, and however he may have reacted to life
as he usually experienced it, this boy, during
that class, had played the part of a person of
high intelligence and had done intellectual
work of very high quality. When we think of
where he started, and where he finished, of the
immense amount of mathematical territory that
he covered in forty minutes or less, it is hard
not to feel that there is an extraordinary
capacity locked up inside that boy·

Other math materials include Dienes blocks and A-blocks, both
mentioned in a letter from Holt that Dennison quotes in his appendix to The Lives of Children (1969). This appendix, incidentally,
includes a lot of additional information about teaching materials.

Silberman (Crisis in the Classroom, 1970, pp. 221-222)
described how the English primary schools often set aside a section of the room as a "math table" for the children to make use of

independently:

> The arithmetic area most likely will have several
> tables pushed together to form a large working space.
> On the tables, in addition to a variety of math texts
> and workbooks, will be a box containing rulers,
> measuring tapes and sticks, yardsticks, string, and
> the like; other boxes, containing pebbles, shells,
> stones, rocks, acorns, conkers (the acorn of a chest-
> nut tree), bottle tops, pine cones, and anything else
> that can be used for counting, along with more formal
> arithmetic and mathematical materials, such as
> Cuisenaire rods, Dienes blocks, Stern rods, and
> Unifisc cubes. There will be several balance scales,
> too, with boxes of weights, as well as more pebbles,
> stones, rocks, feathers, and anything else that can be
> used for weighing.

One of the new ideas most publicized among science teachers
in recent years has been the "discovery method," advocated by Zacharias
and others. In this approach, students are presented with an assort-
ment of scientific tools and equipment, and a problem or a set of
problems. The problem is a real scientific problem which was
originally solved by a scientist using similar equipment. The
idea is to encourage the student to attack the problem by himself,
hopefully in a way similar to the way the 'real scientist' did;
in this way he learns how to think like a scientist.

Most countertheorists prefer this method to teaching out
of a textbook; it provides an opportunity for the student to think
for himself and become involved in the learning process. But some
are quite critical nevertheless. Anthony Barton writes, "The
discovery method, to malign it slightly, consists of attempting
to turn the members of a physics class into thirty Galvanis by
supplying each child with a copper hook, an iron bar and a frog's

leg...and then standing back with narrowed eyes to await the rediscovery of electricity (Repo, 1970, p.201)."

The objection to the discovery method is that it provides an artificial kind of creativity. The child is confronted with a problem that, in the first place, may not matter to him, and in the second place, has already been answered; the teacher simply withholds the answer. Thus, there is little resemblance between what the child does in a "discovery" classroom and what it is hoped he will do with the scientific approach in the world outside.

Barton's criticism appears in an article called "Soft Boxes in Hard Schools," in which he advocates another approach. He described a "Thirties box" with which students are to think and learn about the Thirties; it could be done with science as well. Unlike the discovery method there isn't any special thing the child is expected to do with the box; rather, he's supposed to play around with it, and come up with whatever interests that delight him. Contents of the Thirties box are listed in Appendix 5.

Barton recommends several "don'ts" in planning an educational box. Most important is not to provide any instructions. He also suggests that the maker of the box should plan it by including things that he enjoys personally. Barton rejects the idea that teaching material should be designed for any particular age group. The concept is quite similar to Silberman's description of the math table in English schools.

Classroom Structure

When countertheorists begin to discuss changing classroom structure, many teachers and educators get nervous about the question of order. The fear that the radicals are going to throw away the structure that holds things together, that prevents chaos, that makes possible any useful process at all. Consequently, I begin this section with a passage aimed at allaying this fear. It is from Herndon's _The Way It Spozed To Be_ (1968), and he is arguing that the removal of top-down order need not mean chaos:

> It's really almost impossible for adults, and no doubt especially for adult teachers, to see anything "constructive" going on in a bunch of kids shouting at each other. All the adults can see is just that: kids, all bunched together, yelling at each other. You can't believe they are doing it for anything you'd call a purpose; they are simply creating a problem, something that shouldn't exist at all.
>
> The adults also can't imagine that this problem is going to cease to exist unless they, the adults, make it cease. They feel that unless they issue orders and directions and threats, the kids will never stop making noise, never stop yelling, never get organized.
>
> This feeling is wrong. The adults are wrong on both counts, not because they are stupid, not even because they lack what Grissum called "insight" either. They are wrong because almost no one can stand to wait around long enough without doing anything, so that they can see what all the shouting is about, or what might happen when it eventually is over. They can't stand to, and so they never find out. Never finding out, they assume that there was nothing there. I don't think the quality of insight is unique or even rare, Grissum to the contrary. What does seem to be rare is the ability to wait and see what is happening. (p.176)

I admit 9D could probably outshout the rest
of The Tribe, and The Tribe could outshout
everyone else. There they were, about fifteen
or so kids, all in a cluster, standing, shouting
at each other, Verna in the middle shouting at all
of them --a hundred demands, questions, orders,
all at once. You couldn't make it out at all.
Probably there were a hundred shouted irrelevan-
cies, threats, and insults too. But the fact is
this outcry was orderly in intent and in effect,
for in about four or five minutes it was all over,
readers were sitting down, they had books, the
audience was getting ready to listen. I doubt
very much if 9D could have been organized to read a
play in five minutes, even by an experienced
teacher with a machine gun.

The structure of a classroom is not synonomous with the

structure that a teacher plans and introduces there. It can be less;

it can be more, if the students introduce some ideas of their own.

Countertheorists assume that the conventional classroom, at least

some of the time, imposes too much order, and thereby excludes the

natural creativity and self-designed order that children have to offer

Some innovations that countertheorists propose are in the physical

layout of classrooms. It is assumed that children will introduce some

order of their own into a situation that is not completely defined.

One idea comes from Herbert Kohl's book The Open Classroom

(1969). Kohl says: don't arrange the funiture at the start of the year

If it spends the summer pushed into a corner, leave it there until

the kids arrive. In his own case, he had everything remain all

summer untouched from the end of the last year, right down to the

writing on the blackboard. The point is, Kohl says, that it is both

more democratic and more effective for children to play a part in

designing their own learning environment.

The British Infant Schools offer a variety of possibilities. Recent years have seen a general movement toward less uniform structures in many British infant schools. As these changes have not been programmatically imposed, they differ from one place to another as widely as do the teachers and Heads (principals). But there are some general trends in this movement, as described in Featherstone's report, in <u>Crisis in the Classroom</u>, and in <u>Radical School Reform</u>.

The classroom tends to be physically arranged around the opportunity for various activities. Thus, there is likely to be a "math corner," a "cooking corner," a place to retreat to, and a "book corner"--with just books, not designated as "reading" books or "geography" books. But these things can exist in other, more conventional classrooms; the difference is that in conventional classrooms they are an afterthought. As a result, they are often squeezed into a small out-of-the-way space on the edge of the pre-established rows of desks or tables. And they may remain nearly unused, because of the structure of the school day.

It is impossible to talk about the physical layout of classrooms without discussing the educational process that goes on inside. In the British schools, what goes on inside may look chaotic to an American, at least at first. There isn't a definite beginning to the day; kids just come in and start doing things. And there may never be a time when everyone is doing the same thing at the same time.

Children in these schools get their instruction from themselves, from their classmates, from their teachers in personal conversations and consultation, and in some more formal ways as well. For instance, phonetics may be systematically taught; and displays of words on the wall are common: "words we use in measuring and weighing," or "names of musical instruments," Even in formal instruction, teachers emphasize interests of the children and utilize activities that have been generated by children.

But it is not chaotic. Nor do the teachers, in general, rest easy in the faith that the children will find and introduce all the order they need. Rather, they present some materials that seem promising, see what the kids do with them, and try to shape that. Keeping track of a classroom of kids doing different things requires more alertness and energy than teaching in traditional classrooms. Two things can help ease this burden: first, it's usually more satisfying to work hard at teaching than to work at keeping order. And second, as one teacher said, "I can give all my attention to a child for five minutes, and that's worth more to him than being part of a sea of faces all day."

A key to the success of the British schools is that each has developed a system compatible with the spirit and philosophy of the people in the school. Featherstone has expressed dismay at some of the over-enthusiastic response to his report on the British schools; he feels that many American educators are trying to imitate them too rapidly, without having assimilated the principles, or adapting them to their own local needs and philosophies.

It may be helpful to discuss how one American educator adapted some of these ideas to a peculiarly American situation: a Harlem elementary school. The educator is Lillian Weber, who teaches at City College and consulted at P.S. 123. Her "open corridors" program began in 1968, and was an attempt to bring to P.S. 123 some of the qualities of "in-and-outness" that she had observed in the English schools.

The program, like the English experience, started small and grew. It began by encompassing only one corridor and four classrooms in space, and lasting only three one-hour periods per week. The teachers agreed to let students move around to spend the time in class doing interesting things in which outside students could usefully participate: for instance, learning about a cage full of guinea pigs. Meanwhile, the corridor was stocked with a lot of what might be called "enriched stuff"-- easels, a sandbox, math materials, a water table. Professor Weber's education students watched over corridor activities.

The program, as described in Silberman's book (1970), was a success. Kids liked the period and used it well, to learn and to enjoy themselves at the same time. Teachers found themselves making friends with students, especially students from classes other than their own. Older kids began to teach younger kids some things;

629

imitation is a strong point of the British schools, too. And, as
people saw how it was working, it grew. The next year it was
expanded to one and one-half hours a day, every day, in the same
school; it also began to be imitated in other New York schools,
of different social composition.

One of the nicest features of this whole program --which
was fitted to its environment, then allowed to grow --is how well
the teachers came to like it, and how it changed their view of
the children. "...the teachers were won over as they realized
that their discipline problems had been sharply reduced, and that they
consequently had far less need to exercise conscious control
(Silberman, 1970, p.300).

Wider Structural Changes

Many countertheorists see a need to make changes more
widely than in one classroom at a time. For them, the school-
wide structure within which the conventional classroom exists,
puts that classroom under so many constraints that truly free
teaching is either difficult or impossible. For some, indeed,
changes are necessary throughout entire systems.

An example of a whole school run by a countertheorist
is Neill's Summerhill. The principles of Summerhill are not very
complicated; how they work out in detail is too long a story to
give here. Students at Summerhill do not have to attend any classes
or do any schoolwork except as they wish. The rules with which they
must comply are those made by the whole school in assembly, from six

630

year-olds to Neill, himself, one person -- one vote. The rules are numerous, but are confined to those which make sense to the students; there is no rule, for instance, against going around naked. Classes and various creative activities are attractive enough so that students do spend a lot of time there, even though at the start they may go for months exercising their new freedom not to go to class. Neill, himself, is accessible to, and respected by, all the children.

A less successful school is described in Anne Long's account of her experience at the New School in Vancouver (as given in Radical School Reform, (1969). Here the arrangement looked somewhat similar on paper, but the kids seem (at least for a time) to have displayed absolutely no self-regulation or sense of self-control. It was chaotic and destructive. At least two factors helped make the difference: the different personalities of those in charge, and the different cultural settings in which the schools were established.

Several other models for systems of governance of schools appear in countertheoretical literature, especially in Chesler's "Changing Schools Through Student Advocacy" (1971) and in Silberman's book Crisis in the Classroom (1970). Chesler presents the representative bicameral system, the unicameral system, and the "town meeting" approach to governing schools. In all of these, students have a legitimate voice in making decisions--not just advising. John Adams High School in Portland, Oregon--also mentioned in Silberman's book--is one example of a school operating on a bicameral basis. Students and teaching faculty each elect repre-

631

sentatives from their ranks, who form two policy-making bodies. An executive committee implements them, and runs day-to-day matters.

These are proposals for changing the power structure in schools, for altering how decisions are made. There are also proposals for changing the educational process--the actual teaching part of the school. These changes might be made with or without the institution of student power.

One suggestion is for planning on a wider level than one classroom at a time, by teachers who cooperate with each other. Several plans discussed in other parts of this paper are examples of this. For instance, there is the New York "corridor program," and Kohl's suggestion that teachers can ally to try to make a "school within a school." Much of Herndon's How To Survive in Your Native Land (1971) is a discussion of his experience in working this way with one other teacher. Knoblock's book (1971) describes this same innovation as being helpful in fulfilling teacher's emotional needs. They may experience a sense of community with other teachers, and, thus, overcome their loneliness. And it may also free them to use their talents better; with a more flexible arrangement, they can do things with selected groups of students that would not be appropriate with a whole class at one time.

Postman and Weingartner (1969) have another set of suggestions for loosening the distribution of resources within the school. One of them is to move teachers across subjects, apparently on the theory that a teacher will be more interesting in a field she hasn't mastered.

George Leonard's Education and Ecstasy (1968) suggests that new technology and new knowledge about learning have made the entire concept of classrooms obsolete. He proposes a kind of "learning palace," a technological wonderland in which kids move as they please from computer display screens to artificial environments to Socratic discussions with older people. Learning is so important and so interesting that children will certainly do it, especially if given an alluring and free environment. The idea is attractive, but appears to be removed from all questions of practicality: such as cost, planning, and what to do with the kids who wouldn't blossom in such an environment.

Postman and Weingartner (1969) discuss an assignment they give their own teachers-in-training: to design a high school, from the ground up, with freedom to make it as they would like to have it. They find this assignment stimulates original thought about what education is and how it should be carried out.

At a wider level, Philadelphia has a program which could only be implemented at the level of the whole school system. This is the Parkway Program, in which some students from all over Philadelphia are enrolled. They have a school building, but they do not spend much time there. Instead they go around downtown Philadelphia, using resources of the city itself. They use "educational" resources such as museums and libraries; they also look around and learn from things like businesses and city council meetings. It is doubtful incidentally, whether the resources could accommodate the flood, if the program were extended to include a large fraction of the city's students.

Students in the Parkway Program keep in touch with an academic setting in large part through individual meetings with faculty members who play a supervisory role, similar to the "tutors" of some universities, or advisors in graduate school. This system, as described in Silberman's book, sounds quite successful.

In Britain, one institution has helped the schools to innovate and share ideas, without going overboard or ignoring local conditions. This is the Inspectorate. Inspectors are travelling officials, who visit and consult about schools. Their role has changed from the original one, in which they did, in fact, simply inspect and evaluate; now they are more advisors than inspectors, and they put their expertise, their ideas, and what they have seen in other schools at the service of the schools they visit. As a result, innovations are disseminated; and they are disseminated by people, who not only know "how to do it," but "in what circumstances it was done, and how, exactly, it did work."

In North Dakota, there is an innovation which aims to alter a large fraction of the public education in the state. This is the University of North Dakota's New School for Behavioral

Studies in Education. It had its origin in a legislative study made in 1965, which described a crisis in education: school teachers in North Dakota were poorly prepared, and the students they taught were having trouble making the transition from the rural, isolated setting in which they were growing up to the urban, modern world in which most of them later live. North Dakota planners decided to change the direction of education in the state.

They decided this could not be done within the existing School of Education. So they created a new one.

What the New School teaches is a mixture of many of the innovations and techniques described in this paper, with probably more debt to the English primary schools than any other single source. But it does not slavishly imitate anyone. It does maintain that, to work, a school of education "must itself become a model of the kind of education environment it is promoting (Silberman, 1970). Hence students are taught in informal, individualized ways. They come from the undergraduate school of the university, and from the ranks of the state's experienced school teachers.

The New School does not want to produce a "new breed" of teachers who will plunge suddenly into an unreconstructed, mistrustful school system. So it tries to coordinate, and communicate with, both young and old teachers.

> The New School enrolls regular University of North
> Dakota undergraduates in their junior year, in a
> three-year program leading to a master's degree;
> the school also enrolls experienced teachers, who
> return to the Grand Forks campus for a year or
> more of study leading to a bachelor's degree.
> While they are at the university, the teachers'
> places are taken by the New School's master's degree
> candidates, who spend September to June of the
> master's year teaching, under close supervision
> from the New School faculty.

Some countertheorists conclude that what they really want
is to radically alter the whole society. For instance, putting
together Paul Goodman's <u>Growing Up Absurd</u> and <u>Compulsory Mis-
education</u>, it is easy to conclude that the evils he sees in
schools are inevitably dictated by the evils he sees in society--
most of them stemming from alienation from work, self, and body,
and from the impersonality of bureaucracies. To try to alter the
schools, then, is inevitably to become involved in trying to alter
the society. Education is sick <u>because</u> it trains us appropriately
to function in a sick world. It cannot be improved without
changing that world.

Everett Reimer and Ivan Illich emphasize inequality and
social injustice, and ways that schools help maintain them. Goodman,
on the other hand, maintains that things are pretty bad, even for the
"privileged." Schools are not just shaped by society, but are an
important--and vulnerable--institution that helps maintain the
social structure. Consequently, Reimer is willing to destroy the
institutional status of schools, to see them wither away, in order

to make possible wider changes in society.

While Reimer and Illich want to break the lock-step grip that schools have on Americans, Paolo Freire tried to make a corresponding but opposite change in the Third World. He brought education to those groups who were not supposed to get it -- namely, poor peasants in Brazil--and found that doing so means incurring the wrath of the whole power structure of the country.

Theorists face a complicated situation when they would bring about changes in the educational system which cannot easily be accomodated within the wider society. They must consider how to make their program for the schools a part of a program for the whole society, and how to build an environment in which their ideals can survive. Thus, they must examine the wider society to see just what changes are required there, and what forces will oppose these changes.

In short, the ideals lead one to consider political strategies. This concern led Illich to call for "institutional revolution" and Freire to come forthrightly up against the Brazilian ruling class. And it helps to clarify Goodman's position as a social critic (as well as an educational writer), and Kozol's dedication to schools that aim at changing society.

Any strategy for significant change in the schools has to be viewed as a part of a wider strategy for social change. If you create change in the schools , but not in the environment, you can expect that your efforts will be ineffective. Reimer and

Illich address this point by describing schools as a "weak link"

in the social system--a good place to make an attack on things

as they are. At the other extreme, Bill Ayers, once a teacher

at the Ann Arbor Community School, decided that work within the

schools was not the most fruitful way to try to make an impact;

he then helped to found the Weatherman faction of SDS. Intermedi-

ate positions, of course, are possible.

Special Classes

To some extent the concept of "special classes" loses

meaning when we consider the countertheorists. They see "normal"

classes as being filled with emotional disturbance, or even as

inducing it; so for them, dealing with emotional disturbance in

the schools often means overhauling the whole school system.

But they do have some things to say about "special classes"

as such. One particularly provocative idea is suggested by both

Herndon and Reimer. They suggest that special classes may offer an

opportunity to form "enclaves" of enlightened teaching in an other-

wise hostile school system.

In the first place, they suggest, everyone recognizes

that the children in special classes need a lot of individualized

teaching, as well as smaller classes. This means that there is less

expectation that a teacher will follow a generalized curriculum,

and much more opportunity for her to do whatever she deems appro-

priate for the children. It is impossible for the school system to maintain its established expectations for those very children whom it has excluded.

Administrators are really not very interested in knowing all about what is going on in special classes. They may see these classes as "dumping grounds ." When this is true, an innovative program is not likely to find itself coming under any pressure to conform to anything, as long as it does not make waves.

Finally, Reimer suggests, some of the most interesting and promising children may be found in special classes. If the schools are as anti-human and oppressive as he says, it is quite reasonable to expect that some of the most stubbornly lively and healthy kids will be excluded from the regular classes, for not being able to "make it" on those terms. Hence, a teacher who looks at the special class as an opportunity, rather than as a burden, may find resources among her students that do not exist in the usual classroom.

Reimer has not taught in special classes. Herndon has, but he found it possible to teach successfully without really acknowledging that his students were different from any others. Two other countertheorists, George Dennison and Herbert Grossman, have lessons for us derived from teaching students who were clearly and inescapably different from ordinary kids.

One lesson is that some kids in special classes really are sick; some of their lack of success in regular schools is not to be explained away as the product of institutional pathology or oppressiveness in the schools. This is especially clear in the case of the boys in Grossman's school, who were so disturbed that no other place, short of a residential institution, would touch them. But while he makes this reminder, Grossman does not defend the present system of special classes at all. Most children in them, he says, ought not to be there; those who must be, deserve something better than what special classes are today.

The other lesson is equally simple, and encouraging as well. It is that the same techniques that countertheorists advocate for all children can be successfully applied with "special" children. This is demonstrated in the work of Dennison, a follower of Neill. There is also supporting evidence from Herndon's teaching, from many of the "teaching the unteachable" schools described in Radical School Reform, and in a number of instances cited in Silberman's book.

Survival

Teachers who innovate may get into trouble. The suggestions offered by countertheorists often run so contrary to the usual practices of schools that teachers who follow them ought to be ready for pressure and trouble.

A discussion, in a few pages, of how to handle trouble is at the end of Kohl's The Open Classroom (1969, pp.82-112). Here I will summarize some of Kohl's suggestions, which really deserve to be read in full.

<u>Troubles from other teachers</u>. They are likely to complain about noise. You can try to discuss the problem with the class, try to calm the teacher down, or counterattack by finding a weakness to complain about in return. But it is essential not to deny your children the right to speak freely.

Many teachers don't like dirt and disorder, and open classrooms tend to look disorderly. Reason with them if you can; if you can't, maybe you should paste a drawing over the window of your classroom door.

Your students may cause problems for other teachers, if you encourage them to come alive. Kohl says, "There is no direct way I know of to deal with [the resulting] hostility, but it is important not to be surprised by it (<u>The Open Classroom</u>, 1969)."

Finding an ally, he says, is important. If you have allies in the school, you can start working together, sharing classrooms and students, moving toward having a "school within a school."

<u>Troubles with principals</u>. This depends a lot on the principal. Sometimes a principal is simply not going to put up with what you may want to do. Kohl lists several defenses which may be necessary or desirable: keeping two sets of lesson plans, one real and one "official"; actually creating some authoritarian lesson plans to use when observers come in; keeping quiet at faculty meetings; seeming to comply with orders and directives.

But he doesn't advocate ducking and hiding all the time. Sometimes confrontations are inescapable,unless you want to surrender. For

641

these cases he has advice on how to marshall support, even on how a teacher in Oakland, California, responded to a letter of dismissal with such a barrage of counterattacks and threats of exposure that the letter was withdrawn.

Though it may not be feasible, this is more in tune with what an open classroom _ought_ to be about; it shouldn't involve hiding what you're doing. Kohl's summary words of advice about survival are in this spirit (The Open Classroom, 1969):

> Reporting to Parents, Students, and Supervisors
>
> Document what is happening in your class. Document what you are trying to do. Let the students' work speak for the students. Do not be afraid to admit that you have blundered. Show people what is happening in your classroom, tell them what you are trying to do. Talk about education, learning, young people. When parents ask what is happening to their children let them see their children's work, talk about their children as individuals. Put everything on a personal and qualitative level.
>
> Reporting is fighting for survival. If you care and let people know you care, you may survive. There is no guarantee . (p.112)

Mark Chesler's work is concerned with changing the power distribution within a school, more than with what is good practice in a classroom. He assumes that students, teachers, and administrators are cohesive groups with different interests, and discusses how students may exercise power in a school. Often, he says, they can only achieve legitimate power through the use of their illegitimate power to close the school by not cooperating.

Chesler's work is not directed at teachers. But teachers who want to make the kinds of changes discussed here may find that what they want to do is more in accord with their students' perceived interest than with the perceived interest of their fellow teachers. Consequently, they ought to consider their students, not just as beneficiaries of what they want to do, but also as possible sources of power in the effort to do it.

Outside the public schools, some schools operate on grants; for those operating in such settings, it may be necessary to know a little about how to get grants. Dennison's The Lives of Children includes a bitter discussion of how his school failed to get a grant to continue. The saddest and most important part is the demonstration that packaging is more important than content in applying for money for a school.

Dennison's book also discusses many of the mechanics of starting a school, including especially complying with the rules and regulations of agencies like the Fire Department, Health Department, etc. It is written about New York, but would probably be helpful elsewhere as well.

IV.   SUMMARY

Countertheorists are many and varied, and so are their ideas about education. This paper attempts to compare their ideas in a coherent way.

Part I tries to answer the question: what kind of theory is counter theory? It discusses how countertheorists often are simply radical or unorthodox members of some other theoretical area. It then identifies some of the commonalities among their views, and finally, some of the dimensions along which countertheorists differ.

Part II introduces some leading countertheorists, with the object of giving a sense of who these people are.

Parts IIIA and IIIB attempt to show what countertheorists perceive as their concerns, and what they do about it when they apply their ideas in schools. Both sections treat important issues; Part IIIB treats especially those problems and methods which lend themselves to 'recipe-making,' so that an educator who likes an idea can see what it means to carry out that idea.

It is always difficult to separate philosophy and theory from practice. This is particularly true for counter-theorists. Wherever possible, the reader who is attracted to an idea or method described here, ought to follow it back to its original source.

APPENDICES

TO

COUNTERTHEORETICAL INTERVENTIONS IN

EMOTIONAL DISTURBANCE

(from Ashton-Warner, S. Teacher. New York: Simon & Schuster,
1963, p. 89.)

DAILY RHYTHM

9-10:45   BREATHE OUT

Conversation	Crying	
Painting	Quarrelling	
Creative Writing	Blocks	
ORGANIC Clay		Creative Dancing
Sand		Key Vocabulary
WORK Water		Organic Vocabulary
Paste Paint		Dolls
FOR Doll's washing		Boats
Singing		Chalk
MORNING Day Dreaming		Loving

11-12   BREATHE IN
Key Vocabulary 1/4 hr. for Little Ones
Organic Vocabulary
Organic reading
Organic discussion
Stories, pictures, picture books for Little Ones

1-2   BREATHE OUT
Golden Section
Plastic media for Little Ones   STANDARD

2:10-3   BREATHE IN
Standard vocabulary   WORK
Standard reading
Maori book vocabulary   FOR
Maori book read
Supplementary reading   AFTERNOON
Stories, songs, poems
Letters for Little Ones

(from Goodman, P. Compulsory mis-education and the community of scholars. New York: Random House, 1962, pp. 32-34.)

SUGGESTIONS FOR CHANGE

I. Have "no school at all" for a few classes. These children should be selected from tolerable, though not necessarily cultured, homes. They should be neighbors and numerous enough to be a society for one another and so that they do not feel merely "different." Will they learn the rudiments anyway? This experiment cannot do the children any academic harm, since there is good evidence that normal children will make up the first seven years school-work with four to seven months of good teaching.

II. Dispense with the school building for a few classes; provide teachers and use the city itself as the school--its streets, cafeterias, stores, movies, museums, parks, and factories. Where feasible, it certainly makes more sense to teach using the real subject-matter than to bring an abstraction of the subject-matter into the school-building as "curriculum." Such a class should probably not exceed 10 children for one peda-gogue. The idea--it is the model of Athenian education --is not dissimilar to Youth gang work, but not applied to delin-quents and not playing to the gang ideology.

III. Along the same lines, but both outside and inside the school building, use appropriate unlicensed adults of the community-- the druggist, the storekeeper, the mechanic--as the proper ed-ucators of the young into the grown-up world. By this means we can try to overcome the separation of the young from the grown-up world so characteristic in modern urban life, and to diminish the omnivorous authority of the professional school-people. Certainly it would be a useful and animating exper-ience for the adults. (There is the beginning of such a volun-teer program in the New York and some other systems.)

IV. Make class attendance not compulsory, in the manner of A. S. Neill's Summerhill. If the teachers are good, absence would tend to be eliminated; if they are bad, let them know it. The compulsory law is useful to get the children away from the parents, but it must not result in trapping the children. A fine modification of this suggestion is the rule used by Frank Brown in Florida: he permits the children to be absent for a week or a month to engage in any worthwhile enterprise or visit any new environment.

V. Decentralize an urban school (or do not build a new big building) into small units, 20 to 50, in available store-fronts or clubhouses. These tiny schools, equipped with record-player and pin-ball machine, could combine play, socializing, discussion, and formal teaching. For special events, the small units can be brought together into a common auditorium or gymnasium, so as to give the sense of the greater community. Correspondingly I think it would be worthwhile to give the Little Red Schoolhouse a spin under modern urban conditions, and see how it works out: that is, to combine all the ages in a little room for 25 to 30, rather than to grade by age.

VI. Use a pro rata part of the school money to send children to economically marginal farms for a couple of months of the year, perhaps 6 children from mixed backgrounds to a farmer. The only requirement is that the farmer feed them and not beat them; best, of course, if they take part in the farm-work. This will give the farmer cash, as part of the generally desirable program to redress the urban-rural ratio to something nearer to 70% to 30%. (At present less than 8% of families are rural.) Conceivably, some of the urban children will take to the other way of life, and we might generate a new kind of rural culture.

(from Postman, N., & Weingartner, C. <u>Teaching as a subversive activity</u>. New York: Dell, 1969, pp. 62-63.)

What's Worth Knowing?

What do you worry about most?

What are the causes of your worries?

Can any of your worries be eliminated? How?

Which of them might you deal with first? How do you decide?

Are there other people with the same problems? How do you know? How can you find out?

If you had an important idea that you wanted to let every-one (in the world) know about, how might you go about letting them know?

What bothers you most about adults? Why?

How do you want to be similar to or different from adults you know when you become an adult?

What, if anything, seems to you to be worth dying for?

How did you come to believe this?

What seems worth living for?

How did you come to believe this?

At the present moment, what would you most like to be--or be able to do? Why? What would you have to know in order to be able to do it? What would you have to do in order to get to know it?

How can you tell "good guys" from "bad guys"?

How can "good" be distinguished from "evil"?

What kind of a person would you most like to be? How might you get to be this kind of person?

At the present moment, what would you most like to be doing? Five years from now? Ten years from now? Why? What might you have to do to realize these hopes? What might you have to give up in order to do some or all of these things?

When you hear or read or observe something, how do you know what it means ?

Where does meaning "come from"?

What does "meaning" mean?

How can you tell what something "is" or whether it "is?"

Where do words come from?

Where do symbols come from?

Why do symbols change?

Where does knowledge come from?

What do you think are some of man's most important ideas? Where did they come from? Why? How? Now what?

What's a "good idea"?

How do you know when a good or live idea becomes a bad or
    dead idea?
Which of man's ideas would we be better off forgetting?
    How do you decide?
What is "progress"?

(from Postman, N., & Weingartner, C. <u>Teaching as a subversive</u>
      <u>activity</u>. New York: Dell, <u>1969, pp. 137-140.)</u>

NEW TEACHERS (some suggestions)

1. <u>Declare a five-year moratorium on the use of all textbooks.</u>

    Since with two or three exceptions all texts are not only
    boring but based on the assumptions that knowledge exists
    prior to, independent of, and altogether outside of the
    learner, they are either worthless or harmful. If it is
    impossible to function without textbooks, provide every
    student with a notebook filled with blank pages, and have
    him compose his own text.

2. <u>Have "English" teachers "teach" Math, Math teachers English,</u>
    <u>Social Studies teachers Science, Science teachers Art, and</u>
    <u>so on.</u>

    One of the largest obstacles to the establishment of a sound
    learning environment is the desire of teachers to get some-
    thing they think they know into the heads of people who don't
    know it. An English teacher teaching Math would hardly be in
    a position to fulfill this desire. Even more important, he
    would be forced to perceive the "subject" as a learner, not a
    teacher. If this suggestion is too impractical, try numbers
    3 and 4.

3. <u>Transfer all the elementarv-school teachers to high school and</u>
    <u>vice versa.</u>

4. <u>Require every teacher who thinks he knows his "subject" well to</u>
    <u>write a book on it.</u>

    In this way, he will be relieved of the necessity of inflicting
    <u>his</u> knowledge on other people, particularly his students.

5. <u>Dissolve all "subjects," "courses," and especially "course</u>
    <u>requirements."</u>

    This proposal, all by itself, would wreck every existing
    educational bueaucracy. The result would be to deprive
    teachers of the excuses presently given for their failures
    and to free them to concentrate on their learners.

6. Limit each teacher to three declarative sentences per class, and 15 interrogatives.

    Every sentence above the limit would be subject to a 25-cent fine. The students can do the counting and the collecting.

7. Prohibit teachers from asking any questions they already know the answers to.

    This proposal would not only force teachers to perceive learning from the learner's perspective, it would help them to learn how to ask questions that produce knowledge.

8. Declare a moratorium on all tests and grades.

    This would remove from the hands of teachers their major weapons of coercion and would eliminate two of the major obstacles to their students' learning anything significant.

9. Require all teachers to undergo some form of psychotherapy as part of their in-service training.

    This need not be psychoanalysis; some form of group therapy or psychological counseling will do. Its purpose: to give teachers an opportunity to gain insight into themselves, particularly into the reasons they are teachers.

10. Classify teachers according to their ability and make the lists public.

    There would be a "smart" group (the Bluebirds), an "average" group (the Robins), and a "dumb" group (the Sandpipers). The lists would be published each year in the community paper. The I. Q. and reading scores of teachers would also be published, as well as the list of those who are "advantaged" and "disadvantaged" by virtue of what they know in relation to what their students know.

11. Require all teachers to take a test prepared by students on what the students know.

    Only if a teacher passes this test should he be permitted to "teach." This test could be used for "grouping" the teachers as in number 10 above.

12. Make every class an elective and withhold a teacher's monthly check if his students do not show any interest in going to next month's classes.

This proposal would simply put the teacher on a par with other professionals, e.g., doctors, dentists, lawyers, etc. No one forces you to go to a particular doctor unless you are a "clinic case." In that instance, you must take what you are given. Our present system makes a "clinic case" of every student. Bureaucrats decide who shall govern your education. In this proposal, we are restoring the American philosophy: no clients, no money; lots of clients, lots of money.

13. Require every teacher to take a one-year leave of absence every fourth year to work in some "field" other than education.

Such an experience can be taken as evidence, albeit shaky, that the teacher has been in contact with reality at some point in his life. Recommended occupations: bartender, cab driver, garment worker, waiter. One of the common sources of difficulty with teachers can be found in the fact that most of them simply move from one side of the desk (as students) to the other side (as ''teachers") and they have not had much contact with the way things are outside of school rooms.

14. Require each teacher to provide some sort of evidence that he or she has had a loving relationship with at least one other human being.

If the teacher can get someone to say, "I love her (or him)," she should be retained. If she can get two people to say it, she should get a raise. Spouses need not be excluded from testifying.

15. Require that all the graffiti accumulated in the school toilets be reproduced on large paper and be hung in the school halls.

Graffiti that concern teachers and administrators should be chiseled into the stone at the front entrance of the school.

16. There should be a general prohibition against the use of the following words and phrases:

teach, syllabus, covering ground, I. Q., makeup, test, disadvantaged, gifted, accelerated, enhancement, course, grade, score, human nature, dumb, college material, and administrative necessity.

1. Eliminate all conventional "tests" and "testing."

2. Eliminate all "courses."

3. Eliminate all "requirements."

4. Eliminate all full-time administrators and administrations.

5. Eliminate all restrictions that confine learners to sitting still in boxes inside of boxes.

APPENDIX E

(from Repo, S. (Ed.) <u>This book is about schools.</u> New York:
Random House, 1970, pp. 207-208.)

Soft Boxes in Hard Schools

THE THIRTIES MULTI-MEDIA KIT

Order for packing items in boxes:

1	Dust Bowl Ballads	2x2	Vancouver Police Department Letters
2	German/English Newspapers	2	Help Yourself to our Salad
1x17	Newspaper Pages		Bowl Cabbagetown
1	Jackdaw C13: <u>The Great Depression</u>	2	Investigation of Poverty at Russell Sage Foundation
15	Notes & Quotes 1	2	Notice from CNR & CPR
15	Notes & Quotes 11	2	United Nations
1	Blueprint of Dirigible	2	Classroom of Tomorrow
1	"Guernica"	2x11	Clippings Pages
2	Rivera Mural	1	Prints (1 packet of 20)
2	Adolf & Neville	2	Canadian Paintings of the 1930's
2	Shirley Temple Eating Puffed Wheat	2	Letter to the Editor
2	Bethune	2	Identification Order #1194: Charles Arthur Floyd
2	Pound	2	Hindenburg Folder
2	Hate Page	2	Saint John Hospital Cartoons
2	Relishprobe	9	Phonograph Records
2	Bank of Montreal	1	Bitter Years
2	Garner Interview	1x36	Postcard Reproductions
2	Wanted for Murder	1x22	Slides (1 bundle in elastic band)
2	Calaghan		
2	Ships in the Sky	4	Filmstrips
2	Condemned to Starve.... Compelled to Act	1	Transparency
2	Mass Meeting Tonight & Protest for Justice	1	Sheet of Colored Plastic
2	Quotes	1	Booklist
2	Illusions	1	Guide
1	Audio Tape		
1x80	Literature and Science Cards		
1	Postage Stamps (1 packet of 20)		
1	Mounts for Half-Frame Slides (1 packet of 10)		

655

Ashton-Warner, S. Spearpoint. New York: Alfred A. Knopf, 1972.

Ashton-Warner, S. Teacher. New York: Simon and Schuster, 1963.

Chesler, M., & Lohman, J. Changing schools through student advocacy. In R. A. Schmuck, & M. Miles (Eds.), Organization development in schools. Palto Alto, California: National Press Books, 1971.

Dennison, G. The lives of children. New York: Random House, 1969.

Flesch, R. Why Johnny can't read. New York: Harper, 1955.

Freire, P. Pedagogy of the oppressed. New York: Herder and Herder, 1971.

Glasser, W. Schools without failure. New York: Harper & Row, 1969.

Goodman, P. Growing up absurd. New York: Random House, 1956.

Goodman, P. Compulsory mis-education and the community of scholars. New York: Random House, 1962.

Gross, B., & Gross R. (Eds.) Radical school reform. New York: Simon and Schuster, 1969.

Grossman, H. Nine rotten lousy kids. New York: Holt, Rinehart, and Winston, 1972.

Hentoff, N. Our children are dying. New York: Viking, 1966.

Herndon, J. The way it spozed to be. New York: Simon and Schuster, 1968.

Herndon, J. How to survive in your native land. New York: Simon and Schuster, 1971.

Holt, J. How children fail. New York: Pitman, 1964.

Holt, J. How children learn. New York: Pitman, 1967.

Holt, J. The underachieving school. New York: Dell, 1972.

Holt, J. What do I do Monday? New York: Dutton, 1970.

Illich, I. Deschooling society. New York: Harper & Row, 1970.

Jones, R. Fantasy and feeling in education. New York: New York University Press, 1968.

Knoblock, P., & Goldstein, A. The lonely teacher. Boston: Allyn & Bacon, 1971.

Kohl, H. 36 children. New York: New American Library, 1967.

Kohl, H. The open classroom. New York: Vintage, 1969.

Kozol, J. Death at an early age. New York: Houghton Mifflin, 1967.

Kozol, J. Free schools. New York: Houghton Mifflin, 1972.

Leonard, G. Education and ecstasy. New York: Delacorte, 1968.

Maslow, A. Toward a psychology of being. Princeton, New Jersey: Van Nostrand, 1962.

Neill, A. S. Summerhill. New York: Hart, 1960.

Pearl, A. What's wrong with the new informalism in education? Social Policy. March-April, 1971.

Postman, N., & Weingartner, C. Teaching as a subversive activity. New York: Dell, 1969.

Reimer, E. School is dead: alternatives in education. New York: Doubleday, 1971.

Repo, S. (Ed.) This book is about schools. New York: Random House, 1970.

Silberman, C. Crisis in black and white. New York: Random House, 1964.

Silberman, C. Crisis in the classroom. New York: Random House, 1970.

670

Environmental
  consequences, 168
  cues, direct, 467
  design, 477
  factors, in schizophrenia, 124
  molding, 34
  problems, 416
  transfers, 32
  variables, 465, 479
Environmentalists, 555
  theory, 94
Enzymatic breakdown, 126, 128
Enzyme, 95, 131, 135
  analyses, 99
  intercellular, 137
Epinephrine, 105, 108
Epstein, S., 282
Equipment, operated by child, 475
Erikson, E., 192, 257, 273, 287,
  303, 377
Eskimoes, Netsilik, 320, 606
Ethical issues
  of behavior modification, 241, 243
  of drug use, 115
  of genetic manipulations, 79
Etkin, W., 43
Eugenics, legal aspects, 97, 98
Europe, 33
Exceptional children, 474
  SEE ALSO Special education
      children
Exchange-centered intervention,
  400, 402
Excitor-centered intervention, 399,
  402
Excitor-respondent intervention,
  497
Exhaustion, 142
Existential intervention, 50
Exits, 469
Exogenous
  compound, 127
  mental retardation, 118
Expectations, setting, 522
Experience,
  cultural, 514
  physical, 534

sensory, 548
social, 514
tactile, 479
Experimental
  design, ABAB, 167
  extinction, 215
  study, 352
Exploratory behavior, 194
Expressive
  therapeutic intervention, 351
  therapy, 352, 366
Externalization, 266, 331, 351,
  352, 354, 355, 361, 363
Extinction, 165, 166, 206, 215, 223,
  228, 235, 236
Eye-motor coordination, 120

Fade-out SEE Token, fade-out
Fade-out, attention, 186
Faegre, C., 343
Failure, 284, 311, 313, 314, 342-
  344, 431, 439, 459, 461, 488,
  521
  fear of, 358
  source of stress, 344
  to learn, 338
Fairy tales, 607
Family, 210, 267, 287, 304-308,
  320, 326, 335, 348, 368, 401, 415
  allowance for, 489
  change action in, 481, 484
  contingency, 208
  distorted, 307
  environment, 484
    intervention, 481
  high risk, 101
  history, 99, 102
  inadequate, 306-309
  life, 412
  members, personality of, 484
  neurotic, 306
  prevention of failure, 488
  psychiatric care, 489
  relationship, 557
    intervention into, 517
    with child, 527

671

treatment center, 184
Resocialization, 192, 430, 450
Resolution, of predicament, 41
Respondent-centered intervention,
  399, 400, 402
Response, 168, 194, 200
  assertive, 217
  competing, 216
  cost, 170
    procedure, 227
  facilitation effect, 234
  "I can't", 316
  inhibitory, 234
  social, 175
Responsibility, social, 553
Restorative-supportive intervention, 337
Restraint, physical, 340
Results, of intervention, 503
Revolt, 24
  against care-givers, 63
  against care-giving economics, 64
  against care-receiving investi-
    ture, 62
  against care-taking institutions,
    65
  against melting pot myth, 68
  by labeled groups, 61
  institutional, 637
  of underclass, 67
Reward, 193, 194, 196, 202, 307,
  311, 342, 355, 367, 541, 560
  alternative to, 308
Rezmierski, V., 257, 287
Rhodes, W., 257, 317, 319, 399, 492
  548-551, 555, 560
Riboflavin, 149
Ribble, M., 283
Ricciuti, H., 149
Rimland, B., 150
Rimoin, D., 95, 99, 101, 102
Risk, 608
  taking, 604
Risley, T., 205
Ritalin (Methylphenidate), 109, 114,
  117
Ritter, B., 236

Rituals, 43, 45, 50, 63, 534
  of contact, 53
Robbins, M., 121
Robbins, L., 198
Roberts, J., 91, 93, 99-101
Robins, L., 348
Robson, J., 145, 146
Rogers, C., 245, 257, 357
Role, 333, 354, 364, 446, 452, 501,
  515, 557
  definition of, 512
  model, 275, 290, 368, 369
  of doctors, individual, 442, 443
  of helper, 372
  of intervener, 46
  of nurses, individual, 442, 443
  of parent, 496, 513, 521
  of patients, INU, 441
  of staff, INU, 441
  of Street Club workers, 502-511
  of teacher, 493, 496, 513, 518,
    521
  model, 275, 290, 368, 369
  playing, 189, 318, 323, 354, 363,
    371
  performance, 527
  prescription, 527
  sex, 320, 321
  social, 447
Room form,
  determined by activities,
    474
  significance of, 474
Rosenberg, H., 537
Rosenhan, D., 67, 299
Rousseau, E., 613
Rothman, E., 285, 313, 358
Roxbury, Massachusetts, 277
Ruitenbeek, H., 257
Rules, 340, 354
  Highfields, 451
  classroom, 311
  Gorky Colony, 430
  situation specific, 436
Russ, D., 213
Russia SEE Soviet Union
Rutter, M., 294

693

A STUDY OF CHILD VARIANCE

VOLUME 2